Head and Heart

Praise for Head and HeArt

The incidence and burden of mental health challenges in our modern stressed society is formidable. A limitation of our current medical system's approach to treatment of mental health conditions is that it is focused on pharmaceutical, cognitive and talking therapies. These do not address the many physical, creative and spiritual aspects of these conditions, which, if they were treated, could substantially improve treatment efficacy. This book effectively addresses this limitation by providing a comprehensive and detailed theoretical and practical guide to the skills and behavioral practices from both art and yoga therapy, and is likely to be a valuable resource for both art and yoga therapists as well as conventional mental health providers.

Sat Bir Singh Khalsa PhD
Assistant Professor of Medicine, Harvard Medical School
Chief Editor, *The Principles and Practice of Yoga Therapy*

Yoga therapy, like art therapy, facilitates the emergence of emotion. Dr Horovitz's book conveys how one approach can complement the other, and how their reinforcement can make for more efficient movement of processes toward well-being. This publication will serve to broaden the creative art therapist's understanding of yoga therapy, and how its inclusion may fortify art therapy practice.

Irene Rosner David PhD, ATR-BC, LCAT, HLM
Honorary Life Member, American Art Therapy Association

A unique and groundbreaking classic book. Highly recommended for yoga teachers, health professionals and students.

Larry Payne PhD, C-IAYT, E-RYT500
Author, *Yoga After 50 for Dummies*

Dr Horovitz has combined decades of knowledge and wisdom in yoga therapy and art therapy to create this masterful and informative book. She uses her interoceptive research to help clients and patients open to the strength within. Bravo, Dr Ellen!

Lakshmi Voelker
Founder, Lakshmi Voelker Chair Yoga

Ayurveda, known as the most ancient and complete healing wisdom, teaches that disease begins in the mind. Horovitz's step by step guidance on how to incorporate art, yoga and human warmth in the treatment plan, is a breath of fresh air on the complex journey of healing the mind. *Head and HeArt* provides a complete approach to restoring alignment from its roots – the mind.

Christianne Asper-Contant
Clinical Ayurveda Specialist

Even after retiring from founding a prestigious graduate art therapy program, Dr Ellen Horovitz devotes herself – tirelessly and selflessly – to her therapy patients and senior yoga students. In addition to Hatha yoga, she practices her very own form of Bhakti and Karma yoga. This creative and pragmatic book weaves art – a primary need for humans – with traditional yoga and psychotherapy. In this turbulent 21st century it will do wonders for all looking to alleviate existential angst.

François Raoult MA, ERYT500, C-IAYT
Author, *Lifāsana*

Dr Horovitz's emphasis on patient and professional self-care is highlighted in this comprehensive text through reflective exercises, bracketed by her sensibilities as a therapist, educator, artist, and human being. This masterful text highlights her professional and individual ethos which underscore her genuineness and authenticity while providing information that is rich in scope and visceral in context. As made evident by her riveting case examples, Dr Horovitz imparts a humanistic element that is compelling and pragmatic. This guide will enlighten both the seasoned therapist and novice who seek to juxtapose efficacious therapeutic approaches that truly marry head and heart while promoting health and well-being.

Marica Sue Cohen-Liebman PhD, ATR-BC, LPC
Author, *The Art of Investigation, Forensic Art Therapy*

Through her new book *Head and HeArt*, Dr Horovitz is sending you a ray of sunshine with a creative chromatic bridge of yogic practices and art therapy. Her rich clinical footsteps are displayed vividly to guide practitioners with practical examples along with a comprehensive theoretical foundation to interlace body and mind connections across the lifespan. Read this book and learn from one of the best.

Dr Supritha Aithal PhD, fHEA, MFA, BSc Sp&Hg
Lecturer, School of Applied Health and Social care, Edge Hill University, UK

Head and HeArt: Yoga therapy and art therapy interventions for mental health is a major contribution to the literature of psychotherapy in offering ways to engage the whole person for the most effective treatment. For all psychotherapists, but especially those treating trauma, *Head and HeArt* provides myriad approaches to engage the mind, body and emotions. The beautiful layout, and colorful images of yoga and art-making make this a fun book that also manages to be well-researched. Horovitz generously illustrates the safe treatment of people of all ages, cultures and needs, and provides excellent resources for intake, assessment and practice needs.

Patricia Quinn MS, LCAT, ATR-BC
Author, *Art Therapy in the Treatment of Addiction and Trauma*

This is an incredible book! Dr Horovitz so eloquently brings forth her unique perspective from decades of personal experience as an artist and art therapist, and as a yoga practitioner and therapeutic yoga teacher. Her writing and sharing of insights gained on her path of practice and service helps illuminate the worlds of yoga therapy, art therapy, and psychotherapy, and how they overlap. Her synthesis of these fields is clearly what is lacking in today's approach to mental health. Her holistic and therapeutic view of treatment for mental health and wellness moving forward has the potential to create a self-empowering and sustainable approach that truly incorporates mind, body and soul.

Peter Sterios
Author, *Gravity & Grace*, 2019 Nautilus Book Awards Gold Medal Winner; Founder, Manduka and LEVITYoGA

In her latest creative contribution to the literature of art therapy, Ellen Horovitz has managed to effectively marry two ways of knowing and healing which have been known and honored since time immemorial: art and yoga. While describing a clinical approach authentically informed and enriched by both, she has also incorporated contemporary digital resources. Art therapists can learn a great deal from her open and honest account of this new synthesis.

Judith A. Rubin PhD, ATR-BC, HLM
Author, *The Art of Art Therapy*; Filmmaker, *Art Therapy Has Many Faces*

Head and Heart

Yoga therapy and art therapy interventions for mental health

Ellen G Horovitz

Foreword Amy Weintraub

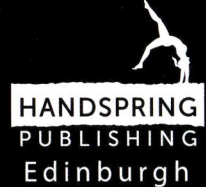

HANDSPRING
PUBLISHING
Edinburgh

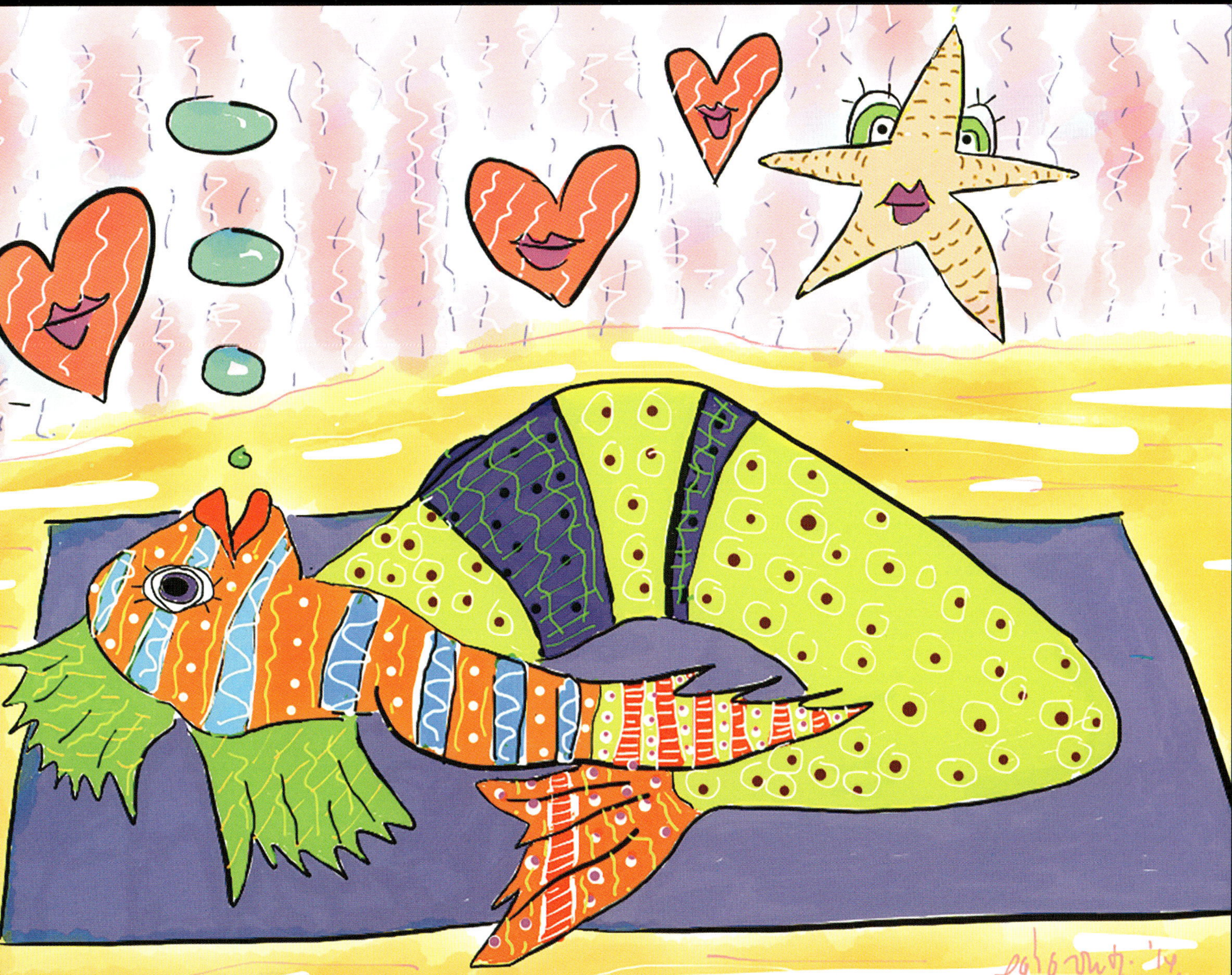

HANDSPRING PUBLISHING LIMITED
The Old Manse, Fountainhall,
Pencaitland, East Lothian
EH34 5EY, Scotland
Tel: +44 1875 341 859
Website: www.handspringpublishing.com

First published 2021 in the United Kingdom by Handspring Publishing Limited
Copyright ©Handspring Publishing Limited 2021

All rights reserved. No parts of this publication may be reproduced or transmitted in any form or by any means, electronic or mechanical, including photocopying, recording, or any information storage and retrieval system, without either the prior written permission of the publisher or a licence permitting restricted copying in the United Kingdom issued by the Copyright Licensing Agency Ltd, Saffron House, 6–10 Kirby Street, London EC1N 8TS.

The right of Ellen G. Horovitz to be identified as the Author of this text has been asserted in accordance with the Copyright, Designs and Patents Acts 1988.

ISBN 978-1-912085-83-5
ISBN (Kindle eBook) 978-1-912085-84-2

British Library Cataloguing in Publication Data
A catalogue record for this book is available from the British Library

Library of Congress Cataloguing in Publication Data
A catalog record for this book is available from the Library of Congress

Notice
Neither the Publisher nor the Author assume any responsibility for any loss or injury and/or damage to persons or property arising out of or relating to any use of the material contained in this book. It is the responsibility of the treating practitioner, relying on independent expertise and knowledge of the patient, to determine the best treatment and method of application for the patient.

All reasonable efforts have been made to obtain copyright clearance for illustrations in the book for which the authors or publishers do not own the rights. If you believe that one of your illustrations has been used without such clearance please contact the publishers and we will ensure that appropriate credit is given in the next reprint.

Commissioning Editor Sarena Wolfaard
Copy Editors Ailsa Laing and Kathryn Mason Pak
Project Manager Morven Dean
Photographer Michele Jenco
Designer Bruce Hogarth
Cover Art Ellen G. Horovitz
Indexer Aptara, India
Typesetter DiTech, India
Printer Melita, Malta
Book printed in Minion Pro Regular 11/13.5pt

The
Publisher's
policy is to use
paper manufactured
from sustainable forests

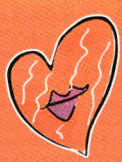
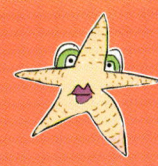

CONTENTS

Dedication	iii
About the author	v
Foreword	vii
Preface: On using this book	ix
Acknowledgments	xi
Introduction	1
1 Creating a safe space	19
2 Assessment for the mind and the body	31
3 The experiential component: the yoga and art process	49
4 Clinical cases: children	77
5 Clinical cases: adolescents	113
6 Clinical cases: adults	153
7 A sampling of *āsanas* for seniors	183
Appendix A Professional practice considerations	205
Appendix B Health history form	211
Appendix C Stages of development	217
Appendix D Practice information	219
Appendix E Cognitive art therapy assessment	225
Appendix F Directional movements of spine and their application	229
Appendix G Movement observation sample	233
Permissions	236
Index	237

DEDICATION

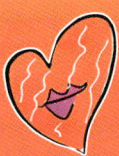 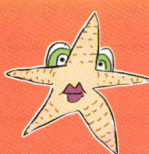

For my wonderful brother-in-law, Orin Wechsberg, who sadly left this plane on Earth Day, April 22nd 2019.

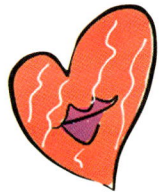 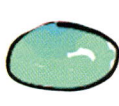 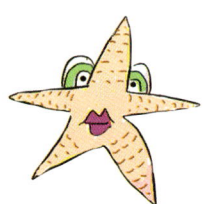

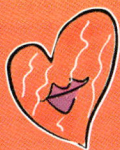 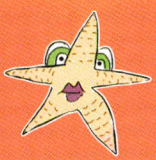

ABOUT THE AUTHOR

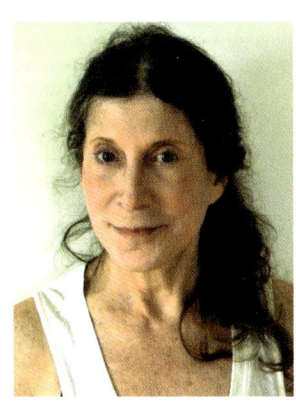

Ellen G. Horovitz is an internationally renowned leader and author in art therapy and yoga therapy, as well as a licensed art therapist, certified yoga therapist and psychotherapist. Ellen currently is the COO of the Open Sky Yoga Therapy Training program in Rochester, NY. She is Professor Emerita and founded the Nazareth College (Rochester, NY) graduate art therapy program, and is past president-elect of the American Art Therapy Association (AATA). She served on the AATA board of directors for 12 years and was responsible for co-writing the national education standards (1992) and manuals for approved graduate programs. In addition, she has served as an expert witness on art therapy education for the US Department of Justice, has won numerous awards and received grants from many organizations, including a graphic consultant grant from the US Department of Defense.

Ellen is also in private practice and works clinically with individuals, couples, and families. She has given hundreds of lectures and workshops nationally and internationally. Currently, she works for Pesi.com as a national speaker and lecturer.

She has authored eight books, on topics ranging from art therapy to yoga therapy to mainstream applications of digital photography, as well as over 50 juried articles and 17 book chapters. Ellen is also an expert in the field of deafness/hearing impairment, and her books, *Visually Speaking: Art Therapy and the Deaf*, and *A Guide to Art Therapy Materials and Methods* have been translated into Korean.

To learn more about her book publications, visit Ellen's Amazon page and her websites at:

yogartherapy.com

https://openskyyoga.com/open-sky-yoga-therapy-training/

FOREWORD

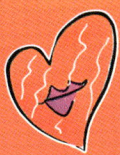
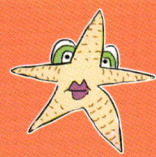

The reader is likely familiar with the ongoing research by Bruce Wampold (2001) which establishes the positive therapeutic alliance, no matter the therapeutic modality, as essential in predicting a beneficial treatment outcome. The many mental health and yoga professionals who have participated in the LifeForce Yoga Practitioner Training over the years have witnessed the powerful effect of the relationship they have with their clients and students. We call it 'the love in the room', and our anecdotal evidence supports Wampold's findings. We humans are often damaged in our earliest relationships through not 'good enough' parenting. Later, we may suffer bullying at the hands of our peers or outright assault by authority figures. It is only logical that to heal from the pain inflicted in relationships, we need the balm a good relationship can provide. The practices and principles of yoga therapy have the potential to enhance the love in the room. When we offer our clients a practice, we join with them, and together move into the spacious, sacred and safe container where healing happens.

The yoga practices offered here help clients and students clear the emotional and mental space to dive more deeply into the work of psychotherapy, accessing the emotions underlying the depressed or anxious mood from a calmer state of mind. Horovitz understands and accessibly describes how a simple yoga intervention can help the student or client dive beneath the constrictions in the physical body, the energy body, the emotional body, and the mental body that in yogic literature are referred to as the *koshas*. When there is physical pain, when there is mental or emotional pain, our access to our larger sense of Self, known in the kosha model as *anandamaya kosha* or bliss body, is restricted. None of these practices cure the pain, but they open a window into a larger space of mind (*anandamaya kosha*) where pain is less gripping.

When we invite those whom we serve into a *pranayama* (breathing) practice for example, and then cue them to stay present to the sensations they are experiencing in the physical body, they are in the present moment, free of judgment about the past and expectation for the future. Through guiding the practice and then the moments of sensory awareness we highlight through our verbal cues, perhaps a tingling sensation in the palms, for example, we open a window through whatever mood state is limiting their access to who they truly are. We help them remember and reconnect with the source of well-being deep inside them, unsullied by whatever may have happened to them. In the beginning of our work with them, it may only be for the few moments after the practice that our clients find a sense of peace, a sense of belonging, a place without shame, depression, anxiety, or the memory of trauma. But as the professional co-creates a home practice (here Horovitz may use it in the homework she sends to clients based on their work in the session), that window of well-being widens. Through continued practice, moments of, 'I'm okay the way I am,' can become hours, days, until there's an established sense of contentment. Anchored in that larger well-being, we and our clients can ride the turbulent waves of life – the disappointments, the betrayals, the failures, and the miscommunications, as well as the achievements and joys.

There is wisdom in the tools to assess that Horovitz provides, some of which she has developed and are used in the wider world of art therapy. Assessment in both yoga therapy and art therapy is vital. In yoga therapy it is essential to meet the client where they are, not just in their capacity to move and stretch into postures and breathe deeply, but also emotionally, culturally, and in ways that are harder to measure but become intuitive as we attune with a client. There is much for the professional to learn here, as Horovitz explains her assessment process. As both a yoga and mental health professional, she communicates her keen understanding of the importance of assessment in establishing the therapeutic alliance and enhancing 'the love in the room'.

Horovitz brings the skills and passion of a creative artist to her training as a yoga therapist and an art therapist, trained by art therapy pioneer Edith Kramer. I am especially moved by the case studies in this book in which art is used to facilitate understanding and better manage family relationships. In one case, we observe Horovitz's work with an 11-year-old boy diagnosed as bipolar and his mother, and appreciate the regular consulting calls she makes to his psychiatrist, always remaining within her scope of practice. To this fraught relationship she brings yoga and art and an attunement to all levels of the family's experience. Because they are religious, she helps them create rituals appropriate to their belief system that brings them closer. There are intense moments that seem life-threatening in and out of session. In the synopsis of the 16 sessions Horovitz spent with mother and son, we see growth in their interactions with each other and a demonstrated reduction in depression, anxiety and stress in the pre- and post-session outcome measurements Horovitz used.

Many years ago, on my final day in a training with the master teacher Menaka Desikachar, a student asked her, 'Madam, what if we give our student a wrong mantra?' She smiled and waved her hand. 'It doesn't matter. It's the relationship that counts', she said, echoing Sharon Salzburg's repetition of words from a psychiatrist. When Desikachar asked him what he thought was the most healing aspect of treatment, he thought for a moment then said, 'I would have to say it's the love in the room'. The book you hold in your hand is not just a manual of principles and practices from the yoga therapy and art therapy traditions, nor is it merely a compendium of research and case studies that illustrate the application of these principles and practices. It is your map for enhancing the therapeutic alliance, the love in the room.

Amy Weintraub MFA ERYT-500 C-IAYT YACEP
Founder of the LifeForce Yoga Healing Institute,
author of *Yoga for Depression* and
Yoga Skills for Therapists

Tucson, AZ, USA
May 2021

Reference

Wampold BE (2001) The Great Psychotherapy Debate: Models, Methods and Findings. Hillsdale, NJ: Lawrence Erlbaum.

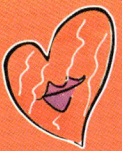

PREFACE: On using this book

Ethical implications of using these modalities and limitations in your practice

This book is envisioned as a resource for all mental health and health professionals and is aimed at: (1) those that assist the therapeutic/healing processes who aspire to incorporate both yoga and creative art therapy interventions into their practice; (2) all health professionals who focus on mental health and/or well-being and want to broaden their understanding of how yoga and creative art therapy interventions can influence mental health approaches, best practices, and efficacy of treatment; and (3) yoga therapy practitioners/teachers and creative art therapists/teachers who wish to deepen their knowledge of integrating yoga and creative art approaches into yoga, mental health and well-being.

I am anticipating that the clinician/reader is:

- professionally trained
- adhering to their professional standards / licensing
- and that their patient is ready to proceed with an established treatment plan.

Nota Bene

In this book, I refer to the word 'patient(s)' since it has a distinct connection to the Latin *pati* for 'suffering', meaning 'the one who suffers'. Though 'clients' can be much more than 'customers' in terms of a word choice, 'clients' are generally connected to legal and/or business contexts, which is not the scope of this work.

While there are numerous models for psychosocial/medical intakes, I have provided my health history form as a resource (Appendix B). Moreover, the reader will find several tables I have developed for ease of comparison and elucidation of the philosophical, developmental and psychological principles behind yoga and art therapy (Chapter 2 and Appendix C). While numerous sources will be offered for the reader to expand their knowledge, I will also offer a brief introduction on the aforementioned systems herein and throughout this book.

Additionally, it is highly recommended that the reader consider using the software program Genogram Analytics and the BetterMind healthcare app to enhance patient outcomes and track efficacy over time. More will be said regarding this in Chapter 2 and other chapters throughout the book, but in sum, Genogram Analytics allows a practitioner to easily design a multi-generational pictograph of the identified patient within their psychosocial system. This information can include intergenerational and psychological conflicts/transitions, medical information, religiosity, occupation, gender identification, racial background and more. It even accounts for pets as family members.

As of this writing, the BetterMind app allows the practitioner to choose from over 60 psychological assessments that can be given to the patient in between sessions and/or in real time. Psychometric data is instantly available to the clinician once the patient completes the assigned assessments. The practitioner can access this information with a 4-digit code (making the app HIPAA compliant) and/or choose to make the results available to the patient. The clinician can use this data as a point of ingress within the sessions and/or tabulate this information to look at efficacy within the sessions over time. It is an incredible psychometric instrument.

Personally, I have been using both of these software applications for over 5 years, and they have allowed me to look at my patients within the context of their family systems (Genogram Analytics) and track the efficacy of my work and patient recovery (BetterMind app) over time.

The Sequence Wiz and YogaMate apps are also excellent resources, and these are discussed in the Introduction for use in your practice.

PREFACE continued

The exercises and patient sample ideas peppered throughout the book can be used exactly as described or as a guide for the reader. Responsibility for treatment resides with the individual therapist/teacher/clinician who understands their patient's specific needs. Thus, this is intended as a resource/guide that will contribute to the well-being of your patient(s).

The information contained herein is written based on current scientific literature available with the understanding that future development in knowledge will always occur. The exercises should be undertaken within the context of the human development cycle (see Chapter 2 and Appendix C) including young children through older adults. It is the responsibility of the reader to determine whether an exercise is age-appropriate or not. For more information on contraindication and benefits of using art therapy materials for specific populations, the reader is directed to my book *The Guide to Art Therapy Materials and Methods: A Practical, Step-by-step Approach*, published in 2017.

For understanding the developmental stages of art, Appendix C provides a useful chart that compares eras and ages of various theorists.

For those who are neither licensed art therapists nor certified yoga therapists, and wish to learn more about those fields, their histories, scope of practice and education requirements, the reader is referred to the Appendices.

In sum, the introduction and presentation of psychological concepts throughout are relevant to the condensed timeline of the presented patient(s). Therefore, the introduction and delivery of psychological concepts, yoga therapy and creative art therapy exercises should be viewed in a flexible manner based on your patient's progress, and treatment response.

So, now, let's begin.

Ellen G. Horovitz PhD ATR-BC E-RYT500
C-IAYT YACEP
Creative Arts Therapy Practice PLLC,
Hilton, NY, USA
Open Sky Yoga Therapy Training,
Rochester, NY, USA

May 2021

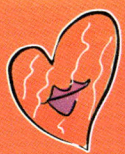
ACKNOWLEDGMENTS
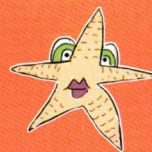

Books percolate, like ideas and good coffee. But in order to get them to a rolling brew, much filtering and consumption informs the process. In this case, there are and continue to be so many people that have held me during the process and influenced its fruition.

First, I need to thank my immediate family members, dear to my heart: Eugene (Jay) Marino, Jr, my husband and constant cheerleader; my children (in no specific order): Kaitlyn Darby (and Grayson Kelly), Bryan Darby, Heather (Foster) Darby, Nicholas (aka Schnickolas) Marino, and Paolo (aka The Paolo) Marino. Additionally, my loving brother, Len Horovitz, MD, and sister, Dr Nancy Bacharach, always have my back when needed. My mother, who still plays bingo and daily bridge, is a constant inspiration; like the Energizer bunny, she just keeps going. I also wish to acknowledge my cousin-sisters and fellow artists, Amy Horovitz Panzer and Cindy Horovitz Wilson. Finally, my sisters, unrelated by birth, but oh so much a part of my fabric, are Karen Armstrong and Dr Irene Rosner-David.

Many yoga teachers have gotten me to the place where I am, and I am eternally grateful for all of their teachings, even my first yoga teacher who patiently endured my endless need to headstand during my adolescence (pitta, pitta, pitta). Specifically, I wish to thank Sri François Raoult, ever my true teacher, and now partner in our new yoga therapy training program (Open Sky Yoga Therapy Training; www.openskyyoga.com). François kindly introduced me to so many notable teachers. I continue to be grateful to all of my teachers, especially Dr Judith Hanson Lasater, Amy Weintraub, Elise Miller, Dr Edwin Bryant, Michael Amy, Carla Anselm, Dr Robert Svoboda, Arthur Kilmurray, Lakshmi Voelker, and Dice Ida Klein at Glo.com for springing me into handstands.

Kelly Birch and Supritha Aithal were particularly helpful in offering feedback in the book's reconstruction/construction and Sarang and Sarju Patel (the Deva twins) were immeasurable in helping me with navigating proper Sanskrit spellings, which vary even amongst the Sanskrit language (thank you, Edwin, for the introduction). Cakra means something in Buddhism, Pali, Hinduism, Sanskrit, Jainism, Prakrit, the history of ancient India, Marathi, Hindi. An alternative spelling of this word is chakra.

In the Yoga Therapy world, I specifically wish to thank Dr Sat Bir Singh Khalsa and the wonderful Dr Larry Payne for aiding me with research pointers and always answering my burning questions. I am also grateful to John Kepner, former Executive Director, Danielle Atkinson, and Dr Lisa Cavallaro, my Accreditation Support Manager at iayt.org. For years, arttherapy.org was my main home, but since finding iayt.org, I have found my inner compass. Between these two organizations and my friends in both places, I am finally at home.

Speaking of which, in the Art Therapy world, I need to acknowledge my dearest tribe members: Dr Irene Rosner David, Dr Michael Franklin, Dr Patricia Isis, Dr Laurie Wilson, Dr Judith Rubin, Dr David Gussak, Elizabeth Stone, Dr Bruce and Cathy Moon (my Moon sandwich), Dr Donna Betts, the late Dr Rawley Silver, and the wonderful Cynthia Woodruff (Executive Director of the American Art Therapy Association), whose boundless energy inspires me. Finally, my greatest mentor and Art Therapy teacher, the Mother of Art Therapy, the late Edith Kramer, who encouraged me to publish and be true to my art.

My friend and photographer extraordinaire, Michele Jenco, is wholly responsible for all the yoga model images. I am grateful for her time and energy and incredible artistic eye. I am also particularly grateful to my dear friend, Dr Jessie Drew-Cates, who patiently modeled for the images in Chapter 2. Also, my quilting friends, specifically Dr Jessie Drew-Cates, Janet Root, Ann Dudek, Marcia Birken, Susan Donovan, Beth Kelly and the 'Fiberistas' hold a huge place in my life. I am anxious to return (full steam ahead) to my quilting/sewing/fiber groups, which admittedly have been on a back burner while this book was marinating. Since art

ACKNOWLEDGMENTS continued

has always been my first love, I have made a promise to myself and my quilting friends to return to my creative urgings (my art) and leave writing in suspension for now. They all laugh at me when I say this and retort with, 'Sure, until the next one.' But I mean it; it is time. Besides, I will be plenty busy with François and OSYTT. Perhaps I can help one of our budding students birth their ideas into writing.

I also need to acknowledge some of my best yogi/yogini buddies: near and dear to my heart are Lori Rivera, the lovely, Julie Hunt, and all my ATT pals at Open Sky Yoga (a special shout out to Dr Monica Javidnia, Eleni Marketos, Karol Thomas, Barb Moran, Becky Lyons, Maxine Ge, and Ream Kidane; you sustained me during our training). I am so grateful that all of you crossed my path and continue to support me as I evolve. And I so miss our contact during our ATT time and since COVID crushed our gatherings. Our Facebook page doesn't quite cut it. But soon we will all meet at Maxine's venture (RAYS - Rochester Accessible Yoga Studio) as we 'ease' back into yoga. And of course, there is ALWAYS the Open Sky (openskyyoga.com).

I am so grateful to Sarena Wolfaard and Andrew Stevenson at Handspring Publishing for believing in me and this book. I also need to thank project manager, Morven Dean; copy editors, Ailsa Laing and Kathryn Mason Pak; proofreader Susan Stuart; marketing director, Hilary Brown; and the incredible design director and illustrator, Bruce Hogarth.

I wish to thank Maureen Howard at Chili Fitness Center and all my 'peeps' in my Senior (if you can call it that) Yoga Class. Your energy, strength, and enthusiasm sustain me. Finally, I need to thank all of my students and patients (past, present, and future). Without you, this work would never have seen the light of day. Allowing me access to your lives has enriched me beyond measure. I am forever grateful.

Ellen G. Horovitz
Hilton, NY, USA
May 2021

Introduction

*I'd rather learn from one bird how to sing
than teach ten thousand stars how not to dance.*

E.E. Cummings

Piecing it together: art therapy

My book concepts come to me as visions during the night; they travel from the undercurrents of my dreams, burrowing a hole into my conscious mind that is so penetrating that they awaken me. What they awaken propels my spirit into the depths of inquiry that quite simply rules me. This inquiry, this mission, gnaws at me like a dog at a bone until it is released. It leaves nothing unturned; instead, it literally chisels me, and I become an instrument to its lead. I don't write the words, they write me. And with each penned entry, I become more enlivened as they captivate and channel my spirit. Not shackled but instead freed to this entity, I ping-pong between its pendulums, this art. It is that flow, that rhythm, that metronome that beats my heart and makes me what I am.

Bullock (1998) coined the word 'uni-verse.' In his definition, he pointed out that uni-verse is indeed our language – one song: all song. Eckert Tolle (1999), in his bestselling treatise *The Power of Now*, described rising from a dream, hearing the voice of a bird and seeing a brilliant diamond in his mind prior to his wakened state of being ever-present. Perhaps what he experienced was the uni-verse that Bullock described: that is, the one song of all kind. Hari Karin Kaur Kalsa in her treatise, *Art and Yoga*, stated that, 'Art is not just a matter of expressing in an outer form what we already know'. She went on to describe that, 'like yoga, art is a union of the known with the unknown… an exploration that steps off the known and moves out to what is beyond' (Kaur Khalsa 2011: vi).

Furtively, humans seek and long for answers to the unknown. Like Kaur Khalsa (2011) and I (Horovitz 1999, 2005, 2017a) have suggested, what emanates from and activates the spirit/Self is not outside you. God, Spirit, Jesus, Buddha, Allah, Animism, or whatever you might call that quintessential creator of the uni-verse, that entity, that energy is in me – it is in all of us – and it innervates every being and all matter on this planet and the universe.

Not a new or novel concept, tapping into this force is as old as time, and the yoga *sūtras*. But it does require firing the Doubting Thomas that runs amok in your mind and replacing it with what was always there – your Self (i.e. creator*)*.

Tolle (1999) talks about honoring that voice that runs amok babbling nonstop by witnessing the transcripts that chatter in your head. He suggests that you stop thinking and embrace the present moment. While I both agree and disagree, force-stopping the incessant chatter is not the answer. Channeling that entity is really what will bring peace, not cutting it off as you would turn off the flow of water from a faucet. Instead, let the floodgates down. Let the chatter, that wellspring, clang through. Give it entry. Offer it passage. Forge an aqueduct if necessary, but don't turn it off. Don't stifle it, squash it, hide it and for Pete's sake, don't ignore it. Instead embrace it, mind it, see it, accept it, and for pity's sake, honor it. *Cittavṛtti* (Sanskrit for the rumination of your thoughts) is on some level your ancestral code; looking at it proactively instead of as something that needs to be banished makes peace with that contemplation and instead rewires it as your contribution, your gift, your creativity, your genetic predisposition, and your art.

As Rumi (2004) wisely said, 'This being human is a guest house. Every morning a new arrival. A joy, a depression, a meanness, some momentary awareness comes as an unexpected visitor. Welcome and entertain them all'.

Heed these inner dialogues. Pay attention to the gurgling of your mind much the way you would pay attention to the orchestration of the acids in your stomach beating the reminder, 'feed me'. These ever-present ramblings that you try to hush while meditating need to be released in other venues. There is a reason that they are trying to break through while you are seeking that state of *nirvāṇa*. Unlike psychotropic uptakes that slowly enter your bloodstream, offer these protestations the deliverance that they deserve. In doing so, you can channel that energy, become enlivened, actually feel lighter and happier and save your Self from a lifetime of enslavement.

Yes, art (and yoga) can heal you. Co-creation is the ticket. It matters little how one travels in order to clean

Introduction

up the baggage of the tattered portions of one's soul. More important is the desire to change and get to that place of harmony, inner peace, soul-making, elemental play, and 'soulution' (Horovitz 1999, 2017a). But knowing and accepting its existence doesn't affirm its placement; practice does. Practicing your art and your yoga transcends the pain – it heals the mind, body and spirit and offers new vision. Bespectacled with a prescription for creative health, you can actually see more and activate your heart. So, permission to co-create becomes the 'soulution', the 'soulution' of heart, mind, body and soul (Horovitz 2005).

While art therapy has never been about the product but instead has always been about the process, I found (like Kramer, 1975) that indeed my patients were working through their issues, but in doing so often their pain, sorrow and losses were being expressed in formed art. Formed art is what Kramer refers to as true art (Kramer 1975). It is the highest form of sublimation, like opera is to classical music, to borrow an analogy, or to put it in Bullock's (1998) terms, uni-verse.

While in this fugue state, your entity is borrowed. You are not the maker but, as Tolle (1999) puts it, 'witness' to the act. To explain this in artistic terms, I give you the apple. In drafting an apple, or any other subject, the artist quite literally dissociates, that is removes themself from the subject, and disembodies. This natural, normal (if you will) state allows for introspection, observation, and accurate delineation of the subject because the artist in this fugue state (as I call it) quite accurately is out of their mind/body experience and becomes one with the subject. They co-create with this other, and become the other while simultaneously separating enough so that the other can be captured and illustrated. Surgeons, musicians, writers – they all do the same thing. They depersonalize in order to liberate the subject in the highest form of art (Fig. 1).

Opening yourself and becoming a conduit to this flow requires trust in the process. And of course, understanding where the art might fall in terms of development is also important, especially if you are dealing with comorbid situations. So, let's explore some of the logistics of looking at the art product itself and safety. While I discuss setting up your environment in

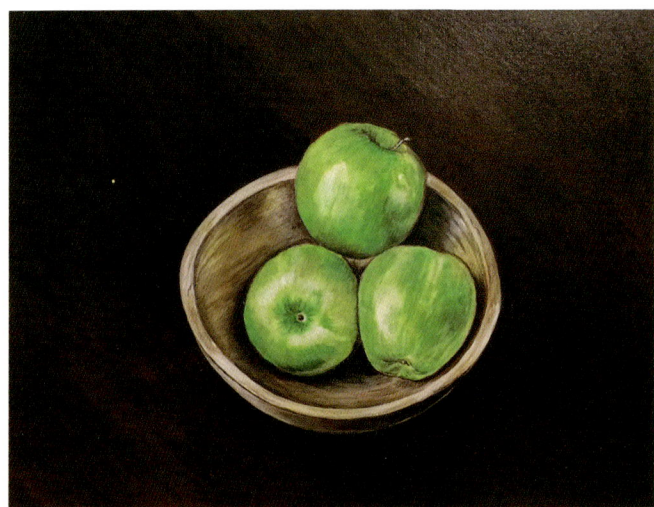

FIGURE 1 Bad apples, illustration by author. (From the collection of Christopher Kisiel, chef and owner of Bad Apples)

Chapter 3, safety is a prerequisite when working with art media.

Artistic development

When I grew up in the 1960s, safety regulations were, to say the least, lacking. But times have changed, and while I still love the smell of many toxic substances that challenge my health and safety, as a therapist I need to protect my patients and/or potential consumers. Thus, it is important to have some facts on hand. For regulation of art materials, I suggest the reader refer to the text (Horovitz 2017b) for information on handling and caring for specific art media. (For a complete compendium, visit the art and craft safety guide at: https://www.nlm.nih.gov/enviro/arts-crafts-and-human-health.html.)

In Appendix C (and also in Chapter 2), I offer the reader a table listing the *normative* developmental stages of art (according to Lowenfeld and Brittain, 1975), and compare those norms against those from other theorists such as Erikson, Piaget, Kohlberg, Fowler, etc. Viewing these artistic stages of development against other developmental theories aids in understanding 'normal' (if you will) artistic expression. Doris Arrington (1991) sums up development by stating, '…from infants to seniors, humans age at different rates, and therefore

Introduction

chronological age is an imperfect indicator of functional age' (Arrington 1991). In her article, Arrington concisely describes the developmental markers in art ranging from preschool to *Thanatos*. But for condensing and synthesizing developmental art levels, nothing beats the art education source, Lowenfeld and Brittain (1975).

Exploring physicality, somatic and traumatic issues, and their impact on development and movement provides the therapist with yet another index for exploring the whole person. Our bodies inform the gut, long considered to be the second brain (Gershon 1999), and as a creative art therapist and trained yoga therapist, I involve the entire person: mind, body and spirit.

Spiritual art therapy and the belief art therapy assessment

In my first book, *Spiritual Art Therapy: An Alternate Path*, now in its 3rd edition (Horovitz 2017a), I laid the groundwork for examining the whole person via the belief art therapy assessment (BATA). The BATA explores issues of spirituality, religiosity and/or belief systems when they arise to the forefront of patient issues.

In the past, religious and spiritual needs were entrusted to the clergy. Baptism, last rites, confirmation, communion, and even prayer are often relegated to religious leaders. This domain has created a fissure for any clinician who has faced a patient's spiritual questions, struggle with faith, and/or desire for forgiveness. Thus, clinicians can choose to:

1. Ignore the spiritual dimension of the patient.
2. Chalk up the patient's thinking as floridly psychotic.
3. Refer the patient to a clergy person without participating in that aspect of care (thus, defeating a systemic approach).
4. Collaborate with a clergy person and work out an interdisciplinary approach to treatment.
5. Attempt to spiritually counsel the patient.

Often, I choose number 5. Thus, I am making the assumption that spiritual care is a legitimate part of healthcare. Even though the clergy has a specified role in this arena, I purport that the spiritual needs of a patient require attention and treatment by the entire healthcare team. Indeed, I have also invoked the clergy to help: years ago, while treating a family that was contending with mourning issues related to the death of their unborn infant, I invited the family's priest to attend the graveside visit so that the funereal process could be recreated and cast in a different light. From a systemic perspective, an interdisciplinary and communal approach to treating an identified patient within a family systems framework is not only essential but also fundamental in the treatment of the whole person. Internal Family System (IFS) enthusiasts would wholeheartedly agree here (see Schwartz 2011).

Moreover, in order to accomplish such a formidable task, incorporating the spiritual, belief and religious components into treatment requires a tool for assessing whatever nodal events contributed to the disorder and dis-ease of the person. While the BATA offers an instrument for estimation, the reader may not be comfortable with continued exploration of a patient's spiritual belief system. If this is the case, then one needs to embrace an interdisciplinary approach and rely on the skills and talents of other professionals within the community.

Nota Bene

It is important to note that I conduct the BATA only when the patient questions or brings up their belief/spiritual dimension on interview or within the aforementioned testing component. Moreover, the BATA is conducted only when the information might lead to an improved understanding of the patient, as opposed to contributing to further deterioration of his, her, or their condition. Even if the patient reveals spiritual struggle by way of the BATA, it is wholly possible that the patient may not be ready to explore the 'spiritual dimension' since this involves abstract thinking. If, in fact, the patient's thinking is formal, rigid and concrete, then the therapist needs to walk this line with trepidation and always respect the patient's lead.

Introduction

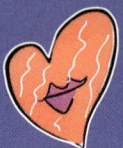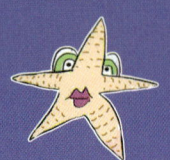

Working with art materials

Working with art materials (including fiber materials) can help relieve stress, depression, anxiety and even diminish pain and other physical symptoms (Horovitz 2017b). Through a series of art activities and creative processes, art therapists can aid people in self-expression and develop a sense of well-being. Often, expressing oneself with art materials facilitates verbal expression. Working with art materials and mastering new skills through visual media enhances self-satisfaction, personal achievement, accomplishment and often mastery. According to Kaur Khalsa, who also combines yoga and art, 'Art and the breath create safe places to be with your feelings and explore them'. She goes on to add this poignant statement: 'drawing is a dialogue between what you know and what you don't know' (Kaur Khalsa 2011: 35).

Working from a studio art therapy perspective

While I discuss assessment in Chapter 2, in 1987 I discussed its importance in the *Journal of Art Therapy* (Horovitz-Darby 1987). In 1988, I published the first edition of the cognitive art therapy assessment (CATA), which was refined in my 2014 publication (Horovitz 1988; 2014). While the CATA is more of a qualitative instrument, it is disguised as a studio activity and therefore is less anxiety-provoking than standardized tests that enforce (for example) drawing a person picking an apple from a tree (PPAT) (Gantt and Tabone 1998).

While the entire CATA is presented in Appendix E, in sum, the CATA can provide a clinician with the following information when deciding what art materials might best assist the patient:

1. Outstanding developmental capacities, deficits, deviations, visual–motor functioning. Developmental stage as seen in artwork. If deficits are indicated, is it possible that they are constitutional and/or emotional, cultural?
2. Self-image: sexual identity, self-esteem, ego ideals.
3. Perception of self in relation to others. Individuation, strong emotional attachments, symbiosis?
4. Sense of reality. Distortions of self and body parts, depersonalization?
5. Thought processes, ability to conceptualize, memory, judgment, concrete or abstract thinking?
6. Defenses — and dangers defended against.
7. Capacity for other gratifications — not art but playful manipulation of materials.
8. Potential to learn, to master, to function on a higher level, environmental or cultural factors that might be influential.
9. Temperamental assessment as seen in art session, mood quality — exuberant, hesitant, overwhelmed by anxiety, etc. Activity level — hyperactive, deliberate, reflective, attention span approach or withdrawal? Adaptability or construction.
10. Capacity for ego gratification through art. Capacity for ego maturation through art.

While theories abound regarding the field of art therapy, I had the privilege to be trained under the great Edith Kramer, long considered the mother of art therapy. While her training hailed from psychoanalytic frameworks, when working alongside her and her patients it was impossible to detect that her mind was interpreting the person from a psychoanalytic standpoint; instead her amazing presence of being an artist, therapist and teacher (all at once) was what I gleaned from her approach.

For example, one day when interning alongside her, a child became overwrought when his painting became darker and darker. He exhibited great distress in his inability to control the paint materials. Edith simply took a large paintbrush, dipped it into white paint and silently offered it to the child. He took the brush, began to add the white color to his muddied work, and as it lightened, so, too, did his mood: he calmed down. These things are not often taught but intuited, much the same way a yoga therapist may see that someone is uncomfortable and would benefit from a *prāṇayāma* bolster to support discomfort and/or physiological need.

Speaking of which, it is also important to understand not just the principles of yoga and its philosophy but how

Introduction

that dovetails with the mental health aspects of holistically treating the whole person. For more about studio art therapy approaches, I suggest that the reader look at the works of my colleagues, Cathy Moon (2010) and Pat Allen (1995, 2005).

Now let's yoke this with yoga and put these aspects together in a psychological framework.

The foundations of yoga philosophy

In order for the reader to have an underpinning in yoga philosophy and its psychology, it is important to understand the five *kleśas* (afflictions/obstacles), the five *vṛittis* (fluctuations of the mind), the eight limbs of yoga: *yama* (abstentions or moral restraints), *niyama* (attitudes toward ourselves and ethical observances), *āsana* (physical postures), *prāṇayāma* (restraint or expansion of the breath), *pratyāhāra* (withdrawal of the senses), *dhārana* (concentration), *dhyāna* (meditation) and *samādhi* (complete integration), the five *kośas* (that make-up an individual), the *cakrá* system (centers of subtle energy located at various points along the spine), and the *nāḍis*.

While some readers may be familiar with these aspects of yoga philosophy, they will be abbreviated herein. Bryant (2009, 2017) offers a comprehensive review of the yoga *sūtras*, the philosophical cornerstones of yoga, and establishes a baseline for understanding that will be welcomed by all serious students of the spiritual heritage of India. The yoga *sūtras*, one of the ancient treatises on Indic philosophy, are considered the basis of classical yoga philosophy (made up of 196 *sūtras* – 'threads' or discourses) and were compiled by Patañjali around 400 CE. The 196 *sūtras* are compartmentalized into four topical books: *Samādhi Pāda* (what yoga is), *Sādhana Pāda* (how to gain a yogic state), *Vibhūti Pāda* (benefits of practicing yoga regularly), and *Kaivalya Pāda* (liberation or freedom from suffering). While the reader may not want to delve into these topics, the following overview will help provide the keystones of yoga philosophy and how these foundations are used in yoga therapy and apply to the field of psychology.

The five kleśas (afflictions or obstacles)

In Hinduism and Buddhism, a *kleśa* is a negative mental state that clouds the mind, causing anguish and the conditions for suffering to arise. *Kleśas* also refer to the obstacles that prevent a person from reaching a state of enlightenment and freedom from *saṃsāra* (metempsychosis or negative mental states). The *kleśas* are viewed as hindrances. In order to understand how the *kleśas* contribute to anxiety and suffering, understanding their meaning and how they affect our interaction in the world is key to understanding anxiety and the *vṛittis* (fluctuations of the mind) according to yogic philosophy. The *kleśas* are: (1) *avidyā* (ignorance), (2) *asmita* (ego), (3) *rāga* (attachment), (4) *dveṣa* (aversion to pain or suffering), and (5) *abhiniveśa* (clinging to life/fear of death).

1. *Avidyā* is a deep spiritual ignorance. In ignorance, any and all obstacles grow and flourish. Having an understanding of what is real and what is not, allows you to work with all obstacles that come into your life. According to Indian philosophy, inside every life-form is spirit that will not die or perish; everything else decays and desists. That fleeting thing that attracts us in the moment often constitutes *rāgas* (attachment to pleasure).

2. *Asmita* literally means ego, but this is false ego. *Avidyā* (spiritual ignorance) is where egos grow. Clearly, you need to have enough strength to create a life for yourself and provide for your family. But *asmita* is the path of how we get in our own way and bring ourselves into disappointment. *Asmitā* mistakes the deep-level Self, *Ātman*, with the body and mind surface-level Self.

3. *Rāga* is attachment to pleasure, that is wanting to repeat things that feel good. While it is understandable that one wants to repeat a pleasurable process, a way of discerning the difference is to ask yourself, what would it be like if you never repeated that thing, experience, pleasure, pose, etc, again? In other words, can you be in the moment, enjoy it, let it go and then be open to whatever comes next? This is where truth and contentment lie. When you can

Introduction

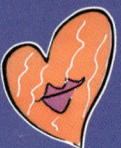 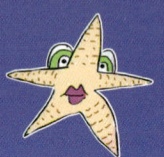

let go of that continual chase for pleasure, understanding breeds what matters. Both *rāga* and *dveṣa* (explored next) exist in the land of wanting, wanting, wanting or fear-based pushing of things (and relationships) away.

4. *Dveṣa* (the flip side of *rāga*) is an aversion to unpleasant things or experiences. While it is natural to avoid unpleasantness or suffering, like *rāga*, *dveṣa* is not wanting to repeat unpleasant circumstances. For example, many people avoid the inevitable aging process, or suffering, illness, or death. *Dveṣa* paralyzes us from walking down new paths, keeps us in our past and doesn't allow us to live fully in the present moment. This leads us to the last *kleśa*, *abhiniveśa*.

5. *Abhiniveśa* means clinging to life. Instinctually, we are all attached to life, to surviving. Even the wisest of sages have trouble with this. After all, bringing a sense of deep acceptance (equanimity) to life is a very difficult process. But according to Indian philosophy, there is a divine spark that will never die. The body dies, but the spirit does not. Meditating on *abhiniveśa* helps us to find sangfroid around the spark, the soul (the part of us that never dies), accepting the body that will die, and understanding the difference.

The five vṛttis

Vṛittis (or active fluctuations of the mind) are the five ways we can have our mind activated: (1) *pramāna* (right perception), (2) *viparyaya* (wrong perception), (3) *vikalpa* (conceptualization, figure of speech), (4) *nidrā* (deep dreamless sleep), and (5) *smṛti* (memory). *Saṃskāras* (unlike *vṛittis*) are inactive, albeit mental imprints, but these are more than merely memories. And this brings us back to *pramāna* (right perception). According to Bryant (2019), we gain knowledge of the world around us through our senses and direct experience. This allows us to apply logic and reason to figure things out. But *viparyaya* (wrong perception) is misconception. As Bryant (2019) puts it, 'We may like to think that we go through life seeing things

Reflection exercise 1

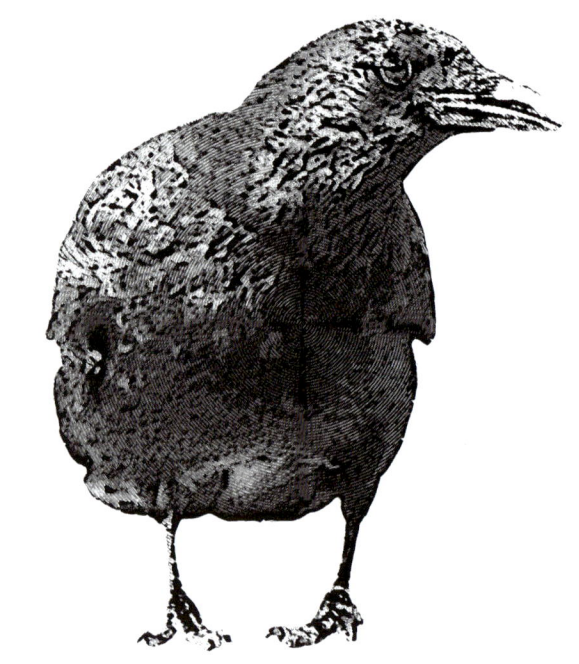

FIGURE 2 Crow illustration by author

In thinking about this concept of *abhiniveśa* and the aforementioned *kleśas*, what is it like for you to pause and consider that this life (as you know it) will cease and that life itself will continue? What would it be like for you to pause once a day (perhaps during *śavāsana*, meditation or artmaking) and reflect on this concept but that also life itself will continue. Perhaps, you could stop and wonder about that or make some artwork around that concept. This is not an easy subject to digest for most people. But in undertaking the yogic path, these are some of the notions that I would like you to think about, for this is the stuff of rumination and anxieties for all humankind.

objectively but in fact, we see the world that we want to see'. As Bryant clarified, '*Viparyaya* is just plain erroneous perception – to think a tree is a person, for example'.

Introduction

So, the question remains: are these *saṃskāras* (mental, subliminal imprints, or epigenetics if you are of more of a scientific bent) or does one have free will? Bryant (2019) answers this by stating:

So, the vṛttis (active mind functions) including smṛti (memory) are considered memory because all thoughts create lasting impressions. So, it can be said that smṛti is the ability to recall a memory. Every memory creates an impression in the mind and these impressions, whether they lead to suffering or freedom, need to be controlled in order to abide in our own true nature – in the state of yoga.

So, what does this all mean? Basically, Patañjali describes these five functions of the mind to ultimately help us reduce our suffering. By being able to recognize these functions and learn how the mind works, Patañjali offers us the foundation to see (our) true nature as separate from the mind. It is almost like stepping out of yourself and observing the functions of the mind, without being attached, upset or frustrated... just simply becoming an observer.

Once you are able to observe without reaction, you will be able to more easily differentiate the mind and all of its fluctuations from your true nature. Patañjali says that 'through sustained practice and the cultivation of dispassion, these fluctuations of mind can be stilled. (Yoga Sūtra: 1.12).

(Bryant 2019)

Bryant (2009) summarizes that the essential point of understanding yoga is that:

... all forms or activities of the mind are products of prakṛti, matter, and completely distinct from the soul or true self, puruṣa, pure awareness or consciousness... Only then can the soul be realized as an entity completely distinct from the mind (a distinction such clichés as 'self-realization' attempt to express) and the process to achieve this realization is yoga.

(Bryant 2009: liii–liv)

It's the getting there that is not so simple a process, and thus the realm of such anxieties has plagued the mind of humankind since the beginning of time.

> ### Reflection exercise 2
>
>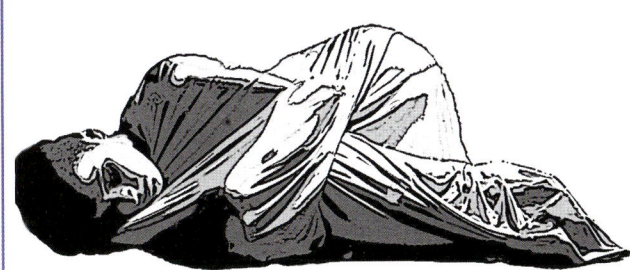
>
> **FIGURE 3** *Vṛittis*, illustration by author
>
> Can you imagine observing your mind without a premediated construct? Place a large piece of paper before you (at least 18" x 24") and place some art materials next to the surface of the paper. Next, close your eyes; feel the parameters of the paper. Feel for a drawing/painting implement nearby and simply create a mark on the paper, either using the entire surface of the paper or whatever you are drawn to. Open your eyes. See what you have created. Perhaps turn the paper in multiple directions. See something within the negative and positive spaces. Embellish it and create more from your mark. This is *saṃskāras* at work. The mental imprints of your own perception are leading your hand and mind. Bask in this interoceptive, mind–body experience.

The yamas and the niyamas

According to Patañjali, the five *yamas* (the first limb of yoga) are considered abstentions or moral restraints. These are: (1) *ahiṃsā* (non-violence or non-harming of all creatures, including ourselves), (2) *sātya* (truthfulness or honesty in words and actions), (3) *asteya* (non-stealing of other's property or time), (4) *brahmacarya* (chastity, which can also be interpreted as restraint or moderation in all impulses, not necessarily sexual), and (5) *aparigrāha* (non-coveting – a practice of letting go of all that is not needed and only possessing what is completely necessary).

Introduction

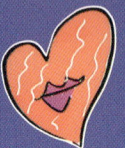 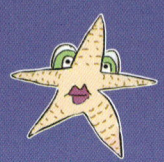

In Patañjali's *Yoga Sūtras*, *niyamas* (the second limb of yoga) are ethical observances, one's own personal discipline and practice. They are: (1) *śauca* (cleanliness), (2) *santoṣa* (contentment), (3) *tapas* (austerity or self-discipline), (4) *svādhyāya* (self-reflections and study of all the scriptures or sacred texts), (5) *īśvara-praṇidhāna* (devotion to God or a higher being). *Īśvara-praṇidhāna* includes dedicating and devoting one's work to a higher power and dissolving ego-focused desires.

Reflection exercise 3

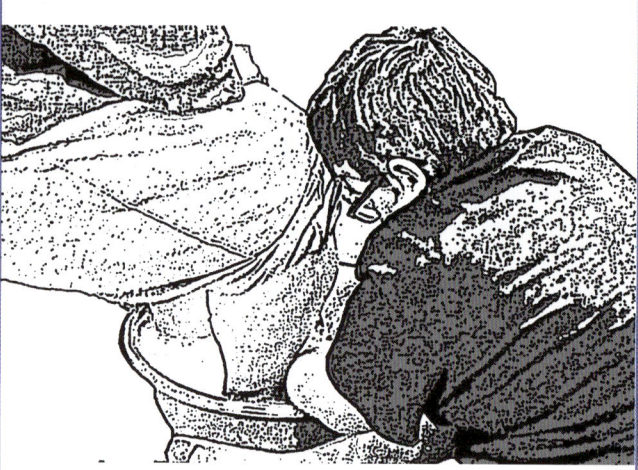

FIGURE 4 *Śauca* (cleanliness), illustration by author

Choose one of the *yamas* or *niyamas* that you relate to or wish to incorporate in your life. Imagine how you can amplify this characteristic either through meditating on this desire and/or creating some artwork or writing to enhance this enactment in your life. For example, suppose you had a patient, which I did, who came to session unkempt, malodorous, and repulsive due to his lack of hygiene. How would you bring this person to the state of *śauca* (cleanliness) in order to not only invite this ethical observance but be able to stomach working with him? While I don't want to give away what I did since this will be covered in Chapter 4, be creative: think about how you might approach this individual with this goal in mind.

The kośas

The *kośa* model consists of five sheaths representing the simultaneous aspects of human existence – physical, breath/energy, emotions, beliefs and bliss or a sense of interconnectedness with all beings. They are referred to as: (1) *anāmaya kośa* (physical), (2) *prāṇamaya kośa* (energy), (3) *manomaya kośa* (mind), (4) *vijnanamaya kośa* (intuition), and (5) *anandamaya kośa* (bliss). These correspond respectively to the physical, vital, mental, intuitive and blissful planes mentioned in Western mysticism.

According to Weintraub (2015), when we practice yoga, there is no mind-body split. It is there that we practice with attention to breath and sensation, move into the present moment and see ourselves as more than our personal stories and dysregulated moods.

Reflection exercise 4

Pick a sheath (*kośa*) that you feel the need to work on in your personal life. Meditate on how that *kośa* will bring you additional protection. Next choose an *āsana* that supports you in that initiative; take that position. Feel the sheath surround you. Next write about that experience or make some artwork that reflects that experience back to you.

The three guṇas

The three *guṇas* refer to the 'quality of primordial nature' (Bryant 2009: 584). According to Bryant's worldview, there are three *guṇas* present in all things and beings: (1) *sattva* (goodness, constructive, harmonious), (2) *rājas* (passion, active, confused), and (3) *tamas* (darkness, destructive, chaotic). According to the *Yoga Sūtra* II.41 (*sattva-śuddhi*): 'upon the purification of the mind, one attains cheerfulness, one-pointedness, sense control and fitness to perceive the self' (Bryant 2009: 490). This is the desired state, but not always achievable since all three *guṇas* are present in everyone and everything. It is the proportion and interplay that defines the innate nature and psychological attributes of the person.

In a lecture, Bryant (2019) explained perception in terms of people looking at a tree and based on their own biases, likes and dislikes seeing different things:

... an artist will see a potential painting, a carpenter sees potential craft possibilities, an environmentalist will contemplate the environmental benefits of the tree and a child will see it as something to climb and explore! So, a tree is not simply what we see with our five senses – we see what is relevant to us which is conditioned by our own biases. So, our thoughts (vṛttis) can be knowledge that is reality as perceived through our senses and interpreted by our minds. However, pramāna (right knowledge) precisely does mean to know that reality correctly... the goal of yoga is to calm these vṛttis; when they are calm, we can start to see things for what they truly are instead of what we perceive them to be.

(Bryant 2019)

> ### Reflection exercise 5
>
> Imagine what it would feel like to be in a *sattva-śuddhi* state of mind and body (one-pointedness, balanced). What *āsana* might this look like to you? Or could you see that state during a meditative state? Maybe practice this in both your meditation and *āsanas*. Journal on what that felt like.

The three doṣas (Āyurvedic constitution)

While Āyurveda is concerned with life's physical bases (not necessarily equated with yoga philosophy), it concentrates on inducing the right relationship of the body with the mind and spirit (Svoboda 1998). At the bare minimum, understanding the three *doṣas*, (*vāta, pitta, kapha* – air, fire and water, respectively) is paramount in discerning how your constitution effects your mind, body and spirit. *Vāta* (the principle of kinetic energy) is

> ### Reflection exercise 6
>
>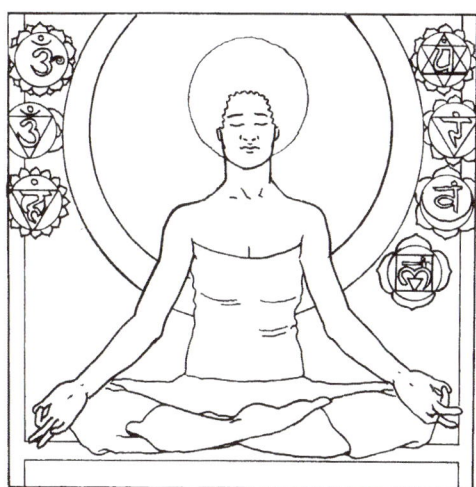
>
> **FIGURE 5** Meditation (from Paolo E. Marino, with permission)
>
> As you begin to comprehend your *doṣa* (*vāta, pitta, kapha,* knowing you have all three components in your constitution) envision how this affects you in your day-to-day interactions. Does this feel balanced or 'out of whack'? Imagine a diet that might make you feel more balanced. Search for something that might calm your system and make you feel more balanced (Fig. 5). Or, try this meditation suggested by Lad (1985):
>
> *Through breathing become aware of the vibration of cosmic sound... this is the soundless sound of aum... (which has) two manifestations, one male, one female. The male manifestation is hum and the female energy is so. During inhalation, you will feel the cosmic sound so. During exhalation, you will feel the sound hum... In the so–hum meditation there is a union of individual consciousness with cosmic consciousness. Listen to the so–hum, hum–so sound through the breath... your breathing will become quiet and spontaneous and you will go beyond thought, beyond time and space, and beyond cause and effect... this merging brings samādhi, the state of highest equilibrium.*
>
> (Lad 1985: 126)

Introduction

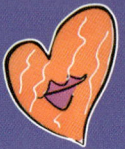

mainly concerned with the nervous system and controls all body movement. *Pitta* (the body's balance of kinetic and potential energies) involves the enzymatic and endocrine systems. *Kapha* (the principle of potential energy) controls body stability and lubrication. Figuring out your constitution is as easy as going online and taking a simple test (Chopra Centre 2020, Doctor Blossom 2020, VPK by Maharishi Ayurveda Products International 2020). But truly understanding the intricacies of Āyurveda is an altogether different subject in and of itself and requires much education and certification in order to become an Āyurvedic practitioner. The Āyurvedic Institute (for example) houses the kingpin of Āyurveda medicine on its faculty and administration, Dr Vasant Lad MASc. Dr Lad is the author of 11 books on Āyurveda as well as hundreds of articles; his work has been translated into 20 languages.

The nāḍi system and the seven cakras

According to Āyurvedic health systems, and in yoga philosophy, all living things function thanks to the life energy known as *prāṇa*, which circulates in the body through the subtle pathways known as the *nadis*. *Prāṇa* can circulate only when the *nadis* are clear and strong. When the *nadi* system is blocked, *prāṇa* cannot flow, and a person's physical and mental health are negatively affected.

The three main *nadis* are:

- *Ida nadi*. Called the left channel, *ida nadi* starts in the *muladhara* (root) chakra, flowing to the left and weaving in and out of the chakras before ending in the left nostril. This *nadi* represents mental energy. Lunar, cooling, *mana shakti*, power of the mind (PNS). *Chandra bedha prānayama* (minus): breathe in left only, exhale right.

- *Pingala nadi*. Referred to as the right channel, *pingala nadi* also starts in the root chakra, but flows to the right, weaving in and out of the chakras in a mirror image of *ida nadi* and ending in the right nostril. *Pingala nadi* is the origin of *prana. Prāna nadi*. Solar, hot, *prāna (shakti)* (SNS). *Surya bedha prānayama* (positive): breathe in right only, exhale left.

- *Suṣumṇā nadi*. The central channel, *suṣumṇā nadi* runs straight up the spine and through the chakras from just below the root chakra to the *sahasrakā* or (crown) chakra. This is the *nadi* of spiritual awareness.

According to Blondon (2019), you should do chakra awakening at least once in your life. We have energy that has great influence on the *doshas*. Blondon suggests that we are not personalities but *dosha* received on the day of our birth (Doctor Blossom 2020). *Cakras* can be too open or too closed but they cannot break. If a *cakra* is really closed, it doesn't spin, and most of the time it has less energy going through. The *nadis* are often compared to the meridians of Chinese acupuncture.

Nāḍis and the vāyus

One way of categorizing *prāṇa* (or breath) is by means of the *vāyus*. *Vāyu* means 'wind' or 'air' in Sanskrit, and the term is used in a variety of contexts in Hindu philosophy. *Prāṇa* is considered the basic *vāyu* from which the other *vāyus* arise, as well as one of the five major *vāyus*. *Prāṇa* is thus the generic name for all the breaths, including the five major *vāyus* of *prāṇa, apāna, uḍāna, samāna* and *vyāna*.

- *Prāṇa*. The exhaled breath (*pra* = 'outward', 'forth') which lives in the lungs.

- *Apāna*. Down and outward energy, most notably the eliminatory systems. It resides in the hips and gut.

- *Udāna*. Rising energy, resident in the throat, but also responsible for lifting kundalini; sound production through the vocal apparatus, as in speaking, singing, laughing and crying.

- *Samāna*. The heat of digestion tract, which resides in the belly between *prāṇa* above and *uḍāna* below.

- *Vyāna*. The energy of circulation that resides throughout the body.

Introduction

The seven cakras

- *Mūlādhāra*. 1st or root chakra, located at the base of the spine.
- *Svādhiṣṭhāna*. 2nd or navel chakra, located below the navel (near the belly button), known for its power in life actions.
- *Maṇipūra*. 3rd or solar plexus chakra, located near the diaphragm; corresponds to personal power, creativity and intellect.
- *Anāhata*. 4th or heart chakra, located near heart; speech, communication and social ability.
- *Viśuddha*. 5th or throat chakra; associated with communication, speech, social abilities, verbal, and emotional expression and the creative arts.
- *Ājñā*. 6th or third eye chakra and is the all-seeing; located between and slightly above the eyes; corresponds to intuition and artistic, creative thoughts.
- *Sahasrāra*. 7th or crown chakra located on top of the head, which is the highest spiritual chakra; corresponds to intuition, spirituality.

Since this is a lot of information for the reader to digest, I have corralled all of the above into a collection of lists (Box 1).

BOX 1 Summary lists

Kleśas Afflictions or obstacles

- *Avidyā* A deep, spiritual ignorance
- *Asmita* Literally means ego, but this is false ego
- *Rāga* Attachment to pleasure, that is wanting to repeat things that feel good
- *Dveṣa* Flip side of *raga*, an aversion to unpleasant things or experiences
- *Abhiniveśa* Clinging to life

Vṛttis Active fluctuations of the mind*

- *Pramāna* Right perception
- *Viparyaya* Wrong perception
- *Vikalpa* Conceptualization, figure of speech
- *Nidrā* Deep dreamless sleep
- *Smṛti* Memory

Yamas 1st limb of yoga

- *Ahiṁsā* Non-violence or non-harming of all creatures
- *Satya* Truthfulness or honesty in words and actions
- *Asteya* Non-stealing of others' property or time
- *Brahmācarya* Chastity, also interpreted as restraint or moderation in all impulses
- *Aparigrāha* Non-coveting

Niyamas 2nd limb of yoga

- *Śauca* Cleanliness
- *Santoṣa* Contentment
- *Tapas* Austerity or self-discipline
- *Svādhyāya* Self-reflections and study of all the scriptures or sacred texts
- *Īśvara-praṇidhāna* Devotion to God or a higher being

Kośas Five sheaths, breath/energy, connection with all living beings

- *Anāmaya kośa* Physical
- *Prāṇamaya kośa* Energy
- *Manomaya kośa* Mind
- *Vijnanamaya kośa* Intuition
- *Anandamaya kośa* Bliss

Guṇas

- *Sattva* Goodness, constructive, harmonious
- *Rājas* Passion, active, confused
- *Tamas* Darkness, destructive, chaotic

Doṣas Ayurvedic Constitution

- *Vāta* Kinetic energy, concerned with the nervous system and controls all body movement

Introduction

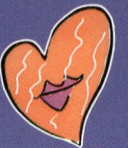
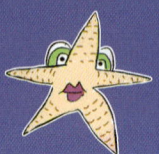

BOX 1 continued

- *Pitta* The body's balance of kinetic and potential energies, involves the enzymatic and endocrine systems
- *Kapha* The principle of potential energy, controls body stability and lubrication

Nāḍis Plural for ~35 million channels thought to pervade the subtle body and chakras

- *Iḍā* **(left channel)** Masculine or logical aspect of each person
- *Piṅgalā* **(right channel)** Feminine aspects of each person**
- *Suṣumṇā* **(central channel)** Central channel of the spinal cord, one of the three principal Nadis of yogic and tantric physiologies. This is the nadi of spiritual awareness.

Vāyus

- *Prāṇa* Exhaled breath, lives in the lungs
- *Apāna* Down and outward energy, most notably the eliminatory systems
- *Udāna* Rising energy, resident in the throat, sound production (speaking, singing, laughing, crying)
- *Samāna* Heat of digestion tract, which resides in the belly between *prāṇa* above and *uḍāna* below
- *Vyāna* Energy of circulation that resides throughout the body

Cakras

1. *Mūlādhāra* 1st, Root Chakra, located at the base of the spine
2. *Svādhiṣṭhāna* 2nd, Navel Chakra, located below the navel (near the belly button) and is known for its power in life actions
3. *Maṇipūra* 3rd, Solar Plexus Chakra, located near the diaphragm; personal power, creativity and intellect
4. *Anāhata* 4th, Heart Chakra, located near heart; speech, communication and social ability
5. *Viśuddha* 5th, Throat Chakra, and is the chakra associated with communication, speech, social abilities, verbal and emotional expression and the creative arts
6. *Ājñā* 6th, Third Eye Chakra and is the all-seeing located between and slightly above the eyes; corresponds to intuition, artistic, creative thoughts
7. *Sahasrāra* 7th, Crown Chakra located on top of the head which is the highest spiritual chakra; corresponds to intuition, spirituality

The Eight Limbs of Yoga

1. *Yamas* Restraints
2. *Niyamas* Observances
3. *Āsana* Postures
4. *Pranāyāma* Breath
5. *Pratyāhāra* Turning inward
6. *Dhārana* Concentration
7. *Dhyāna* Meditation
8. *Samādhi* Openness with all living things

*Saṃskāras (unlike *Vṛittis*) are inactive, albeit mental imprints, but these are more than merely memories.
**Balancing both masculine and feminine aspects will make you more effective in the world, and will enable you to handle life aspects well.

Introduction

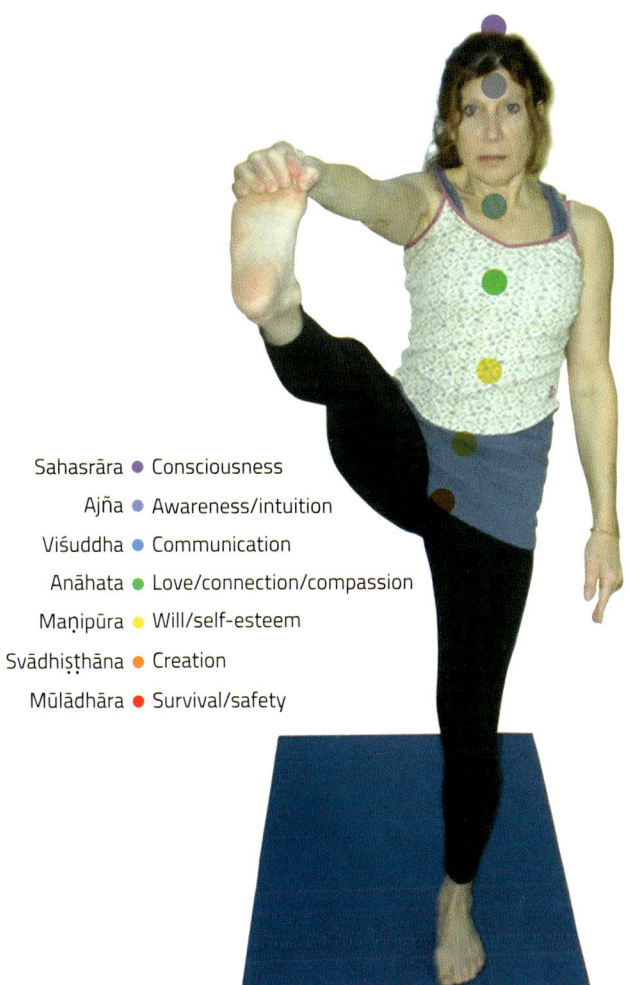

FIGURE 6 Author and chakra system versus Maslow's theory

TABLE 1 Comparison of Maslow's hierarchy with the chakras	
Maslow's hierarchy (read bottom to top)	Chakra system (read bottom to top)
Consciousness	*Sahasrāra* 7th or Crown Chakra, located on top of the head, the highest spiritual chakra, corresponds to intuition, spirituality
Awareness/intuition	*Ājñā* 6th or Third Eye Chakra, the all-seeing, located between and slightly above the eyes, corresponds to intuition, artistic, creative thoughts
Communication	*Viśuddha* 5th or Throat Chakra, associated with communication, speech, social abilities, verbal and emotional expression and the creative arts
Love/connection and compassion	*Anāhata* 4th or Heart Chakra, associated with speech, communication and social ability
Will/self-esteem, or in Japanese terms 'Hara'	*Maṇipūra* 3rd or Solar Plexus Chakra, located near the diaphragm, corresponds to personal power, creativity and intellect
Creation	*Svādhiṣṭhāna* 2nd or Navel Chakra, located below the navel (near the belly button), known for its power in life actions
Survival/safety	*Mūlādhāra* 1st or Root Chakra, located at the base of the spine

While all of the above information might seem daunting, if you view the chakras in psychological comparative terms, they are quite similar to Maslow's theories, as compared in Table 1 and Figure 6.

Note about the *āsanas* (poses), illustrations, and Sequence Wiz and YogaMatePro apps

Sequence Wiz is an excellent resource for yoga teachers and yoga therapists. This software program allows you to individually tailor your 'yoga homework' (with your company logo) and print, download and/or send it out to your patients (see Figs 7 and 8). In the past, I took copious photographic images and then sent these to my patients (via email) with notes regarding the *āsanas* (poses) that were done in the therapy sessions. This consumed precious hours of my time and while this might have been useful

Introduction

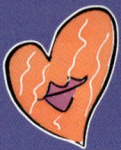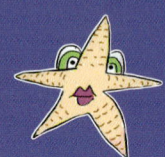

for the individual patient, Sequence Wiz can save your 'favorite *āsanas*' and does this work for you in minutes. Also, instead of sending your patient self-images through the Internet, it is more HIPAA compliant to send a Sequence Wiz sketch instead.

With the YogaMatePro app, you can photograph yourself (or use a model), and place your own photographic images within the described practice. However, while the model might be correctly doing the *āsana*, the fact that it is a model (for which read perfect, or even yourself) can be off-putting. While YogaMatePro is not meant as an 'end-all/be-all' word on yoga therapy, and which *āsanas*, meditations or breathing exercises to employ, it is an excellent platform to use for familiarizing yourself with possible scenarios (both physiologic and psychologic). If you choose the Pro version, the other features are also exceptionally beneficial and the site hosts resources and research from yoga therapists worldwide.

[Note this same information is easily converted in Sequence Wiz and you can add as much information as you decide to include. Note simplicity and ability to add your own logo courtesy of Sequence Wiz when sending as PDFs.]

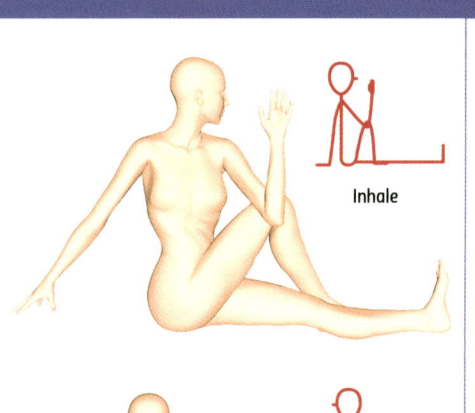

FIGURE 7 Sequence Wiz version of Horovitz homework in Figure 7

Ardha Matsyendrasana
To stretch the neck and strengthen the upper back

Begin in a seated position with the right knee bent and crossed over the extended left leg. Place the left elbow on the outside of your right knee. **Exhale:** Turn to your right, look back. Stay in position. **Inhale:** Lengthen up. **Exhale:** Use abdominal contraction to deepen the twist. Look back for 3–4 breaths, then turn your head and look forward for 3–4 breaths, while maintaining the twist.

Using your legs and arm to resist and twist further; this time instead of touching knee on same side as arm extended in your back area, take the arm to same side knee to open your chest wall even further.
Every breath is an opportunity to go a bit deeper into the twist.

Hold 30 seconds to 1 minute for pose and then another 30 seconds to 1 minute for counter pose. Do on both sides.

Physical benefits
Constipation
Digestive problems
Diabetes
Asthma
Fatigue
Lower back pain
Sciatica
Menstrual discomfort

Mental benefits
Relieves mild depression
Reduces stress and anxiety

Introduction

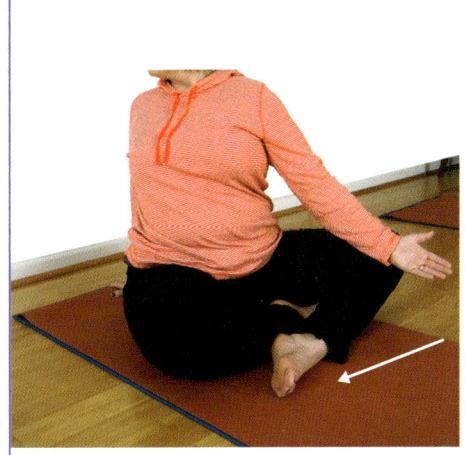

To stretch the neck and strengthen the upper back. Same as spinal twists: removes obstacles (and stress from the system)
- Using your legs and arm to resist and twist further (this time, instead of touching knee on same side as arm extended in your back area, take the arm to same side knee to open your chest wall even further)
- Every breath is an opportunity to go a bit deeper into the twist
- Hold 30 seconds to 1 minute for pose and then another 30 seconds to 1 minute for counter-pose
  Do on both sides
- Same instructions as first homework sheet.

Physical benefits: constipation, digestive problems, diabetes, asthma, fatigue, lower back ache, sciatica, menstrual discomfort
Mental benefits: relieve mild depression, reduce stress and anxiety
Contraindications: high or low blood pressure, migraine, diarrhea

FIGURE 8 Horovitz yoga therapy patient homework instruction (note that patient's face is cropped for confidentiality)

Navigating from your inner road map

For over 35 years, I split my time between the world of academia and my clinical work with patients. Because of my academic research, I was continually granted sabbaticals. While I always had great plans for these sojourns, by some quirk of fate, several sabbaticals ago, a monkey wrench hurled in from the abundant universe. The stars aligned: because a yoga teacher training program did not conflict with my research plans, I enrolled in a training certification with Sri François Raoult, a world-renowned yoga teacher trained by the great BKS Iyengar. Unbeknownst to me, this decision would not only inform my education and clinical operation with patients, but as mawkish as this sounds, it would also profoundly change my life. I returned so changed from this experience, that for over 2 years afterwards, colleagues would ask me, 'didn't you just return from sabbatical?'. I just smiled.

You see, I never fully came back to what I had been and indeed, it exuded from every pore in my body. I was so refreshed from this experience that my encounters with my then colleagues and patients vastly changed. With the Dean's blessing, I began to incorporate my yoga training into my clinical work with patients. Still later, I acquired more knowledge in yoga therapy and incorporated this work into my treatment of survivors of stroke, cancer, ritual and sexual abuse, and emotionally disturbed individuals and their families. In short, I transformed from my yoga trainings and abandoned my previous way of professing and conducting therapy.

At first blush, the work was mostly intuitive, but soon I had the privilege of working under many great yoga teachers and yoga therapists. The most profound influences came from many of my teachers (to name a few: Sri François Raoult, Michael Amy, Dr Judith Lasater, Amy Weintraub, Carla Anselm, Dr Edwin Bryant, Hervé Blondon, Dr. Robert Svoboda, Loren Fishman MD, Elise Miller, and Lakshmi Voelker, all stalwart members of the world of yoga and yoga therapy), and to this day, while quite seasoned as a yoga teacher and a yoga therapist, I find myself continually taking trainings, and workshops. In short, I can never know enough.

Introduction

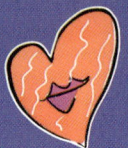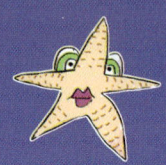

As I attended conferences through the International Association of Yoga Therapy (www.iayt.org), I encountered a new tribe (I had already established my first tribe years earlier at the American Art Therapy Association conferences). Now, it seemed I had two distinct homes. Operating both as an art therapist and a yoga therapist, I truly existed in the very fringes of psychology: I was an outlier.

In statistics an outlier is an observation point that is distant from other observations. An outlier may be due to variability in the measurement or it may indicate experimental error and the latter points are sometimes excluded from the data set. But in this scenario, like previous anomalies, my outside-the-box procedures led to scientific inquiry and most importantly, positive change in myself and my patients. Being an outlier has its rewards since it begs for experimentation that eventually leads to scientific investigation and sound reasoning. I knew I had stumbled onto something important and I wanted to share that with others.

I first began that conversation by presenting at conferences, giving lectures, publishing journal articles, and touring with Pesi.com, leading eventually to the publication of my books, most recently *Yoga Therapy: Theory and Practice* (Horovitz and Elgelid 2015). But herein, I wish to share more practical, accessible methods. I have personally engaged in these constructs and with my patients. It is my hope that you can incorporate these ideas into your clinical work by combining the modalities from the two fields from which I now operate. This is truly a marriage of head and heArt.

Yoga, drenched in somatic experience, feeds into my more cerebral resting place when creating art. Combining both yoga and art informs me as a whole person. When I tune this mirror to reflect my patient's issues, the results are similar: the treatment stems from a holistic perspective, honoring the mind, body and spirit. We both engage as active participants in this therapeutic process.

As you journey alongside me, my *modus operandi* will become clearer through the chapter descriptions, and I hope your own healing path will crystalize. This is healing at its best: the art of changing, adapting, ameliorating, and restoring to a more luminous being.

References

Allen PB (1995) Art is a Way of Knowing: A Guide to Self-knowledge and Spiritual Fulfillment Through Creativity. Boston: Shambhala Publications.

Allen PB (2005) Art is a Spiritual Path: Engaging the Sacred Through the Practice of Art and Writing. Boston: Shambhala Publications.

Arrington D (1991) Thinking systems – seeing systems: an integrative model for systemically oriented art therapy. The Arts in Psychotherapy 18(3): 201–211.

Blondon H (2019) Personal communication.

Bryant E (2009) The Yoga Sūtras of Patañjali: A New Edition, Translation, and Commentary. New York: North Point Press.

Bryant E (2017) Bhakti Yoga: Tales and Teachings from the Bhāgavata Purāṇa. New York: North Point Press.

Bryant E (2019) Personal communication.

Bullock C (1998) The Path to Healing: Experiencing God as Love. Rochester, NY: The Assisi Institute.

Chopra Centre (2020) Dosha Quiz. Available at: https://shop.chopra.com/dosha-quiz.

Doctor Blossom (2020) The Three Doshas. Available at: http://www.doctorblossom.com/the-three-doshas/vata.

Gantt L and Tabone C (1998) The Formal Elements Art Therapy: The Rating Manual. Morgantown, WV: Gargoyle Press.

Gershon M (1999) The Second Brain: A Groundbreaking New Understanding of Nervous Disorders of the Stomach and Intestine. New York, NY: Harper Perennial.

Horovitz EG (1988) Short term family art therapy: a case study. In: Watson D, Long D, Taff-Watson M and Harvey M (eds). Two Decades of Excellence: A Foundation for the Future. Little Rock, Arkansas: American Deafness and Rehabilitation Association (ADARA).

Horovitz EG (1999) A Leap of Faith: The Call to Art. Springfield: IL: Charles C Thomas Ltd.

Horovitz EG (2005) Art Therapy as Witness: A Sacred Guide. Springfield, IL: Charles C Thomas Ltd.

Horovitz EG (2014) The Art Therapists' Primer: A Clinical Guide to Writing Assessment, diagnosis, and Treatment, 2nd Edn. Springfield, IL: Charles C Thomas Ltd.

Horovitz EG and Elgelid S (eds) (2015) Yoga Therapy: Theory and Practice. New York: NY: Routledge Press.

Introduction

Horovitz EG (2017a) Spiritual Art Therapy: An Alternate Path, 3rd Edn. Springfield, IL: Charles C Thomas Ltd.

Horovitz EG (2017b). The Guide to Art Therapy Materials and Methods: A Practical, Step-by-Step Approach. New York, NY: Routledge Press.

Horovitz-Darby EG (1987). Diagnosis and assessment: impact on art therapy. Journal of Art Therapy 4(3): 127–137.

Kaur Khalsa HK (2011) Art and Yoga: Kundalini Awakening in Everyday Life. Santa Cruz, NM: Kundalini Research Institute.

Kramer E (1975) Art as Therapy with Children. New York: Schocken Books.

Lad V (1985) Ayurveda: The Science of Self-Healing. Twin Lakes, WI: Lotus Press.

Lowenfeld V and Brittain WL (1975) Creative and Mental Growth, 6th Edn. New York: MacMillan.

Moon CH (2010) Materials and Methods in Art Therapy. New York: Routledge

Moore T (1992) Care of the Soul: A Guide for Cultivating Depth and Sacredness in Everyday Life. New York, NY: Harper Perrenial.

Rumi J (2004) The guest house. In: Rumi: Selected Poems, translated by Barks C, Moynce J, Arberry AJ and Nicholson R. London: Penguin Books. Available at: https://www.scottishpoetrylibrary.org.uk/poem/guest-house/

Schwartz RC (2011) Introduction to the Internal Family Systems Model. Eugen, OR: Trailheads Publishing.

Svoboda R (1998) Prakriti: Your Ayurvedic Constitution. Twin Lakes, WI: Lotus Press.

Tolle E (1999) The Power of Now. Novata, CA: New World Library.

VPK by Maharishi Ayurveda Products International, Inc (2020) Dosha Quiz. Available at https://www.mapi.com/doshas/dosha-test/index.html.

Weintraub A (2015) Yoga and mental: the crumbling wall. In: Horovitz EG and Elgelid S (eds) Yoga Therapy: Theory and Practice. New York: NY: Routledge Press.

Further reading

Horovitz EG (2020) The Art Therapists' Primer: A Clinical Guide to Writing Assessment, diagnosis, and Treatment, 3rd Edn. Springfield, IL: Charles C Thomas Ltd.

Moore T (1992) Care of the Soul: A Guide for Cultivating Depth and Sacredness in Everyday Life. New York, NY: Harper Perennial.

Creating a safe space 1

Coincidence is God's way of remaining anonymous.

Albert Einstein

Preparing yourself to be a therapeutic container

As therapists, we bank on our patients presenting as they truly are. And we take them at their word. Yet to view participants holistically, a practitioner needs to adapt the inner message that our patients already have everything they need inside. Our role (whether practicing yoga therapy, art therapy or psychotherapy) is to provide the necessary tools to regulate mood management and guide them towards their inner resources. It is our job to assess, cultivate and communicate that subtle awareness beneath their presenting mood/mental state that they are already whole. This is not an easy task. Looking beneath the surface presentation (while assessing mood and mental status) and excavating that pearl is the quintessential component of recovery. This is also the art of yoga.

Yoga therapy and art therapy techniques operate in this realm of body/mind awareness. These somatic-oriented (yoga) and expressive outlets (art) offer another avenue for articulating and directing that wellness. Traditional psychotherapy (or talk therapy) does not always succeed by itself. Combining yoga, art and talk therapies accelerates the process because it calls on the body/mind experience. But adopting yoga therapy into your practice requires a bit of rewiring for the therapist who has never adapted a somatic practice.

I am going to assume that you are already personally engaged in some sort of yoga practice, otherwise you might not be reading this book. And maybe because of your own experience, you have witnessed firsthand the benefits of using this ancient practice and can see the advantage of incorporating yoga with your patients. This is how it began for me. Tapping into my own yoga practice, I personally experienced the benefits and healing process. Instinctively, I knew to trust that inner voice. But I also knew I needed more training and so I sought out many yoga teachers and yoga therapists. Eventually, returning to my inner model, I incorporated what I learned from others and distilled this into my own technique.

As an artist, it is difficult to separate the yoga from art, for they are in many ways one and the same. But as a therapist, when I operate somatically, my head is informed by my heart and the yoga informs the art. Thus, my decision is to work first with the body/breath (yoga) and then express this creatively through art. I see them as integral to each other.

Your true north

Staying clear enough to remember who you are requires a daily yoga, meditation or art practice. If you are going to incorporate this into your practice, you need to adopt some sort of practice every day. In doing so, you clear the space each day for your own healing energy to awaken and flow. At the minimum, this should be 20 minutes of dedicated practice before seeing your patients (if you are requiring your patients to adopt this into their own lifestyle, then you ought to lead by example). Since you will want to feel confident in practicing the yoga and art therapy tools outlined in this book, do what yogis have done for thousands of years: let your body and your mind be your own laboratory! So, be true to your practice and your inner compass: do yoga, make art!

But first, let's look at establishing confidentiality and safe boundaries inherent when incorporating touch with your patients.

Confidentiality, ethical boundaries and the therapeutic bond

A holistic and spiritual practice, be it yoga, prayer, chanting or meditation, should remind us of our wholeness, of who we really are: beings connected to a healing energy greater than ourselves. Hopefully, we exit from our meditation cushions and/or yoga practice, feeling more connected, not less. Creating a safe container for our patients involves the risk of self-disclosure involved in emotional, physical and mental transformation.

Chapter one

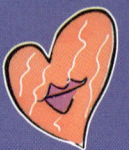 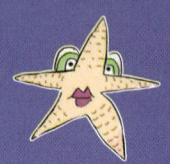

In the Appendices I have reprinted all of my release forms, health forms, informed consent and welcome letters to my practice. Naturally, I have patients sign an informed consent form prior to treatment, but in my welcome letter to all patients (Appendix D), I also state the following:

I will treat with great care all the information you share with me. It is your legal right that our sessions and my records about you be kept private. That is why I ask you to sign 'Informed consent' and 'Authorization to release confidential information' forms before I can talk about you or send my records about you to anyone else. In general, I will tell no-one what you tell me. I will not even reveal that you are receiving treatment from me. In all but a few rare situations, your confidentiality (that is, our privacy) is protected by federal and state laws and by the rules of my profession. Here are the most common cases in which confidentiality is not protected:

1. If you make a serious threat to harm yourself or another person, the law requires me to try to protect you or that other person.

2. If I believe a child has been or will be abused or neglected, I am legally required to report this to the authorities.

3. Sometimes, I consult other therapists or other professionals about my patients. This helps me in giving high-quality treatment (we call this peer supervision). These persons are also required to keep your information private. Your name will never be given to them, some information will be changed or omitted, and they will be told only as much as they need to know to understand your situation.

4. It may be beneficial for me to confer with your primary care physician with regard to your psychological treatment or to discuss any medical problems for which you are receiving treatment. In addition, if you are a Medicare patient, I am required to notify your physician by telephone or in writing, concerning services that are being provided by me, unless you request that notification not be made.

(Appendix D)

While you may know this and set similar stances in your own practice, it is imperative that from the onset, my patients know where I stand regarding my practice since I am ethically bound by my licensing board (New York State), and the ethics and guiding principles of the International Association of Yoga Therapists (IAYT, www.iayt.org), Yoga Alliance (www.yogaalliance.org) and the American Art Therapy Association (www.art-therapy.org).

I also state the following:

I view therapy as a partnership between us. You define the problem areas to be worked on, I use my knowledge to help you make the changes you want to make.

Art therapy/yoga therapy and psychotherapy is not like visiting a medical doctor. It requires your very active involvement. It requires your best efforts to change thoughts, feelings and behaviors. An important part of your therapy will be practicing new skills that you will learn in our sessions. I may ask you to practice outside our meetings, and we will work together to set up homework assignments for you. I might ask you to do exercises, keep records, create art and read to deepen your learning.

(Appendix D)

Thus, from the get-go I have established that like a dance, this is a cooperative process that requires engagement, reflection and work on their part as well as mine.

Regarding the therapeutic bond, Bruce Wampold conducted a meta-analysis of over 400 manualized treatments for depression (Wampold 2001). He suggested that the greatest predictor of beneficial outcome for patients was not necessarily the therapeutic modality used but the relationship between the therapist and patient. Shining through with your own authenticity (which is a secondary gain for the therapist) is the key component in moving your patient toward a trajectory of wellness. I have often said that you need to 'love' your patients and that if you cannot, then you need to refer them to someone who can. And believing your patient has everything they need inside to heal is the foundational belief of all yoga. Believing in and communicating that wholeness

Creating a safe space

to your patient fosters that therapeutic bond. The clinician leads the patient through this via vagal tone. The polyvagal theory, conducted from a clinical standpoint, suggests that the clinician can aid in the re-story of a reptilian state, calming the autonomic nervous system (ANS) through regulation of the vagus nerve. The clinician conducts this return to the ventral vagal system (calm/safety/regulated) from the dorsal vagal system (paralyzed, immobile freeze state) through several variables including vagal tone (Dana 2018). To learn more about the polyvagal theory, see Chapter 6, and Porges (2009, 2011).

Safe boundaries, touch, and introducing yoga therapy and art therapy into treatment

If you are a mental health practitioner, your training may have emphasized not to touch your patients, nor offer tissues (if they cry) and to deviate from any discussion regarding politics and/or God. Having veered off the beaten track (Horovitz 2017a), I never followed that edict.

Functioning as a yoga therapist and/or expressive art therapist is an altogether different approach to working in the manner previously described. I discovered (first-hand) what yoga unearthed in me and knew that extending this work to my patients would enhance their recovery, mobility, verbal expression and in some instances neurolinguistic abilities (more on that in the chapters discussing clinical cases). Using inviting language to introduce yoga therapy and art therapy into your practice requires a bit of practice.

Attention to the environment

As a therapist, you are already equipped in helping your patient feel at ease: this may be done by greeting your patient with a smile, full eye contact, your own calm demeanor and promising to hold the patient in a safe and confidential space. It is also important to offer an inviting space. My office space (approximately 16` × 20`) offers ample space for conducting intakes, psychotherapy, yoga therapy and art therapy with individuals and families. The office houses a yoga swing for inversions, TRX bands and a variety of props, including sandbags, pranayama bolsters, eye pillows, blocks, Co-OperBlankets and Co-OperBands (Fig. 1.1).

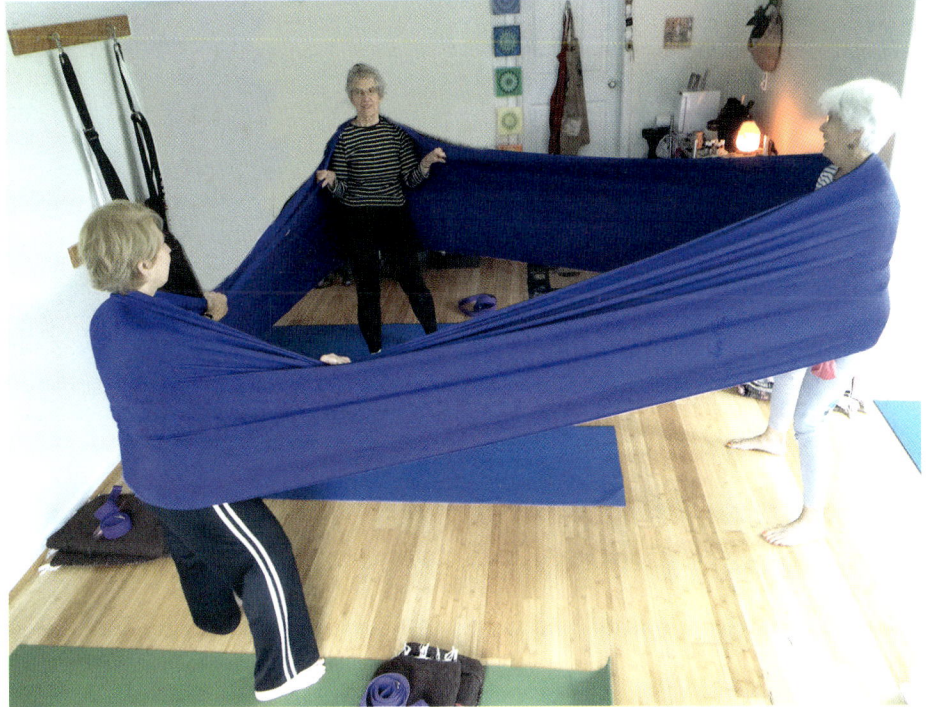

FIGURE 1.1 Sample of group using the Co-Operblanket during yoga

Chapter one

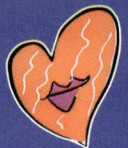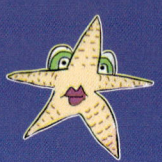

There is ample space to convert the studio for making art with patients (with numerous materials, see Horovitz 2017b) and I have a clay/glass kiln in my basement for firing artwork. For in-depth advice on how to set up an art studio see Horovitz (2017b), which pores over safety regulations, hazards and guidelines. However, below, I am summarizing some important points to consider.

Where to draw the line

When a patient is in a state of dis-ease (Horovitz 1999) it becomes all too easy too pathologize via the diagnosis as well as through the interpretation of the art: unless we look for strengths in the medical and psychosocial histories, we can be trapped in the spiraling mentality of looking at a patient's symptoms and diagnostic classification instead of operating from the viewpoint of wellness.

I caution you to beware of this trap, no matter if an incipient student or a seasoned traveler. It is all too easy to fall victim to the danger of 'fitting in' to this methodology of treatment.

While it is important to understand patient dis-ease (see more on that in Chapter 2), it is often customary to be swayed by diagnostic indicators and definition, both in expectation for course of treatment and expected outcome, thus contributing to failure.

Setting up the studio: important considerations

Regardless of the above, one must consider diagnosis and possibly developmental arrest at the onset of treatment and the subsequent development (and/or regression) that can unfold when the patient waffles in recovery. These things are not easily taught. Over time, therapists come to understand this approach/avoidance dance. Also, there is something that seasoned therapists call 'doorknob therapy'. These are the crystalline moments that generally occur within the last 5 minutes of the session: a patient offers a pearl of insight into their problems or reveals a nodal issue or event and then heads out the door. Fortunately, if this occurs through the art, you have a permanent record of that moment and you can bring it into the next session for both continuity and to pick up where you left off. The importance of this cannot be understated, as well as the need to: (1) date all artwork created in sessions, (2) write process notes immediately following sessions (so the information is fresh), and (3) maintain a portfolio of the artwork so that both the patient and the therapist can review the progress from beginning to end of treatment.

Additionally, in Chapter 3, I will also discuss the importance of recapping/assigning homework to increase emotional and physical regulation, and the use of texting and/or telehealth sessions (via HIPAA-compliant software).

This brings us to setting up the space and the parameters around treatment issues.

Regarding the issue of time in therapy

To lower defenses, Dean (2016) often provides timed warnings with the patient called, 'in through the back door'. It requires the patient to create six images using scribbles or other marking techniques and to mark the back of the paper used, with the time limits (e.g. 1 minute; 1 minute 30 seconds; 15 seconds; 2 minutes; 1 minute) (Dean 2016: 84–85).

While this exercise might allay anxiety, or in fact exacerbate it, I always give 5–10-minute warnings before the session's end, depending on the patient. This is especially important to do if you work with very young children, who often do not want to stop the creative process. Also adding a statement such as, 'I know that it is hard for you to stop, but I will see you again next week' (or whenever the next scheduled session is slated), can allay anxiety and prevent meltdowns. Offering some drawing paper and materials to take home and/or making a journal for patients to use in between sessions can be enormously helpful and provide connection and continuity between sessions. Figure 1.2 is an example of what a 78-year-old client sketched in the journal (that I gave him) in between our sessions. Gifting clients with journals often has illuminated and informed the discussion in subsequent sessions.

Creating a safe space

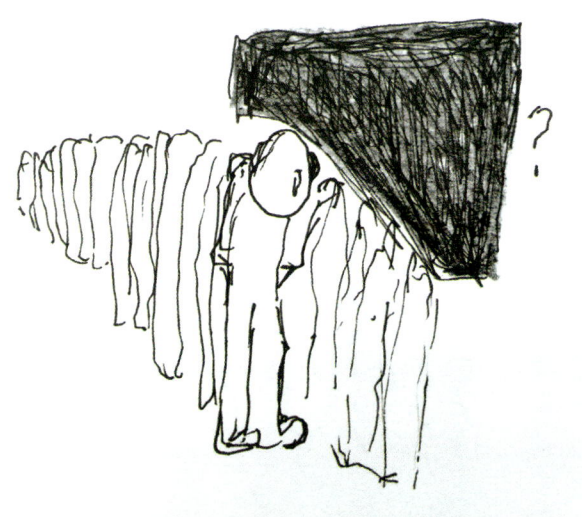

FIGURE 1.2 Journal drawing brought to session by 78-year old patient

It is imperative to try and end on time (and while there may be exceptions, it is often seen as counterproductive to extend the session past the allotted time). There are exceptions to extending the session for the patient's benefit, especially if what arises in those last moments is emergent, critical and would be beneficial to explore. However, taking such actions to a supervisor, whether you are a beginning therapist or advanced, can rule out countertransference on your part. There are some therapists who believe that if you extend past the allotted therapeutic hour that this might be 'seductive' behavior on the part of the therapist. I am just not that rigid; sometimes, overtime is warranted. I make the decisions about extending session time on a case-by-case basis. As Rubin (1998) has stated, flexibility is key for a competent therapist. But if you doubt your actions (if you extend the time with your patient), take it to your supervisor for discussion. To this day, I still meet with peers to exchange supervision. Fresh eyes are always a welcome perspective on particularly tough cases. And I will talk more about basic art materials and digital software programs in Chapter 3.

Vacations

If you are planning a vacation, you need to forewarn your patients so that they are psychologically prepared for the missed time with you. Using or making a calendar for small children or developmentally or neurologically challenged patients is also very useful to concretize the time between appointments.

On attire, clean-up and maintaining the studio

Involving the patient in the therapeutic clean-up of the artwork is also an important ritual in both ownership of the art (and/or mess) created. Furthermore, it is vital that you mirror proper attire and don a smock to protect your clothing so that the patient(s) will do the same. Fundamental is to always be early for your sessions – a half-hour is my bare minimum. The reasons involve setting up the space, re-reading notes and recaps from previous sessions and making sure all art materials are in good working order. This might involve something as mundane as sharpening all colored pencils. No, I am not kidding. These little actions speak boatloads to the patient and metaphorically state that you care enough to offer the art materials in their best working order. There is nothing worse than working with hardened clay when you want it to be pliable.

So, as a result, you need to know all about the materials you are planning to use – not just their properties, but how to maintain them, etc. The old adage that you cannot take your patients any further than you have gone yourself is the maxim. So, this might mean continuing education with a variety of materials. In a pinch, YouTube videos come in very handy for on-the-spot review, but ample preparation (e.g. practicing with the media) allows you to familiarize yourself with the properties and applications of the materials that you are using. I cannot tell you how many of my past students have arrived unprepared with the most basic knowledge of art materials, some never having worked with paint, clay or even papier-mâché! Even learning how to operate and maintain equipment (machines, kilns, etc.) falls under this

Chapter one

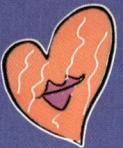

domain. Your job description if you are also an art therapist implies knowing the properties of the art materials you are offering and keeping the safety of yourself and your patient paramount.

Establishing rules and etiquette for groups

In some instances, depending on the nature of a group rules need to be posted. Generally, I prefer to avoid that as it smacks of punitive associations, and instead outline the rules of the group at onset, reinforcing them verbally if needed over time. However, for a rudimentary start, I offer a preliminary example below (especially when working with families):

- Please respect the artwork of others and do not work on anyone else's artwork unless invited to participate.
- Please use all art materials appropriately (e.g. use tarps to protect surfaces, do not throw clay, etc.)
- Please wear a smock (or other equipment, gloves, etc.) to protect yourself from unnecessary spills and mess.
- Listen respectfully to each person discuss their artwork.
- No aggression towards others or others' artwork will be tolerated.
- Be prepared to care for your materials, taking the time to clean up your materials and leave them in good working order for the next person or session.

Obviously, you can alter the rules to state what befits the group that you are working with. For example, let's suppose a patient enters the session in an anxious manner (in yoga this is called the *rājasic state* as described in a multitude of books including the informative website, www.yogapedia.com). You might want to meet the patient's mood, perhaps starting with a simple breathing exercise in order to focus on what is troubling the patient. If this new approach is agreeable, it is important to clarify that the patient can stop the practice at any time and/or ask questions if anything is unclear. Letting the patient know that they are in control (e.g. conducting the train) aids in viewing any approach used as a tool, much like a GPS. The same can be true by offering the patient the use of art materials for self-expression.

Ritual of invitation

Another element to cultivating a safe and sacred space is a ritual of invitation. For example, whenever I conduct a yoga class (as opposed to yoga therapy), I always start off by suggesting that the participants set an intention for the practice by closing their eyes (or averting the eyes to the ground if uncomfortable with this directive). For example, I suggest that perhaps they 'set an intention for their own health, that of another or merely getting through this class' (humor being the most advanced *āsana*).

In therapy, this is no different. Here you might want to invite your patient to breathe beneath their current mood, perhaps beneath the social mask and connect to a fuller, more authentic self. Perhaps suggest that the patient allow that intention to resonate in their life and reveal itself to the heart space. Then you might ask the patient to share that intention with you. Nothing jumpstarts a session better than this initial ritual.

But what if an intention isn't found? Then probe. Perhaps you might wonder about the current emotional state. If truly stuck, Weintraub (2012) suggests:

Alternatively... you can guide your client to invite that which she wishes to enhance in her life to surround her heart on the inhalation, and that which blocks the full manifestation of her vision to be released on the exhale. Finally, you might suggest that she breathe love and acceptance in, and self-judgment out.

(Weintraub 2012: 34)

Suppose your patient is exhibiting a shortness of breath. You might want to use the stair-step breath (which will be outlined in Chapter 3). Also, positioning is important. While these breath practices can be done sitting on a chair or yoga mat, lying supine (on a yoga mat) may be an alternative since it is easier to breathe more deeply when lying down.

Creating a safe space

Other guidelines for the therapist

I always let patients know that I watch them when doing these breathing techniques, since it is my job to watch their breath/body/emotional reaction. Also, unless practicing a particular breath (more on that in Chapter 3), inhalation and exhalation is conducted through the nostrils, not the mouth.

Chanting of Aum ओम्

You could start off with chanting *Aum* (ओम्, Wikibooks 2020), although this might be too difficult for some; but for edification, I am throwing in this definition from Yogapedia (2020):

According to the ancient Hindu and yogic texts, practicing Om (Aum) yoga connects the yogi with the Supreme Being who controls prāna, or life force. Chanting Om (Aum) promotes peace and serenity.

The ideogram of Om (Aum) is a representation of four levels of consciousness: the waking state, dreaming state, dreamless sleep and pure consciousness. 'Mandukya Upanishad' explains that the letters a, u and m in Aum yoga represent three states of consciousness: waking state, dream state and deep sleep state. The fourth state is represented by the silence that exists between the repetitions of chanting Aum.

Although some yoga therapists might insist on chanting *Aum* (ओम्) with patients, I have found that with most patients, chanting is a foreign practice, and at first this can be off-putting. It takes a while to warm up to incorporating this into your practice. If you truly want to include this, first and foremost you need to be comfortable leading this practice or it will fall flat. However, the science suggests that this is most beneficial. According to Mehta (2016):

Chanting of AUM leads to mental and physical benefits to the body, as it slows down the nervous system and calms the mind in a way just like meditation. Through the rhythmic pronunciation, the mind is relaxed, and blood pressure reduces, eventually resulting in an improvement in heart health. In today's scenario, scientific experiments/studies [have] proven the fact that meditation/chanting of AUM is a remedy to stress and therapeutic to many more mental and physical health problems.

(Mehta 2016: 65–66)

Using mudrās or imagery (bhāvana)

Another avenue to create a safe container is using a hand-gesture (known as a *mudrā*). Since the use of *mudrās* is a whole treatise in and of itself, I would recommend if interested that you read LePage and LePage (2014). For example, *apāna vāyu mudrā*, one of the more complicated *mudrās* (known as the *mudrā* of Heart), is often used to strengthen the heart (Fig. 1.3). Along with strengthening your heart and regularizing palpitations, regular practice of this *mudrā* eases gastric issues. Named the '*mrita sanjeevani mudrā*', it was thought to

FIGURE 1.3 *Apāna vāya mudrā* – heart strengthener

This is known as 'The Mudra of Heart' and is often used to strengthen the heart. Along with strengthening your heart and regularizing palpitations, regular practice of this mudra eases gastric issues. Named the Mrita Sanjeevani Mudrā, it was thought to be a 'lifesaver' for suffering from cardiac arrest. It eases pain and improves blood circulation when under angina attack.
Beneficial for: blood pressure, palpitations, arteriosclerosis, and gastrointestinal issues including heartburn and indigestion.

Chapter one

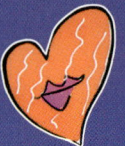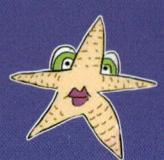

be a 'lifesaver' for suffering from cardiac arrest. It eases pain and improves blood circulation when under angina attack. It has been found to be 'beneficial for blood pressure, palpitations, arteriosclerosis and gastrointestinal issues including heartburn and indigestion' (Schmid and Van Puymbroeck 2019: 190).

Instruction for *apāna vāya mudrā*:

1. If possible, sit in *padmāsana* (lotus pose) or take whatever seat works for simple meditation.
2. Stretch your hands outward and allow them to rest on the thighs. Let the palms face the ceiling.
3. Now, fold your middle and ring fingers towards the palm in such a way that they touch the tip of the thumb.
4. Fold the index finger; it should be tucked near the base of the thumb. The small finger should be stretched outward.
5. Keep your eyes closed and hold the *mudra* as long as you can, preferably for 15 minutes and building to 30–45 minutes per day.

Bhāvana (imagery)

Using imagery to enhance your practice can often lead to calm in your patients. For example, you can suggest that the patient imagine a soothing, serene image or one's own inner resource: a place where they can feel calm and serene. I avoid using the word safe, since if you are dealing with trauma survivors they may resist with statements like, 'Nowhere is safe for me!'. And as an EMDR-trained clinician, a safe place is often referred to as a calm place, since 'safe place' can be triggering to trauma survivors. Sometimes in a session I may lead a patient on an open-ended *bhāvana* and then when they come out, encourage them to create some artwork around the imagery they envisioned.

Therapeutic attitude and body language

Finally, as therapists, we already know the power of body language. When a patient crosses their arms in front of their chest, they are clearly not being open to what is being discussed. As therapists, we should be attuned to what is being presented non-verbally: for therapists with ample experience this is a given, for those with little experience, it may not be so easy to detect.

What you can work on, incipient or not, is how you present your own body language. It is important that you are clear on how you are presenting to the patient (and I am not talking about mirroring the patient's body language, and/or mirror neurons, which is another topic). If your own body language is closed to the patient, they will see it. In the words of Blind Faith (1969) 'Come down off your throne and leave your body alone... Somebody holds the key.'

All of these suggestions are ways in which you can adapt your own practice and create a sense of safety and ease with your patients. To get some sense of putting some of the ideas together, let me offer a snapshot of incorporating yoga therapy and later art therapy (via the homework) in the very first session.

Creating a safe space

Case study

A new private patient complained in a telephone intake that she felt like a 'bug under a microscope' with her previous therapist. When she entered, I welcomed her with a smile, a handshake, offered her tea, explained my process, and my manner of working (even though she had received my welcome letter in advance of our first meeting). In this first session, she presented as anxious, stressed and depressed.

Being mindful of her 'bug under a microscope' fear, I still explained my process: that I wrote detailed session notes post-session and often administered psychological batteries (using the BetterMind healthcare app, see Chapter 2), to evaluate the efficacy of the sessions (in short, to see what was working and what wasn't).

I then gave her the DASS-21 (Depression, Stress and Anxiety Scale, Short Form), a psychological assessment (via the BetterMind app), while she sipped her tea and I reviewed the Health Assessment and Pain Assessment forms I had previously mailed to her (see Appendices). I explained that I often shared the results of the BetterMind app with my patients via text using my HIPAA-compliant Smartline (covered in Chapter 3) along with the homework/recap of our sessions and any other images that I felt might be beneficial to her treatment.

After she completed the DASS-21, I gifted her with a blank-paged art journal to use in between our sessions and I shared the initial genogram (see Chapter 2 regarding Genogram Analytics) which I created based on our phone conversation. We talked more about her present work and living situation, both of which were causing her great stress.

Newly married (although presenting as bisexual), she complained bitterly about two additional male roommates, friends of her husband, who had been living with them for over 2 months. Neither roommate contributed to the cost for rent, food or housekeeping.

After learning more about her present living condition, and ascertaining how anxious she was becoming, I suggested that we try a calming, belly breath breathing technique. First, I demonstrated this by placing my right hand on my belly and my left hand on my heart. Belly breath requires inhaling through the abdomen and exhaling through the lungs, opposite of how most people breathe, as chest breathers. By demonstrating this with my eyes closed and offering her the option of closing her eyes and/or averting them to the ground, I took some of the edge off. Next, she tried and was able to successfully relax using this method of breathing for ten counts.

I then taught her coherent breath (as taught by Elliott, 2005). Autonomous nervous system (ANS) breathing is facilitated by the diaphragm and intercostal muscles. In coherent breath, you consciously guide the ANS, and the relative sympathetic/parasympathetic nervous system. For example, by inhaling for four counts, and then holding the breath in the glottis region for two counts and then slowly exhaling for four counts, you can begin to change the heart rate variability (HRV, the rate at which the heartbeat changes). So, instructing her to do this for 10 breaths, she noticeably relaxed. Then we increased her range to 6–2–6 (six counts inhaling, two counts holding, six counts exhaling).

I suggested that we take this a step further. I demonstrated *tadāsana* (mountain pose, Fig. 1.4) and then asked her to replicate what I had demonstrated. I asked permission to adjust her shoulders and arms, aiding her in the pose. (It is important to always ask permission when touching a patient since touching a patient without express permission (especially if connected to previous trauma)

Chapter one

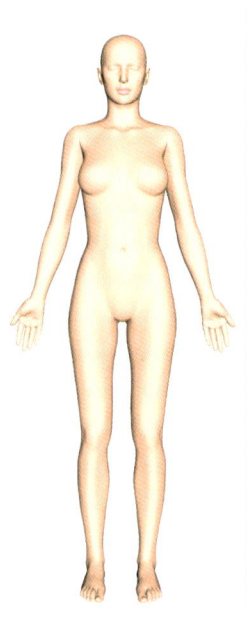

FIGURE 1.4 Mountain pose (*tadāsana*) with instructions: stand with feet parallel, spine elongated with shoulders back, diaphragm in, head ascending as if on a string towards the ceiling

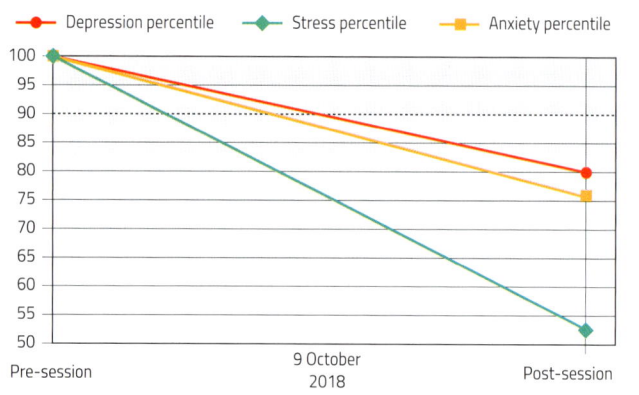

FIGURE 1.5 Chart of DASS-21 from Session 1: pre- and post-session

can markedly detract from forming a therapeutic relationship; more importantly, it allows the patient to be in the driver's seat.) When she stood in mountain pose (*tadāsana*), I suggested that she repeat the following mantra to herself, 'I am strong, stable and secure'. Using the Sequence Wiz (2020) app, I later sent this to her electronically since I had not yet secured permission to take images of her in therapy. She did this for about 3 minutes.

I asked her to take the DASS-21 again, from the vantage of how she was feeling after our session. Indeed, her DASS-21 results, pre- and post-session, accurately reflected what I had witnessed: there was a marked decrease in depression, anxiety and stress (Fig. 1.5). I later sent a snapshot of this result along with a recap of our session via my HIPAA-compliant Smartline. I view this part of the work as my responsibility/homework post-session, in addition to writing detailed session notes, which I review before our next session. As earlier stated, I see this as a partnership.

Pre-session DASS-21 scores

Relative to the sample population, this patient was in the:

- Extremely severe range for depression
- Extremely severe range for anxiety
- Extremely severe range for stress.

Post-session DASS-21 scores

Relative to the sample population, this patient was in the:

- Mild range for depression
- Mild range for anxiety
- Normal range for stress.

Before leaving, we discussed the notion of talking to her husband about preparing their roommates (his friends) to vacate their apartment. I suggested posting a physical calendar that literally marked off the days before they needed to go. I recommended the end of the month to offer the roommates an opportunity to find new quarters.

Creating a safe space

Here is the recap along with the DASS-21 information that I sent her at the end of our first session.

Recap:

1. Use the journal I gave you to write down anything that bubbles up between now and our next session. Feel free to collage, draw or just write in there.

2. Practice belly breath breathing as well as the coherent breath. Try and work up from inhaling in 4 counts, holding for 2 counts exhaling for 4 counts to 6–2–6 and then 8–2–8. The slower you breathe in and out, the less anxiety you will feel.

3. Mark that physical calendar so your husband's roommates literally see the writing on the wall. Discuss with your husband: they cannot continue to stay with you as it is worsening your relationship with him and causing you undue stress.

4. Speaking of which, talk with your husband about your feelings regarding the roommates and make a plan (as a couple) to get them out of your home so the two of you can start your lives anew.

5. Text me when you know your schedule, so we can move forward with your therapy. And hang in there!

As she left the session, I inquired how she felt about our work together and if she felt at all like a 'bug under a microscope'. She responded, 'Not at all!' and relayed that she would text me when she knew her new schedule. We have worked together since then for over a year. Clearly, trust was established.

In sum, while writing up session notes and then creating a recap to send to my patients requires additional time (sometimes up to an additional hour of my time), I consider this my homework. When my patients text me between sessions, I also consider it my responsibility to respond to these inquiries. I do not charge for this service as I see this as part of the therapeutic journey and container that I am holding for that relationship. In fact, if a patient sends me a URL, YouTube, book suggestion or the like, I too must engage in that process as a means of better understanding my patient and deepening our therapeutic relationship.

References

Blind Faith (1969) Can't find my way home. Los Angeles, CA: Atlantic Records.

Dana DA (2018) The Polyvagal Theory in Therapy: Engaging the Rhythm of Regulation (Norton Series on Interpersonal Neurobiology), 1st Edn. New York, NY: WW Norton & Co.

Dean ML (2016) Using Art Media in Psychotherapy: Bringing the Power of Creativity into the Practice. New York, NY: Routledge Press.

Elliott SB (2005) The New Science of Breath: Coherent Breathing for Autonomic Nervous System Balance, Health and Wellbeing. Allen, TX: Coherence Press.

Horovitz EG (1999) A Leap of Faith: The Call to Art. Springfield, IL: Charles C Thomas Ltd.

Horovitz EG (2017a) Spiritual Art Therapy: An Alternate Path, 3rd Edn. Springfield, IL: Charles C Thomas Ltd.

Horovitz EG (2017b) The Guide to Art Therapy Materials and Methods: A Practical, Step-by-step Approach. New York, NY: Routledge Press.

LePage J and LePage L (2014) Mudras for Healing and Transformation. Sebastapol, CA: Integrative Yoga Therapy.

Mehta S (2016) Aum: the healing power. In: Roy S, Mishra GC, Nanda S and Jain A (eds) Conference Proceedings of the 2nd International Conference on Public Health: Issues, Challenges, Opportunities, Prevention, Awareness. New Delhi, India: Krishi Sanskriti Publications.

Chapter one

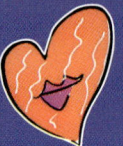 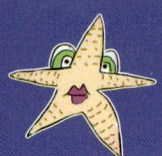

Porges SW (2009) The polyvagal theory: new insights into adaptive reactions of the autonomic nervous system. Cleveland Journal of Medicine 76(Suppl 2): S86–S90.

Porges SW (2011) The Polyvagal Theory: Neurophysiological Foundations of Emotions, Attachment, Communication, Self-Regulation. New York, NY: WW Norton & Co.

Rubin JA (1998) Introduction to Art Therapy: Sources and Resources. New York, NY: Routledge.

Schmid A A and Van Puymbroeck M (2019) Yoga Therapy for Stroke: A Handbook for Yoga Therapists and Healthcare Professionals. Philadelphia, PA: Singing Dragon.

Sequence Wiz (2020) Sequence Wiz Home Practice App. Available at: https://sequencewiz.com/

Wampold BE (2001) The Great Psychotherapy Debate: Models, Methods and Findings. Hillsdale, NJ: Lawrence Erlbaum.

Weintraub A (2012) Yoga Skills for Therapists: Effective Practices for Mood Management. New York, NY: WW Norton & Co.

Wikibooks (2020) Hinduism/Religious Symbols of Hinduism. Available at: https://en.wikibooks.org/wiki/Hinduism/Religious_Symbols_of_Hinduism

Yogapedia (2020) Om Yoga. Definition from Yogapedia. Available at: https://www.yogapedia.com/definition/5471/om-yoga.

Assessment for the mind and the body 2

Yoga does not just change the way we see things; it transforms the person who sees.

B.K.S. Iyengar

Disclaimer

While you may decide that assessing a patient is the farthest idea from your practice, knowledge is a powerful tool. You may decide to use some of the suggested apps and assessment tools after viewing their presentation herein, or not. It is a personal choice as to whether you decide to use any of these tools for assessing your patients. I use them to ascertain not just clinical information but also efficacy in my practice. But I want to provide you with options for your practice, thus their presentation herein; it also gives you a glimmer of how I use yoga therapy, art therapy and psychotherapy.

Much to my surprise, many of my yoga colleagues disdained the notion of using a goniometer (and the Morris–Payne method presented further in this chapter). Because my yoga training is Iyengar-based (long considered the medical model of yoga because of its emphasis on alignment, safety and using props), as well as doctoral-level, clinically based therapeutic training, I have always looked at a patient's 'dis-ease' (Horovitz 2020) through somewhat of a medical lens. Thus, I feel that it is important to present assessment options and let you decide what works best for you in your practice.

As of this writing, many yoga therapists are purporting the idea of tracking electronic medical record- (EMR) keeping with your patients (Zador et al 2019). While I have been using SOAP notes (subjective, objective, assessment and plan) for years, many may be unfamiliar with this process. So, it is important to be abreast of what this form of record-keeping is to decide whether or not you wish to implement this in your treatment of patients. Since the SOAP note has been around for over 50 years, it might be worth considering, based on its acceptance in clinical settings (Jacobs 2009). At the very least, I encourage clinicians to take the time to write up notes for themselves post-session (as well as to do a host of other things, which will be presented in great detail in Chapter 3.

If you decide to forgo using assessments altogether, than you may want to skip this chapter. But between you and me, if I went to a medical doctor (or any kind of therapist) and they prescribed medicine and/or advice without first ascertaining causation, diagnosis or assessment, I would be suspicious at best.

Understanding genograms, assessments, anatomy and physiology

As in any medical profession, the use of assessments is crucial in order for the therapist to understand the patient's psychosocial, psychological, cognitive/developmental, physiological, genetic, cultural, emotional and spiritual states. Armed with this information, you can then track the patient's progress over time (using a biopsychosocial model) and throughout the entire therapeutic journey.

For me, standardizing genogram (familial) information is as necessary to the validation of every instrument as is diagnosis and treatment. This information allows for multiple disciplines to understand and value inherent data that can be used in an interdisciplinary format. The many factors that may influence the outcomes of your treatment and assessment are of import for best practices (for example: one needs to consider culture, race, gender, age, religion, and sexual orientation (to name a few)).

There are many different apps out there, but prior to apps, I laboriously created genograms first in Microsoft Word, and then Adobe Illustrator. This was unsatisfactory and fortunately now there are genogram applications available for the practitioner. In this book, I am using Genogram Analytics software since it creates a visual schematic that allows you to consider the 'whole' person as opposed to the 'identified patient' (IP). Indeed, the patient's strengths and weaknesses can be 'seen' from a generational perspective where transitional conflicts (and/or epigenetics) may have been handed down from generation to generation. Having this visual map can serve to elucidate familial information. Systematizing genogram and timeline information also allows for multiple practitioners to understand and value inherent information that can be shared in an interdisciplinary format. This app will become more understandable when viewing case studies presented in this chapter and throughout the book.

Chapter two

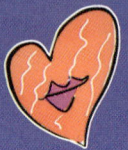

It seems that there is a mobile phone application for almost everything – from financial transactions to multi-player games. But now, you can use your smartphone for psychological testing. I use the Better Mind app since to date there are over 60 psychological assessments (some also physiological in nature) that track changes over time and, therefore, the efficacy of my sessions. This is a powerful tool that saves me boatloads of time (e.g. I no longer need to crunch the numbers and data as the app does all of this instantly for me). I can send these to my patients before they walk in the door, and thus have a barometer of where they are before I see them in my office. They can take these assessments on their phones, tablets or computer, making it very accessible. While there are many other assessments and applications out there, this is how I track my patients' psychological and physical progress over time.

Countless books have been written on anatomy. Although it is not the premise of this book to rehash anatomy for the reader, arming yourself with knowledge of the workings of the body (and the mind) is paramount. Some variations might include Bainbridge-Cohen (2014), Hanna (1970), Myers (2014), and Robins (2002). Speaking anatomically, the more you understand the workings of each system, synergistically working together and their effects, the better armed you will be. Although I am not a medical doctor and while I dissected bodies (before there were regulations), I can never know enough about anatomy and/or how the body works or doesn't. To be perfectly candid, I am a science junkie. Hey, there could be worse addictions!

It is important to note that there are a number of anatomy apps that are particularly useful in exploring physiology. One that I recommend is Essential Anatomy 5 (3D4Medical 2014). It has over 8,200 structures, is highly accurate, immersive, has quizzes to test your knowledge and is visually stunning. The professional version also offers videos for more in-depth learning.

So now let's explore some of these assessments and how they work.

Case study: 23-year-old female

Let's take a look at how applications informed me in this specific scenario combining both yoga therapy and art therapy. Let's begin by reviewing the issues of a patient's genogram (Fig. 2.1). For this purpose, we will call her identified patient (IP).

Intake information and current living situation

The IP saw a psychotherapist around age 19–20 years. That therapist suggested medication. The patient refused to take medication. Currently, she stated that she might be open to medication. When in college her anxiety increased. She self-disclosed as an introvert (e.g. she has difficulty reaching out to people to make doctor appointments, dentist appointments, etc.). She described having difficulty in college (she found the curriculum in high school easier).

She recently located her biological father on Facebook. She had no contact with him prior to this contact (he had just remarried). While he offered child support, there was no communication with him during her childhood. Her biological parents divorced when she was 3 years-of-age. IP described both of her biological parents as depressed.

Her mother (around age 40 years at patient's intake) remarried at IP's age 12 years. The stepfather was around at IP's age 8 years. The stepfather is now 51 and was described as verbally abusive towards IP. He was stated to favor chores over education and was described as a 'neat freak with obsessive compulsive disorder', and overly critical towards her. Essentially, her mother and stepfather disagreed with her choice to further her education through college and 'threw her out' of her home. So, she moved in with her maternal grandparents (MGPs).

Assessment for the mind and the body

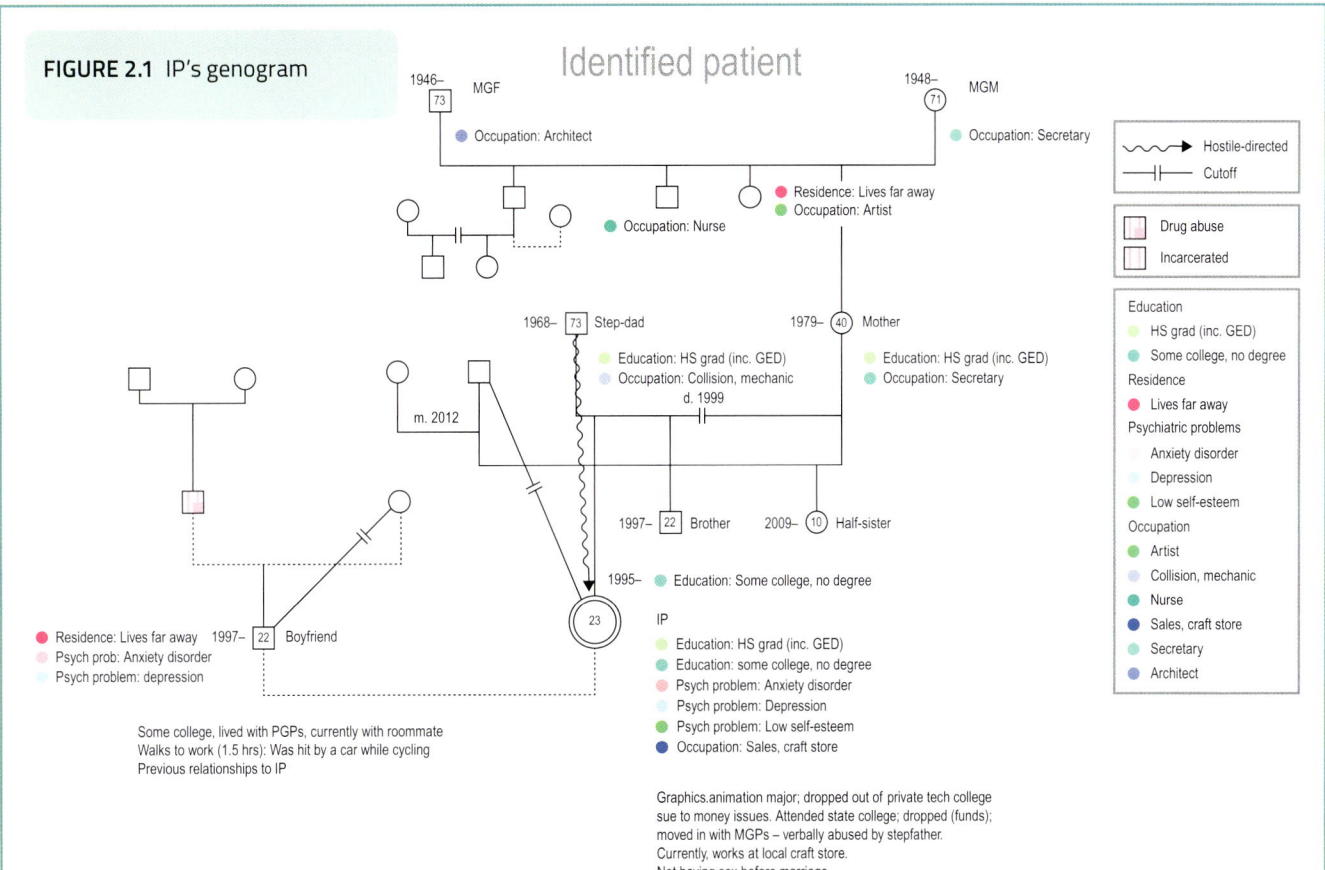

FIGURE 2.1 IP's genogram

IP has a younger brother (14 months her junior) who excels in academics and there is also a half-sister, now aged 10 years.

IP dropped out of private college due to the expense. She has been working at a local craft store for about for 3 years. Last year, she decided to return to college again and was majoring in Animation and Graphics. Her grandparents worked (MGF was an architect, MGM was a secretary), although both are retired.

Stated goals: to move out of her MGP's home and move in with boyfriend

She described being in a relationship with her boyfriend for over a year, although they were not having sexual intercourse (both wanted to wait until marriage). The boyfriend had experienced multiple relationships before and had recently withdrawn from college, as did IP. While they lived 4 hours apart, she drove to see him as often as possible. Her boyfriend walked to work (requiring 1.5 hours) since being hit by a car while biking. He was described as both depressed and anxious (specifically about driving, walking and biking).

Session 2

The IP reported that her job had been less stressful. She had to get up at 04:00, although now she could arrive by 06:00. She reported feeling underappreciated at work despite her seniority there; some people lauded their superiority and that truly bothered her. She seemed to present as a true introvert and I gave her the book, *Quiet: The*

Chapter two

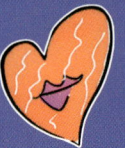
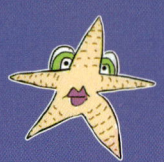

Power of Introverts in a World That Can't Stop Talking (Cain 2012), since I thought it might help her. (I learned about this book years earlier through one of my yoga teachers, the great Dr Judith Hanson Lasater.)

We talked a bit about her boyfriend who (currently) didn't have a license or a car and was afraid of driving on the highways. His grandparents were aiding him, and she was attempting to get him to feel more secure on the roads. She mentioned things they liked to do together (grocery shopping and the like). She seemed to have a nervous tic (right eye), but upon creating artwork (the kinetic family drawing or KFD assessment), she immediately calmed down and the tic subsided. For those unfamiliar with the KFD (Burns and Kaufmann 1972), the procedure is very straightforward: using an 8" x 10" (20.32 x 25.4 cm) piece of white paper, ask your patient to draw a picture of their self and their family doing something. The direction is quite specific: 'I want you to draw yourself and your family doing something'. Be careful not to say, 'together', at the end of the sentence as you are trying to assess if the patient and the family actually interact with one another. The instruction calls for a number two pencil and an eraser.

I am not that strict with the materials offered; if a patient asks for colored pencils or markers, they become available. Just remember color causes affect and this veers from the instruction.

The kinetic family drawing (KFD) assessment

The KFD was very revealing: her work with pencil had very pronounced lines (despite her artistic qualities) and screamed of anxiety and underlying issues (Fig. 2.2). When we talked about the art, it led to discussion of how little she knew of her biological father, including the divorce proceedings, whether or not there was joint custody, etc. (her memory of numerous events appeared to be vague).

She then mentioned that when she tried to pick up her half-sister at her mother and stepfather's home, the house was locked up like 'Fort Knox'. She also stated that she could not access the house, even with her key, which made her feel truly shut-out, since they had literally changed the locks, denying her access to the home. The fact that she drew herself in her childhood home and part of this family also underscored her hurt regarding expulsion from the family system.

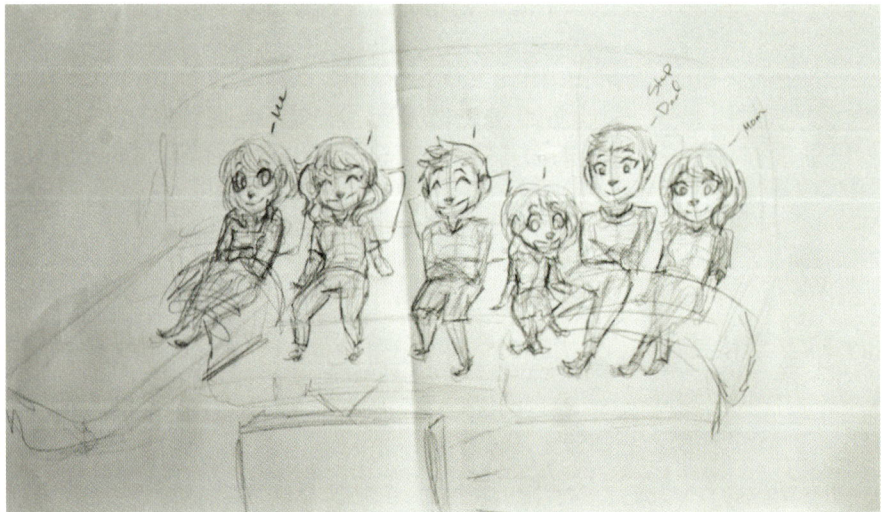

FIGURE 2.2 Kinetic family drawing (KFD) from patient IP

Assessment for the mind and the body

Of interest was the half-sister under a blanket with the mother and stepfather. She referred to her as the 'golden child'. While she was pictured to the left also under a blanket, her clear sense of displacement shone through this artwork. Indeed, her need to blanket and/or comfort herself was apparent through this picture.

Session 3

I suggested that in time perhaps she might ask her mother specifically about why she (and her brother) were not able to visit their father and why her mother was so adamant about their not seeing him. IP stated further that she had a visceral reaction to not going, which is what prompted me to suggest that she ask her brother and her mother about their memories of those times.

At this point, she began to cry. For the first time, she calmed down. I mentioned a quote by Swami Kripalu ('One who cries knows yoga') and also talked about how crying serves to dispel cortisol, engages the parasympathetic nervous system (PNS) and aids in neurotransmitter connection (i.e. crying is actually a good thing).

All this unfolded from the kinetic family drawing. She was able to state that she was afraid to ask her mother about the issues, since she thought if she did that her mother, 'would no longer love (her)'. This led to her fear of abandonment, and the homework that I suggested between our next session.

Homework

- Journal your feelings about approaching this subject (the divorce proceedings) with your mother.
- Explore the feeling about your mother 'no longer loving' you.
- Draw something connected to that abandonment feeling regarding your mother.

Next we will look at how psychological assessments dramatically affected the outcome of this care.

Psychological assessments

The beauty of using the psychological assessments which I employ is that the results become available immediately should you want to look at them while in session. Also, a PDF file of the results are immediately emailed to the practitioner so that you can store the results in your records. Indeed, all assessments are digitally backed up by the system. This also allows you (the practitioner) to glean the efficacy of what you are doing and what is working (for example, art therapy, yoga therapy, psychotherapy or combinations of all three). Also, if you ask the patient to take the same assessment (pre- and post-session) and answer how they are feeling post-assessment (as I sometimes do), you have more feedback on session efficacy.

Fig. 2.3 is a snapshot of the Center for Epidemiologic Studies Depression Scale, Revised (CESD-R) (Eaton et al. 2004) results post the session conducted with IP. The CESD-R is a self-report questionnaire used to measure symptoms of depression and is particularly useful for tracking symptoms over time. This assessment taps into different symptom groups of Major Depressive Disorders, as defined by the DSM-5 (American Psychiatric Association 2013). The results following the session where I conducted the CESD-R were extremely helpful. The results (the amount of responses of 2, 3 and 4) indicated possible suicidal ideation, which was not obvious either from the patient's presentation or affect. However, after reviewing the results I immediately called the patient to ascertain her mental state (whether or not she had a plan for suicide) and to assure her that if she felt unsafe, we could arrange for an emergent session.

Chapter two

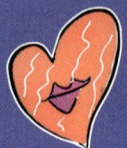
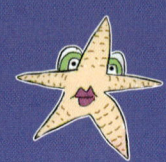

		Not at all/ less than 1 day	1–2 days	3–4 days	5–7 days	Nearly every day for 2 weeks
1	My appetite was poor	**0**	1	2	3	4
2	I could not shake off the blues	0	1	**2**	3	4
3	I had trouble keeping my mind on what I was doing	**0**	1	2	3	4
4	I felt depressed	0	1	2	3	**4**
5	My sleep was restless	0	**1**	2	3	4
6	I felt sad	0	1	**2**	3	4
7	I could not get going	0	1	2	**3**	4
8	Nothing made me happy	**0**	1	2	3	4
9	I felt like a bad person	0	1	2	3	**4**
10	I lost interest in my usual activities	0	1	2	3	**4**
11	I slept much more than usual	0	**1**	2	3	4
12	I felt like I was moving too slowly	0	**1**	2	3	4
13	I felt fidgety	0	**1**	2	3	4
14	I wished I were dead	0	1	**2**	3	4
15	I wanted to hurt myself	0	1	**2**	3	4

FIGURE 2.3 Responses on the Center for Epidemiologic Studies Depression Scale – Revised (CESD-R)

As treatment continued, I tracked her results using the DASS-21 (Henry and Crawford 2005). This allowed for continual reframing of what was working (or not) in sessions.

Figure 2.4 shows the improvement of the patient from the beginning of treatment through termination (the practitioner should be aware that often, verbalization of feelings can lead to heightened scores as seen here by the rise in anxiety score). At termination, the DASS-21 results were well in the normal range of functioning.

While there are some practitioners who prefer not to use assessments at all, for those who want to track efficacy and change over time, the use of the aforementioned batteries to record efficacy and evidence-based change is key to gaining increased acceptance by Western practitioners. More will be stated on that as we look at varying tools to assess art therapy, yoga therapy and psychotherapy. For a more complete look at art therapy assessments, the reader is directed to Horovitz (2017, 2020), Horovitz and Elgelid (2015).

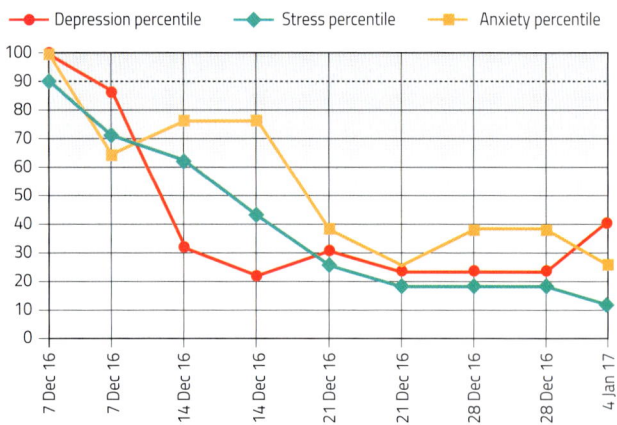

FIGURE 2.4 DASS-21 results over time

Assessment for the mind and the body

Assessing and understanding the art

Based on the Formal Elements Art Therapy Scale (FEATS) Assessment (Gannt 2001, Gannt and Tabone 1998), publication of Gussak's (2013) and my own (Horovitz 2020) subjective assessments can now be tied to the American Psychiatric Association's DSM-5 using the FEATS Assessment's 14-point rating scale. This scale is affixed to specific personality disorders of the DSM-5. Being able to link subjective artwork to personality disorders verifies the efficacy of using art therapy diagnostically and for treatment (Gussak 2013, Horovitz 2020). I have also explained that adding the Crayola multicultural markers (to the prescribed Mr Sketch markers) for artistic assessment allows for multi-cultural differences in skin color, so the reader would be wise to add these to the actual FEATS Assessment (Horovitz 2020, Horovitz and Elgelid 2015).

In order to look at the normative values of development as pertains to the art produced in sessions, see Table 2.1.

Stages of art development comparison chart

It is important to be able to understand the normal stages of art as outlined by Lowenfeld and Brittain (1987), but the comparison which have I created in Appendix C aids in understanding these norms in terms of the eras and ages of development according to Erikson, Piaget, Kohlberg, Fowler, and Gannt and Tabone. I added in adult and artistic stages of development, as well as brain injury or traumatic brain injury (TBI), so that the reader has a sense of what that would look like. Should the reader not be familiar with these normative artistic stages of development, I would highly recommend browsing through

TABLE 2.1 The Horovitz-adapted formal elements chart for non-standardized assessments

Formal element scale	HTP	KFD	ATDA	BATA	CATA	'Road'
Prominence of color	✓ chromatic	✓ chromatic**	✓	✓	✓ chromatic**	✓
Color fit	✓ chromatic	✓ chromatic**	*	*	*	✓
Implied energy	✓	✓	✓	✓	✓	✓
Space	✓	✓	✓	✓	✓	✓
Integration	✓	✓	*	*	*	✓
Logic	✓	✓	*	*	*	✓
Realism	✓	✓	*	*	*	*
Problem-solving	✓	✓	*	*	*	*
Developmental level	✓	✓	✓	✓	✓	✓
Details of objects and environment	✓	✓	*	*	*	✓
Line quality	✓	✓	✓	✓	✓	✓
Person	✓	✓	*	*	*	*
Rotation	✓	✓	*	*	*	*
Perseveration and environment	✓	✓	✓	✓	✓	✓

HTP, House–Tree–Person test; KFD, kinetic family drawing; ATDA, art therapy dream assessment; BATA, belief art therapy assessment; CATA, cognitive art therapy assesment; Road, 'draw a road'.
*This scale may or may not apply based on the client's response (e.g. abstraction, etc.).
**While the KFD and the CATA (drawing subtest) are achromatic assessments, often art therapists allow for color usage in this battery. Donna Betts has adapted her own version of the FEATS for use with the face stimulus assessment (FSA).

Chapter two

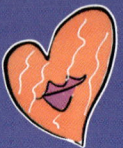
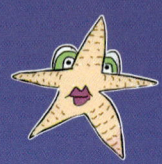

Lowenfeld and Brittain (1987), long considered the 'bible' of art education and art therapy.

Regarding the stages of development as outlined by Lowenfeld and Brittain, they did not describe brain injury as a 'stage', and while it is not a stage, brain injury can occur at any age. I have described this as consisting of organic qualities, where objects float on the page (e.g. lack of order and ungrounded quality to the artwork is pervasive in the representations, be they 2- or 3-dimensional in design). Also, since Lowenfeld and Brittain do not cover the adult or artistic stages of development, I feel that these stages vary dramatically from the adolescent period, the last stage which Lowenfeld and Brittain describe. Therefore, all three of these stages (brain injury, adult and artistic stages of development) are covered in my comparison (see Appendix C). In Table 2.2 I have placed art samples next to each stage for ease of comparison and clarification.

More will be stated about artwork and the use of art therapy combined with yoga therapy in subsequent chapters which highlight case studies.

TABLE 2.2 Stages of artistic development with art samples

Eras/ages	Lowenfeld and Brittain	Horovitz	Art samples	Example art
Infancy (0–1.5 yrs)	Scribble stage: beginning of self-expression (0–2 yrs)		**Random scribbling**: kinesthetic images which are pleasing to the child **Controlled scribbling**: 6 months past random scribbles, connection between marks on paper and page movements **Named scribbles**: child relates to outside world	
Early childhood (2–6 yrs)	Preschematic stage: first representations (4–7 yrs)		Schemas of person Representational symbols Variations of houses, trees, people are common Child is at the center of their world	
Childhood (7–12 yrs)	Schematic stage: formed concepts (7–9 yrs) Gang age: dawning realism (9–12 yrs)	Adult stage: formation in the world (8 yrs – adulthood)	Representational objects supercede the human figure Child can judge left/right visual space (age 4 and up) Artwork may reflect intellectual functioning X-ray presentations common	

Continued

TABLE 2.2 continued

Eras/ages	Lowenfeld and Brittain	Horovitz	Art samples	Example art
Adolescence (13–21 yrs)	Pseudo-naturalistic stage: age of reasoning (12–14 yrs) Adolescent art: period of decision (14–17 yrs)	Artistic stage: formed art any age (generally in adolescence through adulthood)	Perspective becomes important Moral development is strong More details appear in the human figure and clothing Child uses additive method in clay or other 3D materials	
Young adulthood (21–35 yrs)			Schema disappears, work often banal, commonplace Sexual characteristics often exaggerated Strong peer pressure to conform Interest in more complex art media	
Adulthood (35–60 yrs)			The period of decision Increased attention span Mastery of a variety of media Naturalistic, abstraction, and cartooning occurs in the art	

Continued

TABLE 2.2 continued				
Eras/ages	Lowenfeld and Brittain	Horovitz	Art samples	Example art
Maturity (60+ yrs)		Adult stage: formation in the world (8–adulthood)	Not necessarily an artist but enjoys working with art materials	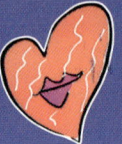
		Artistic stage: formed art Any age (generally in adolescence through adulthood)	Highly skilled in 2D and 3D media Capable of realism, abstraction, surrealism, and metaphoric thinking Prolific, self-motivated	
		Brain injury	Everything floats, ungrounded artwork, nothing looks like you think it should	

Assessment for the mind and the body

Assessing joint range of motion using a goniometer

Joint flexibility is defined as the range of motion (ROM) at a joint. A joint's ROM is measured by the number of degrees from the starting position of a segment to its position at the end of its full range of the movement. The most accurate techniques for measuring ROM (particularly active ROM) include measurements of joint angles from arthrography, radiographic images, photographs and video. However, these techniques require expensive, complex equipment and extensive training.

The easiest method is to learn to measure ROM using a protractor goniometer, which is simply a protractor designed for use on the human body. A stationary arm is placed parallel with a stationary body segment and a movable arm moves along a moveable body segment. The pin (axis of the goniometer) is placed over the joint. When anatomical landmarks are well defined, the accuracy of measurement is greater. If there is more soft tissue surrounding the joint area, measurement error can be more frequent. In addition to stationary goniometers, now there are digital goniometer apps, such as the Goniometer Pro.

ROM can be measured as either active or passive. Active ROM is created by the person using their muscles to move that joint. Passive ROM is created by an external force (e.g. partner, therapist, piece of equipment) pushing on the body around the joint in order to move it. Passive ROM is always greater than active ROM.

In musculoskeletal injury (MSI) prevention, a goniometer is used to measure either active or passive joint ROM. This is pertinent to functional reach and workplace design. A goniometer can also measure progress in return of ROM during recovery. This is what the Morris–Payne (Payne and Morris 2013) technique aims to do.

A traditional goniometer is a fairly simple protractor with extending arms. To use a goniometer (Wellness-Keen 2020):

1. Align the fulcrum of the device with the fulcrum of the joint to be measured.
2. Align the stationary arm of the device with the limb being measured.
3. Hold the arms of the goniometer in place while the joint is moved through its ROM. The degree between the endpoints represents the entire ROM.

Important tips in using a goniometer are:

- Stabilize the stationary portion of the body. This is the part of the body that is proximal (closer to the midline of the body) to the joint you are testing. It is important that the patient does not move their body while moving the joint; this step isolates the joint movement for a more accurate measurement.

- Look at the reading on the goniometer before removing it from the patient's body. Ensure that you take an accurate reading of the degrees of motion on the goniometer, and that you consistently use the same stationary and movable landmarks on the body when measuring (and re-measuring) to ensure consistency.

- Be sure to record the range of motion for the joint. The free goniometer evaluation chart shown in Figure 2.5 from the Washington State Department of Social & Health Services (www.dshs.wa.gov) is useful for evaluating these measurements.

The free images in Figure 2.5 are extremely helpful in understanding how to use a goniometer. If you choose to use a goniometer for measuring musculoskeletal injury and/or ROM pre-session, post-session or to look at efficacy over time, it is important to be able to compare the measurements of the patient's body from an accurate standpoint. Thus, knowing the average range of rotation, lateral flexion, hyperextension, abduction, adduction, and the like for each body part you are assessing is paramount. And as stated, while many of my yoga teachers, also physical therapists, prefer not to do these measurements, I believe that one should be armed with the knowledge should you choose to add this to your practice. Even if you decide not to use a goniometer to measure physical change over time, it is important to at least understand the instrument's measuring system.

Chapter two

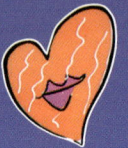
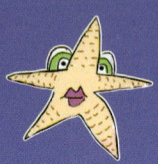

NAME OF PATIENT | CLIENT IDENTIFICATION NUMBER

INSTRUCTIONS: For each affected joint, please indicate the existing limitation of motion by drawing a line(s) on the figures below, showing the maximum possible range of motion or by notating the chart in degrees. Provide a complete description of all affected joints in your narrative summary. If range of motion was normal for all joints, please comment in your narrative summary. If joints which do not appear on this chart are affected, please indicate the degree of limited motion in your narrative.

1 Back

Extension 25°	Flexion 90°
Degrees	Degrees

2 Lateral (flexion)

Left 25°	Right 25°
Degrees	Degrees

3 Neck

Extension 60°	Flexion 50°
Degrees	Degrees

4 Neck (lateral bending)

Left 45°	Right 45°
Degrees	Degrees

5 Neck (rotation)

Left 80°	Right 80°
Degrees	Degrees

6 Hip (backward extension)

Left 30°	Right 30°
Degrees	Degrees

7 Hip (flexion)

Left	
Knee Flexed 100°	Knee Extended 100°
Degrees	Degrees
Right	
Knee flexed 100°	Knee extended 100°
Degrees	Degrees

8 Hip (adduction)

Left 20°	Right 20°
Degrees	Degrees

9 Hip (abduction)

Left 40°	Right 40°
Degrees	Degrees

10 Knee (flexion)

Left 150°	Right 150°
Degrees	Degrees

Assessment for the mind and the body

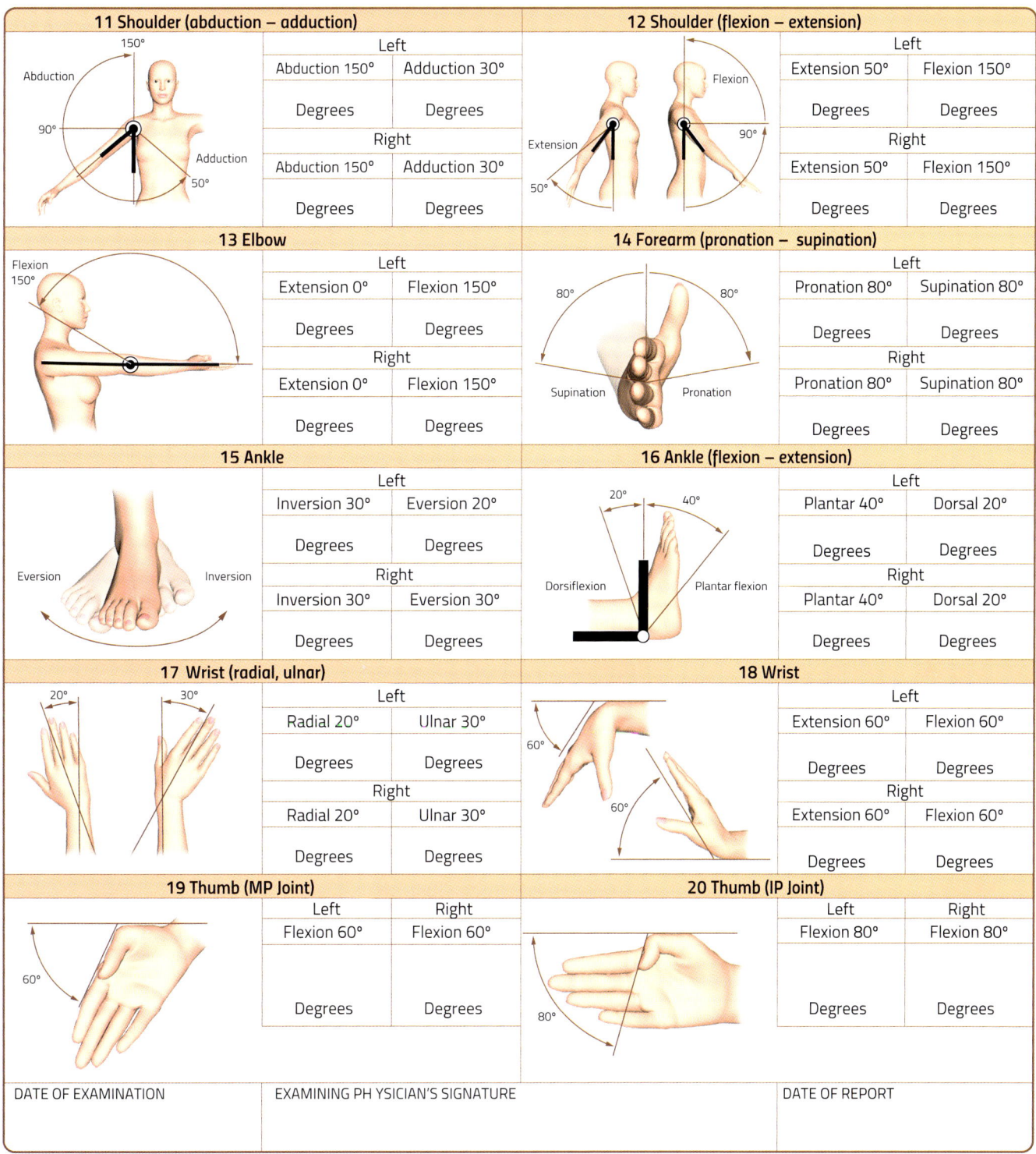

FIGURE 2.5 Goniometer evaluation chart from the Washington State Department of Social and Health Services (www.dshs.wa.gov)

Chapter two

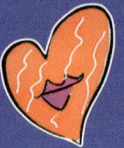 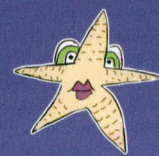

There are three typical methods used today for flexibility training: static, dynamic (ballistic), and proprioceptive neuromuscular facilitation (PNF) stretching.

> **Nota Bene**
>
> Because temperature affects the extensibility of the soft tissues around the joint, completing 5 minutes of warm-up (light aerobic exercise) is recommended before performing flexibility exercises.

This is the reason to start with warm-up exercises whether assessing the patient's ROM or conducting yoga (see Chapter 3 for more on this).

Static and dynamic stretching are both effective means of increasing flexibility, but generally static stretching is considered safer and results in less soreness of muscles. Dynamic stretching recruits the muscle spindle to reflexively cause contraction just after the fast stretch. This may result in small muscle tears due to a fast/forceful transition that may not be timed perfectly. The slow or static stretch also recruits the muscle shaft, but at a lower response intensity so that tearing is minimized or eliminated. Holding a stretched position for 10–30 seconds is usually effective. PNF is considered the most effective method that results in the least amount of post-stretching soreness (Luttgens and Hamilton 1997).

Improving joint flexibility is essential for injury prevention. One may increase joint flexibility (ROM) by regular stretching. Table 2.3 summarizes the average ROMs published. Compare your measurements with these values. Are they in similar ranges or not? If not, why not? What are the factors affecting flexibility of a joint? Recording of the measurements several times (as suggested by Luttgens and Hamilton, 1997) allows for increased accuracy.

Pain assessment for patients using the five kośas

According to Weintraub (2015):

TABLE 2.3 Normal range of motion (ROM) (according to www.dshs.wa.gov).

Body part	Movement	Normal ROM
Back	Extension	25°
	Flexion	90°
	Flexion (lateral)	25°
Neck	Extension	60°
	Flexion	60°
	Flexion (lateral)	45°
Hip	Extension	100°
	Flexion	100°
	Adduction	20°
	Abduction	40°
Shoulder	Extension	50°
	Flexion	150°
	Adduction	30°
	Abduction	150°
Forearm	Pronation	80°
	Supination	80°
Ankle	Extension	40°
	Flexion	20°
	Eversion	30°
	Inversion	30°
Wrist	Extension	60°
	Flexion	60°
	Deviation (radial)	20°
	Deviation (ulnar)	30°
Knee	Flexion	150°
Elbow	Flexion	150°

Yoga practice itself can often be a cathartic experience. When I ask a group at the beginning of a workshop or training, how many people have cried on their yoga mats, nearly everyone who practices yoga raises a hand. The tears we shed on the mat are most often not about the story, but rather are a release of a physiological or emotional constriction for which we may not have words. Even a simple breath may activate feelings.

(Weintraub 2015: 155)

A constriction in one area of the body–mind may simultaneously affect other aspects of our being. For example, a

Assessment for the mind and the body

tightness in the chest (*anāmaya kośa*) may affect the heart, breath and lungs (*prāṇamaya kośa*), as well as the emotive or mood state of the person (*manomaya kośa*). This constriction may also affect the person's belief about their Self (personality) and/or their surroundings (*vijnanamaya kośa*). And if, through a *prāṇamaya* breathing practice or a simple posture held with attention to sensation and breath, a release occurs, then all of the *kośas* are affected. In fact, there may even be a momentary experience of bliss and/or opening (*ananadamaya kośa*). This opening to the present emotion/moment may allow the person to feel that, although experiencing the emotion, they may be more than that emotion, and so much more than that self-limiting belief about how they operate within the world.

Whether an individual carries the label of depression or anxiety (the psychology model) or *tamasic* or *rājasic* (the yoga model), there are yoga strategies that can move us back into balance (*sattva*). With training, both yoga therapists and health professionals can offer a set of practices that meet the current mood and empower the person to find a way back to a more *sattvic* (or balanced) state.

Figure 2.6, by artist Paolo E. Marino, is a simple illustration (which was first created for my book *Yoga Therapy: Theory and Practice*, Horovitz and Elgelid 2015). Here, the *kośas* are illustrated as they surround the body like a protective sheath, much the same way a parent surrounds and protects a newborn child.

I use the Sequence Wiz app (Sequence Wiz 2020) to help in pain assessment (Sequence Wiz 2017) and to send yoga drawings (as will be seen throughout this book) post-sessions. The reasons are multifold: the drawings and wordage can be edited, the practitioner's logo can be inserted into the downloaded PDF file, and the sketches are HIPAA-compliant when being sent electronically post session.

Final thoughts

As can be seen, there are multiple ways of assessing a person, which include using applications and assessment techniques that offer physiologic, psychologic and diagnostic information. But in the words of Michael Amy (2019) (one of my yoga teachers and also

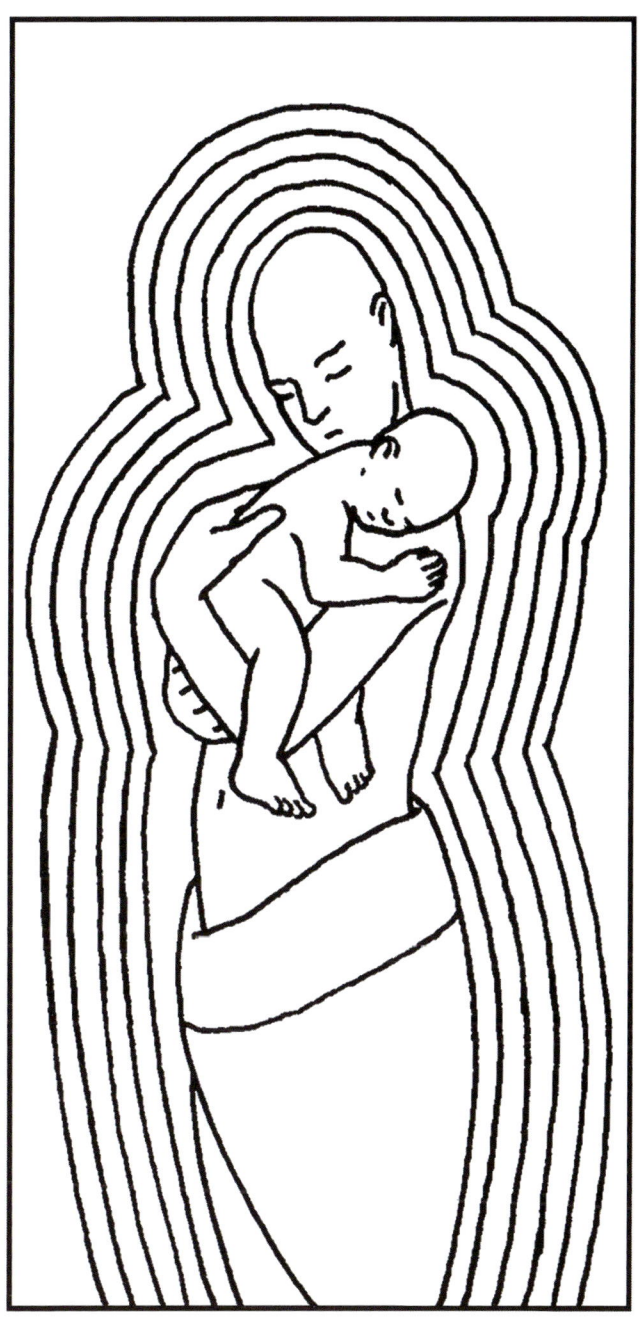

FIGURE 2.6 The kośhas by artist Paolo E. Marino

Chapter two

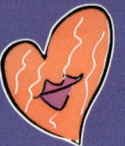 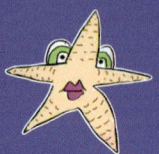

a physiotherapist), you can just simply watch the gait, breath, posture and presentation of the person and proceed from there. In a personal communication, he wrote:

> *A practitioner will be 'intuiting'/assessing from the very beginning. It starts with the initial contact (phone, meeting, handshake) and builds from there. I feel like relying solely on rudimentary measurements (goniometry as an example) falls way short of giving one adequate information. How do you look, see, and sense the person as a whole? It will be an ongoing process/dialogue. One of the reasons as a practitioner it is vital to practice self-care is to stay grounded and open to that.*
>
> **(Amy 2019)**

So, no matter how you decide to assess patient outcomes, via tracking efficacy through apps and/or diagnostically utilizing goniometers or similar scientific instruments, like Amy, the most important assessment that I rely on is my intuition. Often, this direction comes from within, deep within the recesses of my own energy system as I am affected by the person(s) in my space.

Regarding that, my friend Richard Burger, who is a meticulous housecleaner, always urges me to 'cleanse' my studio/therapy space before and after seeing patients. The reasons are multifold. One is to clear the room of the previous energy so that what I am picking up is of that person and not the 'residue' of the preceding patient. While this might not seem necessary, I too use this space for my daily practice and to create my own artwork. And so, it is all-important to 'clear the space' so that I am not affected by any negative energy that is left behind. More will be stated about that in 'clearing the space' in Chapter 3.

References

3D4Medical (2014) Essential Anatomy 5. Available at: https://3d4medical.com/apps/essential-anatomy-5.

American Psychiatric Association (2013) Diagnostic and Statistical Manual of Mental Disorders, 5th Edn (DSM-5). Washington, DC: American Psychiatric Association.

Amy M (2019) Personal communication.

Bainbridge-Cohen B (2014) Sensing, Feeling and Action: The Experiential Anatomy of Body–Mind Centering. El Sobrante, CA: Burchfield Rose Publishers.

Burns RC and Kaufman, SH (1972) Actions, Styles and Symbols in Kinetic Family Drawings (K-F-D): An Interpretive Manual. New York, NY: Brunner/Mazel.

Cain S (2012) Quiet: The Power Of Introverts In A World That Can't Stop Talking. New York, NY: Crown Publishing Group.

Eaton WW, Muntaner C, Smith C, Tien A and Ybarra M (2004) Center for Epidemiologic Studies Depression Scale: Review and Revision (CESD and CESD-R). In: Maruish ME (ed) The Use of Psychological Testing for Treatment Planning and Outcomes Assessment, 3rd Edn. Mahwah, NJ: Lawrence Erlbaum: 363–377.

Gantt L and Tabone C (1998) The Formal Elements of Art Therapy: The Rating Manual. Morgantown, WV: Gargoyle Press.

Gantt LM (2001) The formal elements art therapy scale: A measurement system for global variations in art. Art Therapy: Journal of the American Art Therapy Association 18(1): 50–55.

Gussak D (2013) Art on Trial: Art Therapy in Capital Murder Cases. New York, NY: Columbia Press.

Hanna T (1970) Bodies in Revolt. New York, NY: Holt, Rinehart & Winston.

Henry JD and Crawford JR (2005) The 21-item version of the Depression Anxiety Stress Scales (DASS–21): Normative data and psychometric evaluation in a large non-clinical sample. British Journal of Clinical Psychology 44: 227–239.

Horovitz EG and Elgelid S (eds) (2015). Yoga Therapy: Theory and Practice. New York, NY: Routledge Press.

Horovitz EG (2017). The Guide to Art Therapy Materials and Methods: A Practical, Step-by-step Approach. New York, NY: Routledge Press.

Horovitz EG (2020) The Art Therapists' Primer: A Clinical Guide to Writing Assessment, Diagnosis and Treatment, 3rd Edn. Springfield, IL: Charles C Thomas Ltd.

Jacobs L (2009) Interview with Lawrence Weed, MD: The father of the problem-oriented medical record looks ahead. The Permanente Journal. Kaiser Permanente. Summer, 13(3): 84–89.

Lowenfeld V and Brittain WL (1987) Creative and Mental Growth, 8th Edn. New York, NY: MacMillan.

Luttgens K and Hamilton N (1997) Kinesiology: Scientific Basis of Human Motion, 9th Edn. Madison, WI: Brown & Benchmark.

Assessment for the mind and the body

Myers TM (2014) Anatomy Trains: Myofascial Meridians for Manual and Movement Therapists, 3rd Edn. New York, NY: Elseveir Health, Inc.

Payne L and Morris R (2013) Yoga Therapy RX: Morris–Payne Yoga Therapy Evaluation. Los Angeles, CA: Samata International.

Robins M (2002) A Physiological Handbook for Teachers of Yogasana. Tuscon, AZ: Fenestra Books.

Sequence Wiz (2017) Pain Assessment Handout. Available at: http://sequencewiz.org/wp-content/uploads/2017/09/Pain-assessment_handout.pdf.

Sequence Wiz (2020) Sequence Wiz Home Practice App. Available at: https://sequencewiz.com/

Weintraub A (2015) Yoga and mental health: the crumbling wall. In: Horovitz EG and Elgelid S (eds) Yoga Therapy: Theory and Practice. New York, NY: Routledge.

WellnessKeen (2020) Don't Know How to Use a Goniometer? Now You Will. Available: https://wellnesskeen.com/how-to-use-goniometer.

Zador V, Zador L and Anderson M (2019) Design and implementation of Electronic Medical Record (EMR) templates for yoga therapy. Yoga Therapy Today, Spring: 32–35.

3 The experiential component: the yoga and art process

1.2 Yogaś citta-vṛtti nirodhaḥ: Yoga is the stilling of the changing states of the mind.

Bryant (2009: 10)

On being in the zone

I started practicing yoga at age 14 – my brother and I used to do headstands in our living room after going to our weekly yoga class. Truthfully, our yoga teacher seemed uninterested in cultivating our adolescent practice, and we were all about the *āsanas* and stretching the limits of the poses. Our practice waxed and then waned – we lost interest. Other activities commandeered my yoga practice, specifically swimming and art. I religiously swam, sometimes daily, and continue this practice as often as I can. I had always been physical and found that I completely relaxed when I was 'in the (corporal) zone'.

Sometimes, when swimming in open water and gazing at the fish below me, I simply 'forgot' to come up for air and breathe. It wasn't until much later that I discovered why: apparently, our ancestral attributes are often, but not always, preserved in an organism's development. For example, both chick and human embryos go through a stage where they have slits and arches in their necks like the gill slits and gill arches of fish. Human embryos do not have gill slits, they have pharyngeal pouches. In fish, each gill slit has an accompanying set of blood vessels that filters out food and water intake. But according to Held (2009), human embryos make five pairs of aortic arches (which once sent blood to five pairs of gills). Later, the embryo destroys two of them completely. The remaining aortic arches become the vessels that take oxygenated blood to the lungs, head, and body. This Sisyphean lunacy only makes sense as an evolutionary artefact: it was only genetically possible to adapt by reconfiguring the existing plumbing, and not to scrap it altogether and start again. So developmentally we harbor some sort of gill system, and perhaps it is for this reason that I feel so at home in water. Floating and weightless, the buoyancy of the water sends my mind and body adrift.

And while Colangelo (2003) argues that we were 'built to walk', and that we were 'not designed to lift weights, nor swim, nor cycle, nor sit', here I contend with that theory (Colangelo 2003: 181). Other than that postulate, I found her book refreshing and very relevant. And while sitting too much has been touted as the 'new cancer' (Laskowski 2018), horizontality, as Colangelo suggests (think *śavāsana*), is clearly a better choice.

What is so interesting to me is that when in a yogic mind/body state, I feel exactly the same way as I do when I swim. Initially, when in my formative yoga trainings, I complained about my inability to meditate to my teacher, Sri François Raoult (http://www.openskyyoga.com/teachers). He commented: 'but Elena (his pet name for me, pronounced el-en-ah), when you are in *āsana*, you are meditating'. Bryant (2009) would agree. Contrary to popular belief, he states: 'Yoga is not to join but to unjoin, that is to disconnect *puruṣa* (the soul) from *prakṛti* (primordial matter), (Bryant 2009: 5) In other words, in *yogāsana*, I was 'in the zone'. I can't tell you how much relief this provided for me. These days, while I actively try and meditate more, I find that my mind frees when I am 'in the zone' no matter what physical form my body makes. Perhaps the movement surrounding my body, be it air or water, provides the necessary buoyancy that I once experienced when in the womb. While I will never know for sure, on a proprioceptive level, intuitively this makes abundant sense to me.

This takes me to the creative process. The great thinker Mihaly Csikszentmihalyi (2008) connected the creative process to a 'flow state' or being 'in the zone'. For most artists, writers, poets, composers, musicians, dancers, and even scientists, when absorbed in their activities, they fall into this state of flow.

My sister, author Nancy Bachrach, used to remark that oftentimes she would pass me and many hours later I was still engrossed in creating my artwork, had not finished my morning cup of coffee nor taken a bathroom break. She was the same when writing. As the saying goes, time is meaningless in the face of creativity. I literally become lost in the process. And when I am in '*yogāsana*', swimming or like activity, the same is true for me. For all intents and purposes, I am lost to the ages, happily entrenched in what I am doing, unjoined from *puruṣa* (the soul) and *prakṛti* (primordial matter). For a more comprehensive review of the yoga *sūtras* and philosophical underpinnings as outlined in the Introduction,

Chapter three

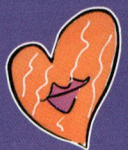 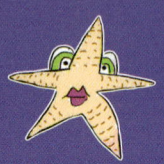

it is suggested that, for starters, the reader review Bryant (2009) and Iyengar (1979, 2005).

Rumination and anxieties have no bearing while in this flow state. It is for these reasons, that I try to get my patients to experience this first-hand. I suggest becoming completely absorbed, but not in an egoistic manner.

Avidyā (the mother of all *kleśas*) is where egos grow. In Sanskrit, 'a' means not and 'vid' is related to seeing, so this literally means not seeing clearly or not having correct knowledge (e.g. spiritual ignorance). In ignorance, obstacles flourish. This is not the path of yoga nor what the mother of art therapy and my mentor, Edith Kramer (1977a, 1977b, 1979, 1993) referred to as 'true' or 'formed art'. It is the absolute antithesis, which I refer to as 'dis-ease' (Horovitz 1999, 2005, 2014, 2017a, 2017b). Moving away from this stance and into a trajectory of wellness is harder than you might think (Fig. 3.1). For many, the homoeostasis of 'dis-ease' is what is known, safe if you will. And shaking up that system and changing is the real work. The vision *('vid')* is in the knowing and the doing. And that is the work ahead.

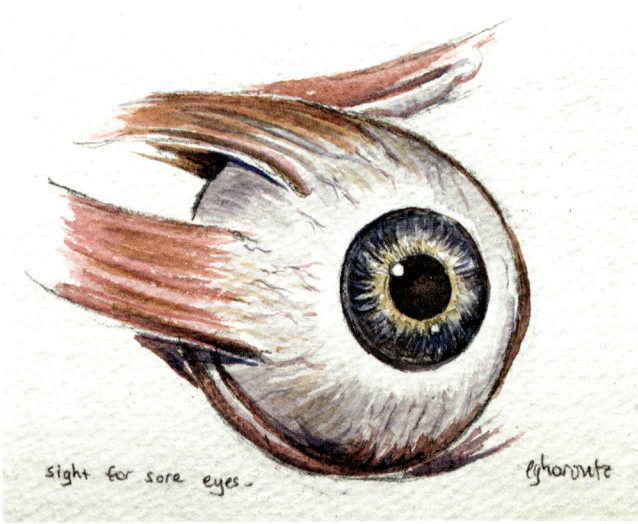

FIGURE 3.1 Sight for sore eyes, by the author (collection of David Klein MD, with permission)

Clearing the space

In Chapter 2 I mentioned Richard Burger, a meticulous housecleaner, who urged me to 'cleanse' my studio/therapy space before and after seeing patients. His recommendation addressed the all-important topic of residue and clearing the space in between seeing patients. While that is an important consideration, which will be raised repeatedly throughout this book, here we are talking about cleansing, or in yogic terms *śaucha* – cleansing and purifying the mind, body and the spirit.

Many years ago, my good friend and colleague, Dr Shaun McNiff, wrote an important book called *Earth Angels: Engaging the Sacred in Everyday Things* (McNiff 1995). At the time, this book had an enormous influence on me. I am not certain if it appealed to my artistic sensibility (or pack-rat mentality – for months, I saved a perfect specimen of a dead fly to paint) or because of those things that I hold dear. As an artist, I am constantly repurposing things, sometimes creating from by-products. This leads to an inability to throw anything out since I see potential even in discarded items. While it might lead to hoarder mentality, I periodically try to purge my stash and discard items that I have not used. Throughout my life, I have become attached to certain things. Attachment, while seemingly healthy when one is an offspring and dependent on others for survival, can later prove a hindrance in life. If speaking about this in terms of the *kleśas*, it is called *abhiniveśa* (clinging to life).

Instinctually, we are all attached to life, to surviving. But if you can bring a sense of deep acceptance (equanimity) to life, within that is a divine spark, that the body dies yet the spirit goes on. Meditating on *abhiniveśa* helps us to understand that the body will die, and to find tranquility around the spark that remains, and to begin to see the difference. Because of my life experiences and losses at an early age, I talk about death all the time. I see it as a natural progression of life. However, the constant joke among my children is my absolute inability to have a dinner conversation without bringing up the subject of death. Guilty as charged.

But *Earth Angels* is not about the letting go, but rather the holding on. All of us hold onto things of import in

The experiential component: the yoga and art process

our lives. It is how we build a home, a hearth, comfort ourselves and our loved ones. In McNiff's treatise, he is not suggesting *abhiniveśa* or the clinging onto of life. Rather, it is about looking at those everyday things that become a sacred part of our lives.

When I moved into the new home from which I am presently writing, I spent 6 luxurious months with nothing on my walls. Marie Kondo, the present-day guru of declutter, would then have been happy to walk into my space. Kondo's maxim is to 'discard anything that doesn't spark joy'. It is in the discarding or 'letting go' that we really delve into the reasons why we can't let something go. According to Kondo (2014), there are only two reasons: 'an attachment to the past or a fear for the future'. This pretty much sums up our reasons to cling so tightly.

But when you clear the space you make room for expansion, acceptance, creativity and growth. In Carbonetti's (2001) book, *Making Pearls: Living the Creative Life*, she talks about the nature of waiting. She suggests that this state of going within ('transpersonal consciousness') is really a kind of research (and expansion towards others) that every creation begins with – whether making art or curing a disease (Carbonetti 2001: 22). This is where I tend to go when I enter that creative zone but first, I need a *tabula rasa*, the blank slate. It is there that I can imprint my internal wanderings. This form can take on multiple states and it can be influenced by multiple wanderings. It might start with cleaning the space, leafing through my art materials for inspiration, glancing out my studio window to see the river moving past my studio and home, walking in nature, yoga, writing, playing an instrument, or striking a simple movement/dance. Once I engage in the heightened state of creation, if you enter my lair, it may look like a tornado hit my studio. For it is in the mess, the chaos, that the creativity flows. But the clean-up process, as Ulman and Dachinger (1976) espoused, births order out of chaos. It is here that Kondo's concept shines, but it is in the chaos (whether creating or decluttering) that the real work begins. When in this artistic state, one is in a state of *tapas*, which according to its yogic principle involves self-discipline, austerity, and the attempt to achieve union with the higher Self. According to Iyengar, 'life without *tapas* is a heart without love' (1979: 38). *Tapas* may relate to three types: the body, the mind, or speech. Raman (1998) stated that 'every artist is imbued with the quality of tapas ... inner inspiration, which apparently is sourceless, [and] is what makes for a successful artist in any field' (Raman 1998: 132). Raman goes on to state that 'when in this state of mind, the artist excels, as he or she is totally identified with the object of work' (Rahman 1998: 133).

No matter what it takes to clear your space, know that in the clearing you will be getting rid of that sticky residue that prevents your cleansing and moving not just yourself, but also your patients into the highest form of art and creation itself. That higher realm of existence (in yoga) is known as *īśvara-praṇidhāna*. It is in that state that the artist achieves both union and humility as they devote themselves to a higher power and dissolve ego-focused desires (a tall order that could take a lifetime to achieve). Herein we will focus on steps toward that end.

To illustrate how that clearing can occur, I will offer an example from my own life. In my advanced teacher training (ATT) my yoga teacher, Sri François Raoult, declared the need for us to have a talent show at graduation. At first I bemoaned the situation, but I know there is always a method to François' madness. Generally, I am better for following his edict and bending to his whims. I went full-hog on this assignment – it interrupted the writing of this book and required months of creation. I decided to create two puppets (from foam, a material with which I was completely unfamiliar) of François and BKS Iyengar, his teacher and master guru. The reasons were multifold, but the idea was sparked over a glass of wine with my husband. Because François' checkered past involved a decade of touring Europe with an *avant garde* puppet theater, composing music for their plays and manipulating the string puppets, my husband thought maybe I could do something around puppetry. Of course, François had established a 'theme' for the talent show: inner and outer travels. With this in mind, I embarked on the idea of having the puppets sing Frank Sinatra's song *My Way*, albeit with the lyrics rewritten (by me) for comic effect. I joined forces with my yoga mates (or 'yoganauts' as François called us) Maxine Ge, who played the violin and Ream Kidane, who helped

Chapter three

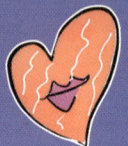

operate the Iyengar puppet. This overtook my life as I got into the flow of making the puppets (Fig. 3.2), their outfits, the curtained stage and our matching T-shirts sporting François and Iyengar's images (Fig. 3.3). But I so enjoyed the process, once again, lost to the ages.

So now it's your turn. Perhaps you can give yourself a similar assignment based on what is going on in your life at this moment (Fig. 3.4). Or try the space-clearing exercise in Reflective exercise 3.1 to get the juices flowing.

Warm-up techniques

As discussed in Chapter 1, creating a safe space is all-important in aiding your patient (and yourself) to feel comfortable and engage in a therapeutic environment. To summarize, some of the ways of doing this are:

- Lighting of and gazing at a candle or oil wick (*trātak*)
- A hand gesture (*mūdra*)
- A simple yoga breath (*prāṇayāma*)
- A soothing image of sanctuary or peace (*bhāvana*)

Reflection exercise 3.1

Space clearing exercise for the reader

Pause, perhaps during *śavāsana*, maybe in *sukāsana* (simple cross-legged pose) or gazing at a candle (*trātak*) and reflect on your surroundings both inside your person and outside. Perhaps in assessing this inside/outside space, make room for your creativity, ponder this and then clear into the urgency of the creativity that this unearths. Try not to censor anything that bubbles up: embrace it all.

Reach for some art materials. Create that urgency; allow it to swim forth onto paper, clay, paint, fabric, your iPad software programs, or whatever calls your spirit.

After its creation, sit with this creative offspring. Let it be your guide and set your intention with it as you go out into the world.

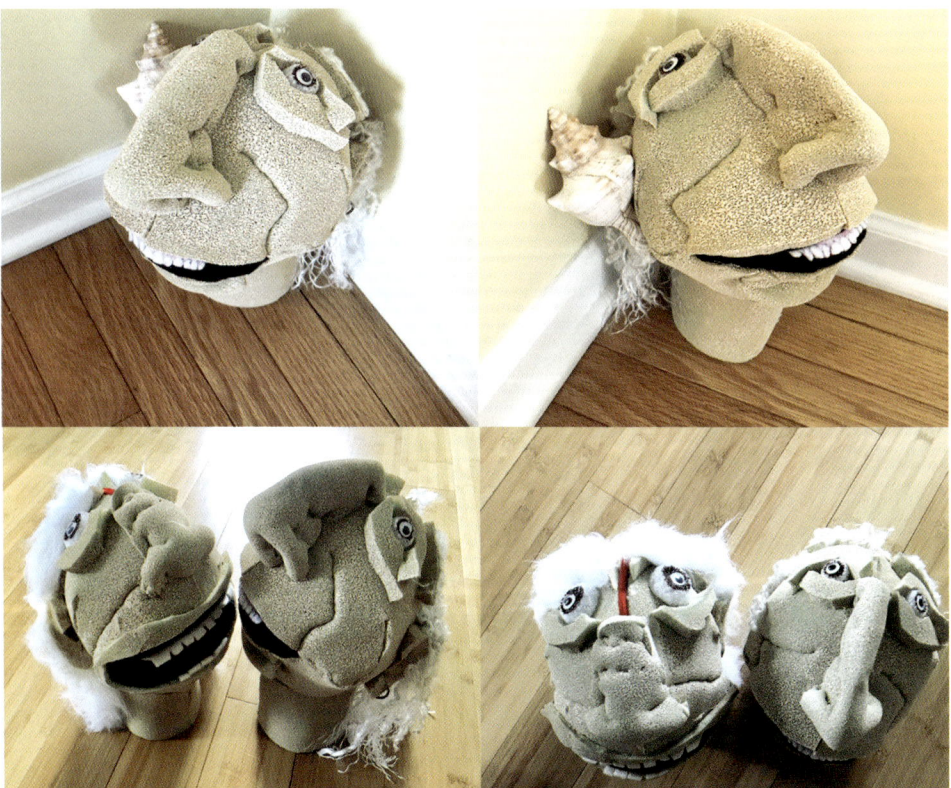

FIGURE 3.2 François and Iyengar puppet heads, artwork created by author (note: François is well known for an image of him holding a conch shell next to his ear)

The experiential component: the yoga and art process

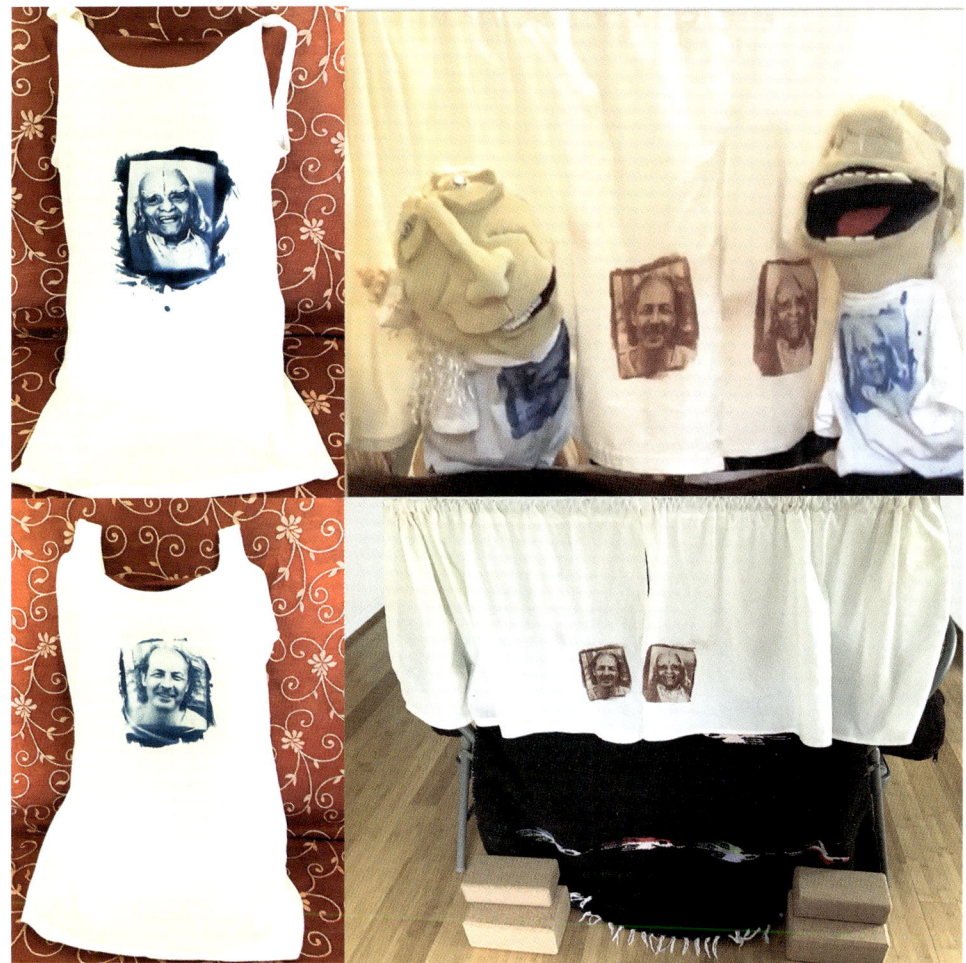

FIGURE 3.3 T-shirts, (left) puppets in action (upper right), and curtains and puppet stage (made with yoga props) (lower right). Artwork created by author

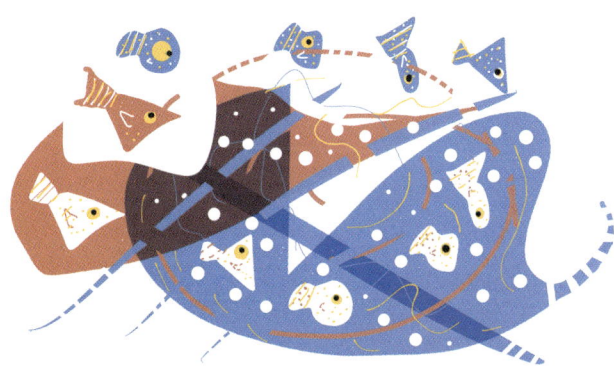

FIGURE 3.4 On being sick (fish jumping out of water): 'Creating order out of chaos,' by the author. Digital artwork created in Paper53 app

- A soothing universal tone (*māntra*) (e.g. you could chant *so ham*: this signifies that there is no separation between the energy that surrounds you and the energy that you are – it means, 'I am that')

- A cleansing breath (*kriyā*)

- Client's intention (*sankālpa*) perhaps for a positively oriented *saṃskārā* (driven by beneficial experiences and deeds)

- Playing a sound such as a singing bowl or like instrument to clear the space

- Chanting *Aum* with your patient if this seems appropriate to the situation and the person (perhaps try toning *nāda yoga*, as the sound used does make a difference – the fluid vibration goes through

53

Chapter three

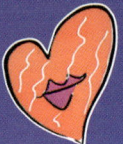
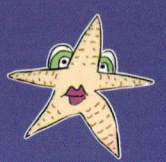

the body, stimulating the parasympathetic nervous system and calming the automatic nervous system).

In addition, you can also add the following:

- Hula hooping can be a great ice-breaker and warm-up activity, especially with young children and their families
- Moving on the mat to a favorite song, especially helpful with pubescent and adolescent populations.

Yogic breathing and meditation techniques for mood management

Examples of meeting the mood: understanding the guṇas

In the Introduction we looked at a person's constitution in relation to the *guṇas*. For example, *rājasic*, in emotional terms, would be anxiety, mania, hypomania or like symptomatology. While your first instinct might be to calm your patient down when in this state, a paradoxical approach is key. Instead of downplaying the hyperactive mood, and trying to quiet your patient, instead you need to meet the *rājasic* state with vigor – then, when ready, move your patient to a more calming practice. While this may seem antithetical, according to one of my teachers, Amy Weintraub (2012), this approach truly serves your patient. My own experience as a practitioner is in complete agreement with this theory. While it took my mind some time to wrap around this paradoxical approach, given my past psychological teachings, I have found that meeting the mood works.

Additionally, Arora and Bhattacharjee (2008) suggest that one of the goals of yoga is to achieve quietude of the mind. In turn, the authors suggest that this instills well-being, relaxation, improved self-confidence, and restores an optimistic outlook on life. A yogic practice generates energy vital to immune system functioning, which optimizes the body's sympathetic responses to stressful stimuli and restores autonomic regulatory reflex mechanisms associated with stress. According to Desikachar et al (2005), yogic practices inhibit the areas responsible for fear, aggression and rage while stimulating the reward/pleasure centers in the median forebrain. This inhibition results in lowering anxiety, heart rate, respiratory rate, blood pressure, and cardiac output in those who practice yoga and meditation. Moreover, Streeter et al (2012) purport that yogic practice is correlated with increased functioning of GABA (gamma-aminobutyric acid). GABA supports higher brain structure by inhibiting signals and activities of fear-based networks (Mason and Birch 2018). And according to Timothy McCall (2018), 'when the breath changes, it affects every component of the autonomic nervous system'. He goes on to purport that 'if we can change how a person breathes, it can lead to changes in short order' (McCall 2018).

So, returning to the *rājasic* patient, one way you could 'meet the mood' is to fire up the patient's system using *kapālabhāti* breath, which literally means skull shining breath. However, it should be noted that according to Iyengar, *kapālabhāti* breath invigorates the liver, spleen, pancreas and abdominal muscles, and should not be practiced by persons with poor lung capacity or a weak constitution (Iyengar 1979: 450).

Nota Bene

A great resource for looking at dis-ease, be it physical and/or emotional, is to turn to the works of Iyengar (1979), Raman (1998) and Mason and Birch (2018).

Steps of kapālabhāti padmāsana

- First, sit on the floor in *padmāsana* (lotus pose or if not capable, simple cross-legged pose) and close your eyes and keep the spine straight.
- Now, take a somewhat shallow breath (inhaling) through both nostrils.
- Next, exhale through both nostrils forcefully, so your stomach will go deep inside. Bring the diaphragm towards the back of the spine as you do this.
- When doing *kapālabhāti padmāsana*, it almost sounds like a dog's breath when panting. Generally,

The experiential component: the yoga and art process

you should aim for 60–80 breaths-per-minute, which might seem difficult for beginners. Remember that the inhale is shallow, and the exhale comes out of both nostrils.

Looking to the *guṇas* again, next let us review meeting the *tamāsic* state. In emotional terms, this would be dysthymia (mild, chronic depression), lethargy and/or major depression. In this instance, it is advised that you meet the *tamāsic* state with a slow, restorative practice, then build to a more energizing practice.

For example, you could meet your patient with slow coherent breathing (count 6 to inhale, count 2–4 for breath held, count 6–8 to exhale, repeating this for up to a minute or longer). Doing this a few times would meet your patient's mood, then to energize your patient you could move to a more active pose such as *tādāsana* (or *Samasthiti*) (mountain pose, Fig. 3.5).

Steps of tādāsana (or samasthiti) (mountain pose)

- Stand erect with the feet together (or parallel and residing under hips) and rest the metatarsals on the floor, stretching all the toes flat.
- Next, tighten the knees and pull the kneecaps in, contract the hips and pull the muscles in at the back of the thighs.
- Keep the stomach in, chest is forward, spine is stretched skyward and the neck is straight.
- Keep the arms outstretched at the side. Doing this pose actively in this manner is essential to the art of standing correctly. If done actively in this manner, it will increase the patient's energy.

You could move on to *adho mukha śvānāsana* (otherwise known as downward-facing dog), that is if your patient does not suffer from high blood pressure. If your patient does have high blood pressure you can offer modifications, such as placing lengthened arms at the wall (Fig. 3.6) and backing up until the spine and arms are straight, drop the head between the arms but not lower than the waist, keep the legs stiff and do not bend the knees.

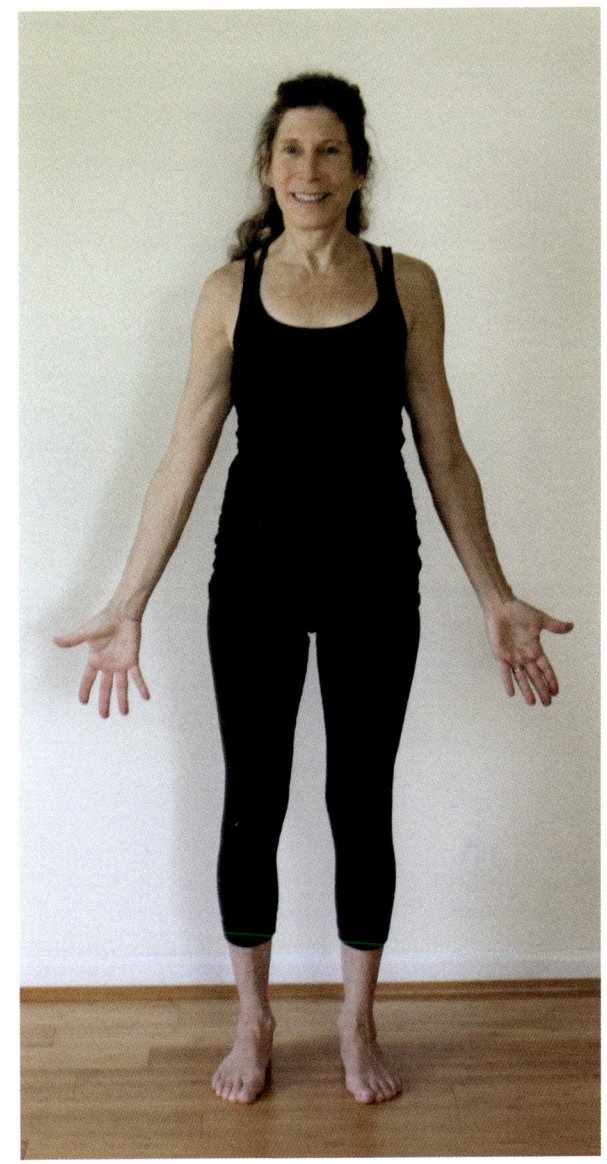

FIGURE 3.5 Author prepares for *tādāsana*, mountain pose

Heels and toes should be completely flat on the ground. Note that the patient in Figure 3.6 has had two shoulder replacements, and at this juncture, straightening her elbows was not an option; so careful attention needs to be paid to specific poses.

According to Iyengar (1979), staying in *adho mukha śvānāsana* for a longer time may eliminate exhaustion

Chapter three

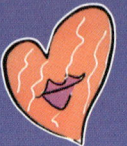
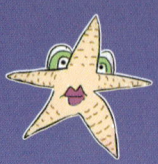

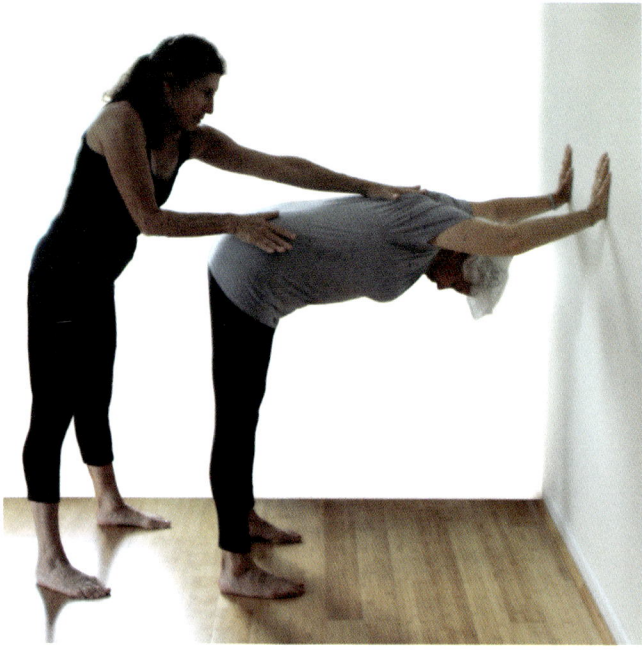

FIGURE 3.6 Author adjusting student in *adho mukha śvānāsana*, modified at the wall

Steps for stair-step breath

- Sitting in simple cross-legged pose or *padmāsana* (lotus pose), close your eyes and inhale through the diaphragm, bringing the air back towards your spine and taking small breaths in through your mouth, sipping the air much like you would water through a straw. While doing this imagine taking an elevator up the mountain of your spine.
- Hold it at the top for 3–4 counts, then exhale the out-breath from your nose in a smooth continuous breath, while imagining an elevator descending down the mountain.
- Repeat at least 10 times.

Steps for bellows breath

- Stand in *tādāsana*, inhale and raise your arms overhead and exhale as you take them out wide to your sides (Fig. 3.7).
- Inhale again and raise your arms over head, exhale as you bring your torso down over your thighs and exhort at the top of your lungs, 'HA!'.
- Repeat 10 times and then stand again in *tādāsana*, close your eyes and feel the effects of your practice.

Nota Bene

Do not have patients with unmedicated high blood pressure lower their head below their hearts – others can descend their heads forward to their thighs.

(depression) and fatigue and restore lost energy (Iyengar 1979: 110). While there are great physiological benefits to doing this pose (e.g. eradicating stiffness in the shoulder blades, relieving arthritis in the shoulder joints), emotively it can lead to exhilaration and rejuvenation of the brain cells (Iyengar 1979: 111) – not bad for one simple *āsana*.

If you care to further invigorate your patient a bit more slowly, you could move toward a meditation practice, offering a 'stair-step breath', and then move to *tādāsana*. Once in *tādāsana*, you can easily move your patient into 'bellows breath', which literally can change the mood when the final exhale of bellows breath is exhorted into a loud 'HA.' Churning the breath in these ways prepares the mind for acceptance and less rumination. For example, I had a patient who came into my practice complaining that some days he could barely arise from bed. I suggested trying bellows breath to rev up his engine on those mornings. Once he completed this practice, he was visibly lighter and laughing as we performed the 'HA' outbreath together.

It should be noted that oftentimes people who suffer from mood disorders may find a meditation practice especially difficult. For example, depression is often accompanied by a lot of negative self-talk, therefore making a quieting practice difficult to achieve. This does not mean that meditation cannot be achieved, only that the practitioner should proceed by taking cues from the patient's baseline and building meditation into the practice over time.

The experiential component: the yoga and art process

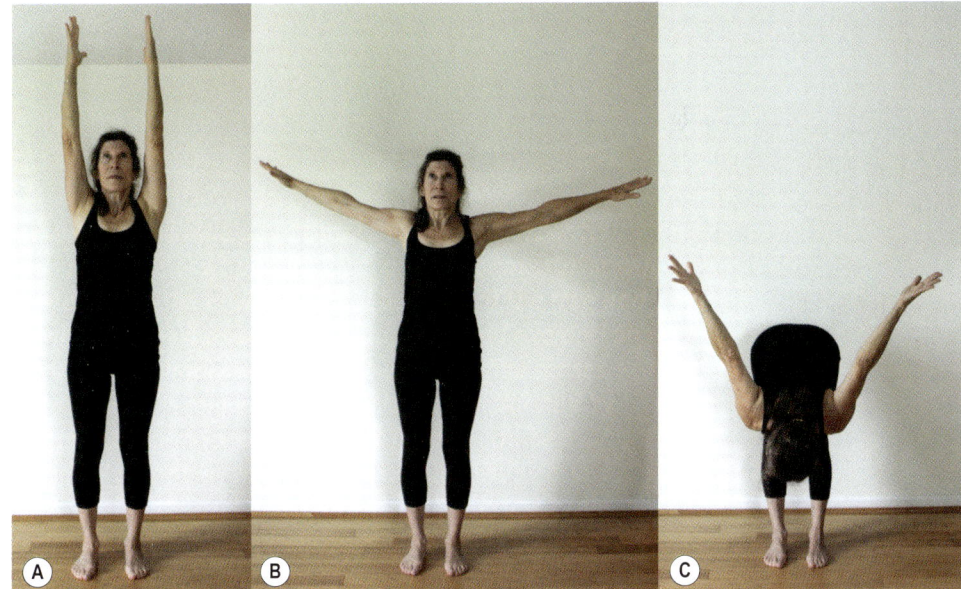

FIGURE 3.7 Author doing bellows breath

According to Weintraub (2012), establishing an observer's mind, or the 'seer' as Patañjāli (Bryant 2009) puts it, through regular mindfulness (or mantra-based practice when not depressed) and then meditating can aid in detaching from those self-critical thoughts. Tantric and Buddhist traditions of nondualism provide a number of meditation techniques that offer the busy mind a method of slowing down and decreasing negative self-talk and rumination.

Modifications and sequencing of poses

Modifying for a yoga class or yoga therapy session

Whether conducting a yoga class or private yoga therapy session, it is essential to have an idea of how you are going to sequence your class or session. In both instances, taking cues from the people in front of you is paramount. Practitioners refer to this in a variety of ways; Garner (2018) refers to this as the biopsychosocial care model which incorporates an 'allostatic load'. Garner describes this 'allostatic load' as a heuristic model (observational/ intuitive) which is a result of 'genetic, environmental, biographical, psychosocial, behavioral (lifestyle choices)

Reflection exercise 3.2

Breath and creative exercise

It is always my practice to be comfortable in what I am asking my patients to do, so if you have never done stair-step breath and/or bellows breath, practice both so that you can comfortably lead your patient through these exercises.

Make sure you have some paper and paint out ready to use as soon as you complete the breath practice. Then checking your internal barometer, choose one of the breath practices and repeat the sequence 10–20 times.

Move immediately to the paper and the paints. Without censoring, pick up a brush, dip it into the first color that attracts you and just paint, moving with the paintbrush as if it were an extension of your breath. Do this until you feel satisfied with the result.

If you want to take it a step further, write a paragraph about what you are feeling at this very moment as you look at the created artwork.

Chapter three

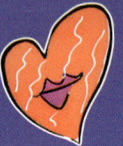 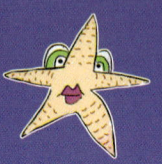

factors', that contribute to the clinical variables of the individual (Garner 2018: 9). In previous publications (Horovitz 2017a, 2017b), I have referred readers to Bronfenbrenner's (1994) ecological theory of development where one looks at a chronosystem, which links individuals and families by social interdependence, sociohistorical influences, environmental events and transitions over the life-course and factors in both culture and time (Figure 3.8). Basically, the chronosytem model is similar to Garner's biopsychosocial system and like that system incorporates the concept of the five kośas (sheaths) of the individual.

Let's now look at how you incorporate a chronosystem model of thinking with yoga teaching and/or yoga therapy.

At the YMCA near my home, I teach an active yoga class (advanced). The students that come are diverse in age and skill, and although I have 'regulars' that have attended the class for years, the constituency is ever-changing. As a result, this is a constant challenge to me. Being a seasoned teacher, it takes vision and creativity to adapt advanced poses and modify them for everyone in the room, especially when limited by only having yoga blocks, belts and mats. Also, sometimes the class size mushrooms to 52 people – I am not kidding!

Towards the end of my advanced class, if we have done enough back-bending preparations, one of the poses that my very advanced students like to do is *eka pāda rājakapotāsana* or pigeon pose. This is because I have sequenced the class so that their limbs are ready to attempt this pose. However, some are incapable of taking this position and so modifications are key, and all kinds of variations can be offered (Figure 3.9). Some may be able to adapt into an advanced version called mermaid pose, others may just use their yoga belts to hold onto one leg, and still others may just remain in the preparatory first step of the *eka pāda rājakapotāsana* pose. Being able to offer the variations to your students and/or patients takes inner practice and knowledge. For example, in Figure 3.10, a student who has multiple physical issues (including two shoulder replacements and arthritis in her hips) is offered props in order to attempt this pose, which she loves to do.

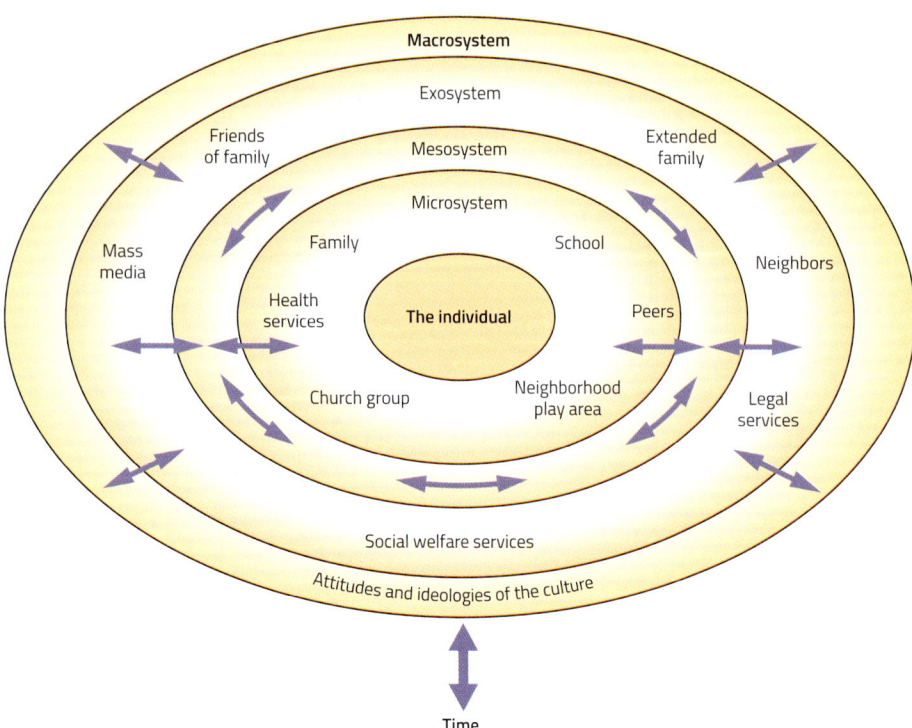

FIGURE 3.8 The chronosytem patterning of environmental events and transitions over the life course: sociohistorical conditions

The experiential component: the yoga and art process

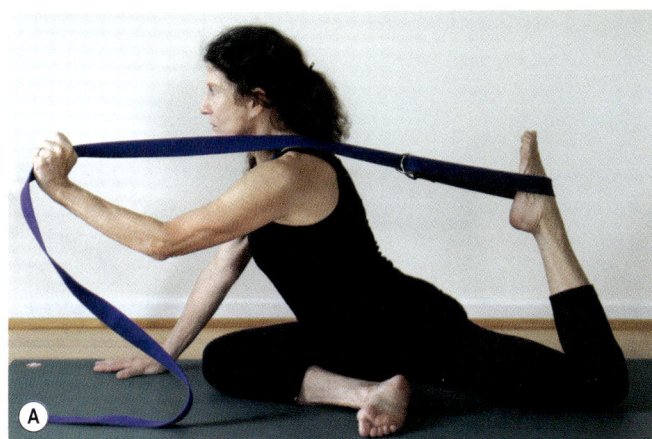

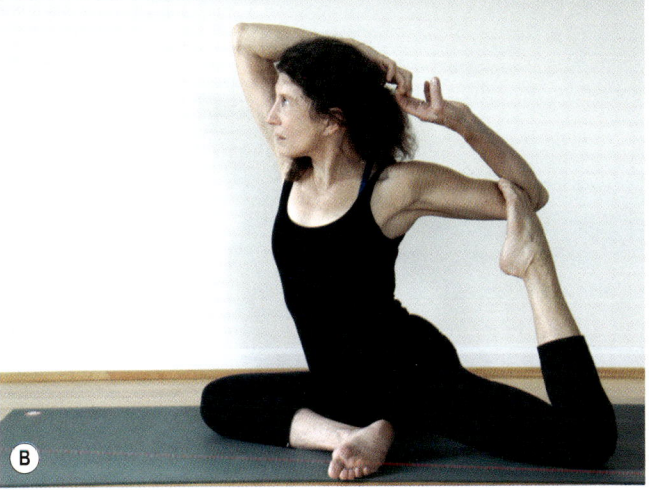

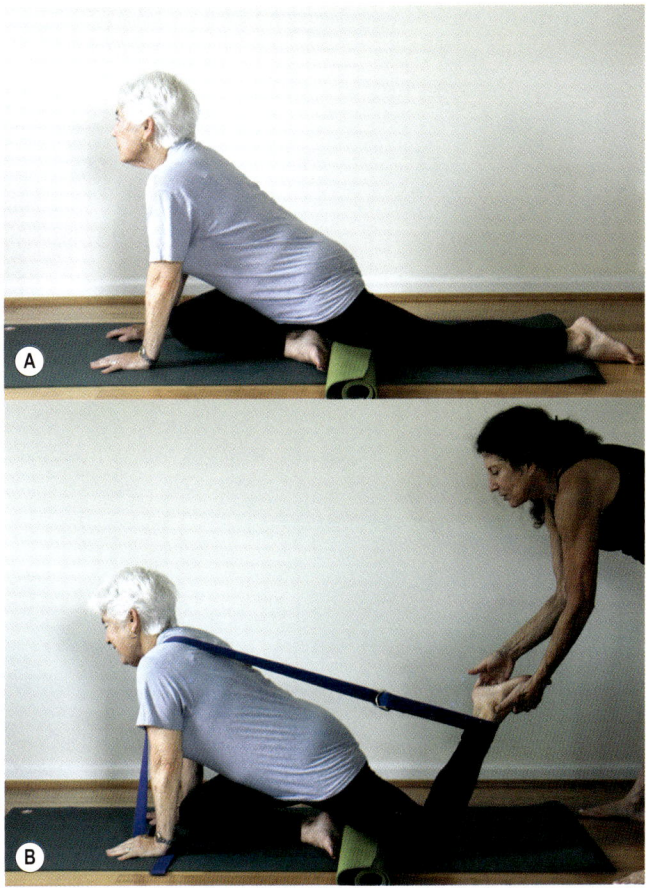

FIGURE 3.9 Author doing warm up for *eka pāda rājakapotāsana*, adapting with a yoga belt into mermaid pose

FIGURE 3.10 Student doing modified *eka pāda rājakapotāsana*, with prop and yoga belt assist by the author

I also teach at a local fitness center (Chili Fitness Center, CFC). Both settings are completely different. At the CFC the class is geared towards seniors (students are aged 80–94) and while it is billed as a Silver Sneakers Yoga class, I teach it very differently to the traditional Silver Sneakers classes (even though I am also certified as a Silver Sneakers teacher) (see Chapter 7 for more on this). One of my teachers is the chair yoga master Lakshmi Voelker. Her course deviates from anything I have ever read, such as the work of Shifroni (2014). But as François has taught me, it is important to put my own spin on these teachings to make them genuinely mine.

In this class, the last 15 minutes is the time when my students sit in the chair. Other than that, I might use it only as a prop (unless someone needs to use the chair for the entire class). Also, Lakshmi taught me to incorporate weights in chair yoga. Sometimes, I add them during standing yoga sequences or when sitting. Furthermore, recent research points out how important weight-bearing exercises are for seniors to reduce the risk of falling, and can in fact cause changes in the brain (Brown et al 2008, Brody 2018, Reynolds 2019). I always offer the option not to use the weights, but this class has grown over the last 3 years by word-of-mouth and there are newcomers every week. Generally there is a minimum of 24 people and of late the seniors want to use their voices and sing *Aum*.

Chapter three

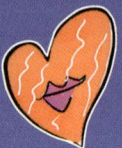 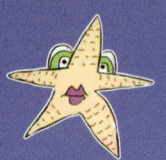

Of course, true to yoga, whether at the Y or CFC class, I start everyone with an intention, a small meditation and always finish in mediation and *śavāsana*. At the end of class, I offer aromatherapy via Young Living essential oils and a cranial–sacral massage. For many of these seniors (widowed and/or touch-deprived) this is the only touch they might receive until the next class. Of course, for those who don't want this added feature, it is skipped.

Use of essential oils in therapy

While many may see essential oils as a 'fad', the reality is that there is medicinal science behind the use of essential oils derived from plants. Here are some facts as presented by the pioneer Jean Valnet MD (1990):

- Aromatic essences are volatile, oily, fragrant substances which are derived from plants via pressing, tapping, separation (using heat) and enfleurage (absorption of the grease and separation).
- Aromatic essences generally pre-exist in plants, and are soluble in alcohol, ether, and some are insoluble in water. Boiling points vary from 140–240°C.
- Egyptians prepared essence of cedarwood over 4000 years ago. Arabs distilled plants in the middle ages. In the 16th century, the perfume industry in Provence produced essences of lavender and aspic, which flourished in Montpelier, Narbonne and Grasse. In the 19th century came the first analyses (Valnet 1990: 26–28).

According to Valnet (1990), in spite of the research, phyto- and aromatherapy underwent a period of neglect and is now emerging as a science (Valnet 1990: 29). While I could elaborate more on the chemical and scientific benefits of pure essential oils and their application, it is important for the reader to know about the history and science of essential oils if planning to use them in your practice. I highly recommend reading Valnet's work – it is replete with stories and cases.

From my personal life, I am a firm believer. For example, one day, I stupidly grabbed something from a 375°F (190°C) oven without protection. I ran my hands under cold water, but then remembered one of Valnet's stories where in a laboratory accident he also burned his hands and placed them in a vat of lavender oils (distilling in his lab). I did the same thing – I placed Young Living's lavender essential oils on my terribly burnt hands. No burns, swelling or blisters formed.

I dipped into the subject further and read that frankincense oils (taken orally and topically) were suggested for cancer (Life Science Publishing 2018, and now there is also an app). I developed basal cell carcinoma on my nose before knowing about these oils. A Mohs surgeon removed the first round of cancer (requiring two passes to excise the cancer) and left a scar on my right dorsum nasi and ala area of my nose. When a second basal cell carcinoma appeared 6 months later in the same area but on my left dorsum nasi and ala area, I had by then read about the benefits of applying both frankincense and copaiba oils to eradicate cancer. I had to wait 2 months before I could get to the Mohs surgeon after my dermatologist's biopsy revealed the second carcinoma. I figured I would give it a try: every day, I applied both frankincense and copaiba oils topically to the fold of my dorsum nasi and ala as well as in the inside of my left nostril. When the surgeon went in for the first pass, like the time before, I had to wait an hour before the lab results were returned to let me know if he excised it all or had to go for a second pass.

Much to my surprise (and delight), when I went back into the surgical room, the doctor stated that he couldn't explain it, but the lab results yielded no cancer at all. I just smiled as he cauterized me and sent me home. With his blessing, I went swimming the next day. I tell you these anecdotes because they are true. And to this day, I use frankincense day and night on my face as a preventative.

The experiential component: the yoga and art process

I often turn to Valnet's work and the *Essential Oils Desk Reference* (Life Science Publishing 2018) and app to look up certain maladies and medical suggestions (both emotive and physical) for aromatic, topical and/or oral applications. While I welcome Western medicine's views, and embrace all scientific remedies, I also use medicinal plants (as Ayurvedic science recommends) as a natural mode for healing. I welcome it all.

Sequencing

Sequencing a class and/or a yoga therapy session is an important feature. As already discussed in the Introduction and Chapter 1, setting an intention establishes the directions for the practitioner and the patient(s). Intentions can be structural, energetic, emotionally and/or physically based. For example, let's suppose someone enters with the intention of relieving sciatica pain. Perhaps you could address this issue via the *kośas*: (1) *annamaya kośa* (physical), (2) *prānamaya kośa* (energy), (3) *manomaya kośa* (mind), (4) *vijnanamaya kośa* (intuition), and (5) *anandamaya kośa* (bliss).

You could establish the yogic tools for each of the aforementioned dimensions: (1) *asanas*, (2) breathwork/*prāṇayāma*, (3) text study/chant, (4) meditation, and/or (5) ritual, prayer.

In this case, based on the patient's sciatica and desire for relief, perhaps after establishing the intention, you might start with breathwork (*prānamaya kośa*, energy) and emphasize a continual connection to the selected breathwork during the movement in order to minimize the risk of injury. Your supporting elements might be breath awareness and visualization. But these need to course through the entire practice to support the intention.

In terms of visualization, threading the awareness of the physical element (lower back area) throughout the practice is key. For sciatica, Iyengar (1979) recommends starting in standing positions (in this case *samasthiti* or *tāḍāsana,* and like poses that lengthen the back, see Figure 3.5), followed by *supta pādāṅguṣṭhāsana* (most likely modified and using a yoga belt, Figure 3.11), and perhaps modified doing this supine with one leg crossed over the other, using props to support the overhanging leg (Figure 3.12). *Adho mukha śvānāsana* (downward facing dog) may need to be modified at the wall (see Figure 3.6) and if possible, a twist (*paripoorṇa matsyendrāsana*, Figure 3.13 and 3.14). Obviously, you would add appropriate warm-ups as needed for the patient or physical situation.

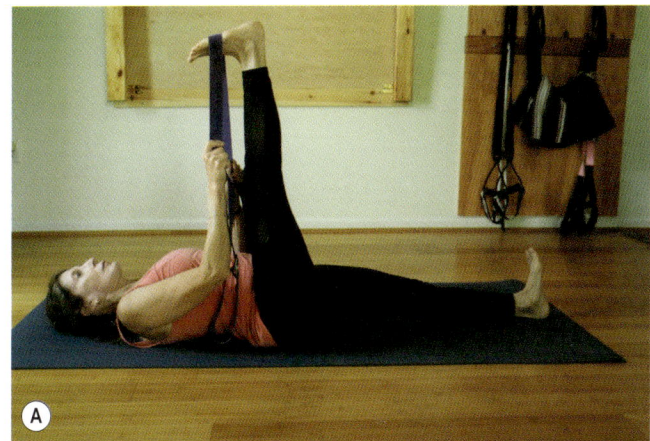

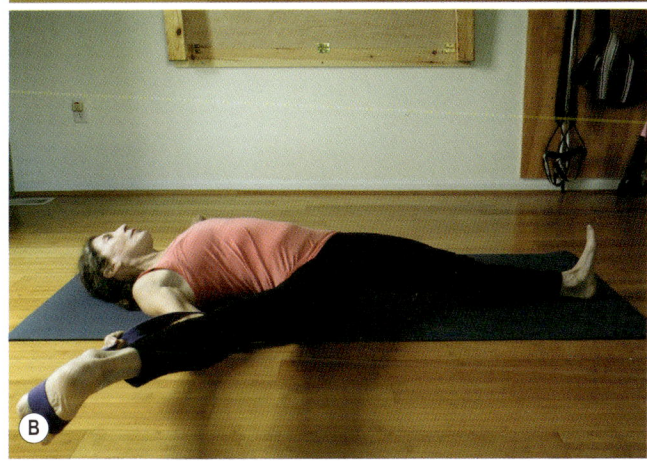

FIGURE 3.11 Author doing *supta pādāṅguṣṭhāsana* using the belt and to the side

Chapter three

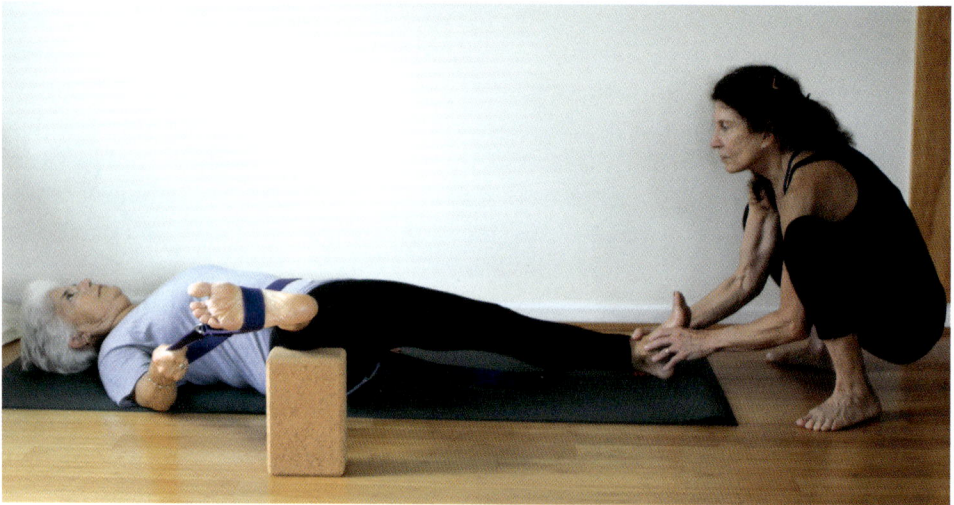

FIGURE 3.12 Author supporting student with a block doing *supta pādāṅguṣṭhāsana* to the side

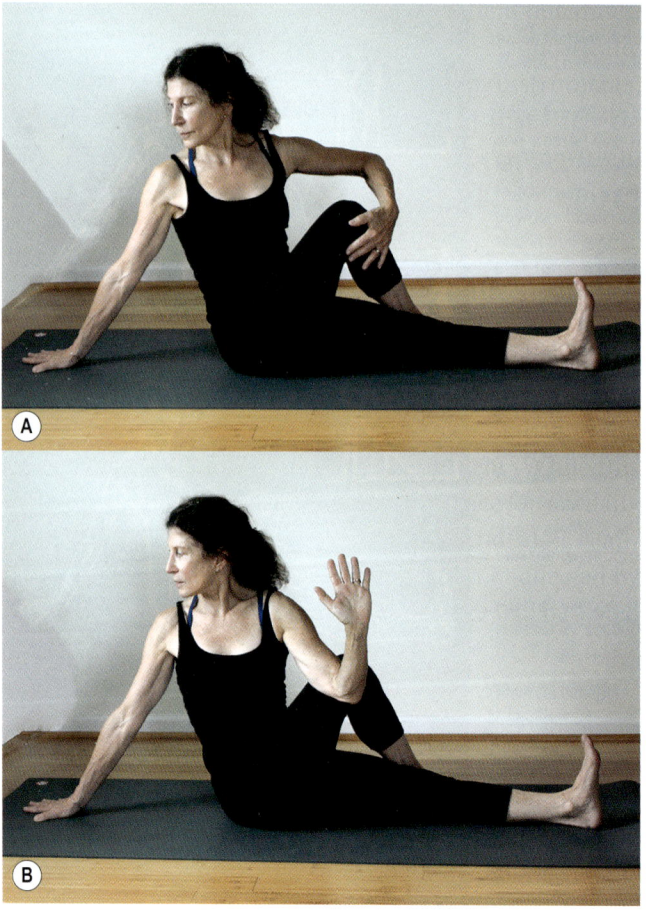

FIGURE 3.13 Author doing *paripoorṇa matsyendrāsana*, modified

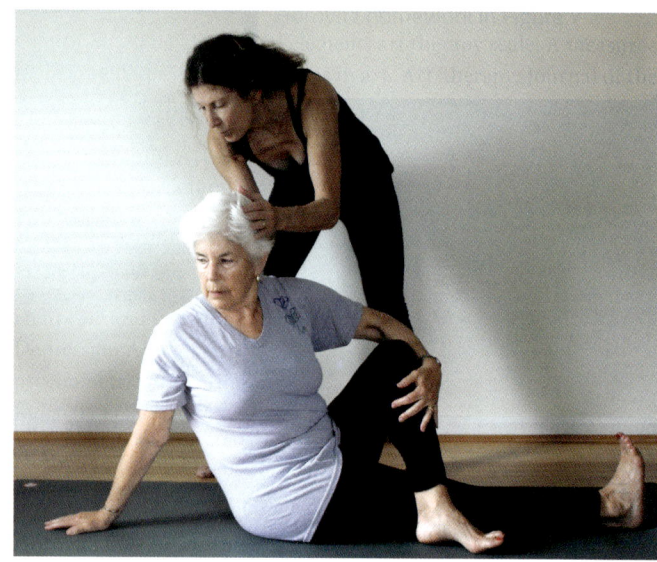

FIGURE 3.14 Author adjusting student in *paripoorṇa matsyendrāsana*, modified

Visual imagery to address mood management

In Horovitz (2017b) I addressed a wide range of media that can be used with varying patient populations, along with the benefits and contraindications for each. Just like in yoga, some materials may be inappropriate for a specific population. For example, when individuals are angry in a *rājasic* state, using clay can be calming and may offer

The experiential component: the yoga and art process

an instrument that allows the anger to be sublimated in a healthy, constructive manner. However, if working with inmates in a prison population, specific art materials are not allowed (e.g. clay, paint, scissors, etc). Specifically, David Gussak (1997) offers wonderful ideas on how to use art with this population. Years ago, I invited Dave to give a workshop on this subject to my graduate students. One of his exercises was to take a piece of white paper (9" x 12") and using only your hands, construct a 3-dimensional model. The results were stunning and required out-of-the-box thinking. In a facility when almost all materials are banned, the use of most art materials (as well as yoga belts, blocks and similar props) might not be allowed. It is for these reasons, that yoga and creative art therapists need to be resourceful in their work.

Case study 3.1

Let's look at some issues that might show up in your office or studio space. While Chapter 4 will go into specific clinical cases, we'll cover a few here. For starters, one of my patients presented with pressured speech (often referred to as verbal diarrhea), a history of panic attacks, and was riddled with anxiety. As discussed earlier, I needed to meet her mood, allowing for her constant chatter until some of this was literally expunged. After engaging in breathwork practice such as bellows breath (see Figure 3.7), we next moved to clay. The reason was multifold. She wanted to create items for her shrine, but in this instance, even if the clay is amply prepared and ready for use, I might instruct her to knead the clay, much like one does when kneading bread, although I always teach the Japanese spiraling method (Lin 2010) of kneading clay.

Even if this is all we do during the session and do not make an actual product, just the simple act of kneading the clay (via the Japanese spiraling method) produces a calming, meditative effect. This might be equivalent to restorative yoga poses, as the continual spiraling of the clay produces a meditative, medicinal effect (Figure 3.15).

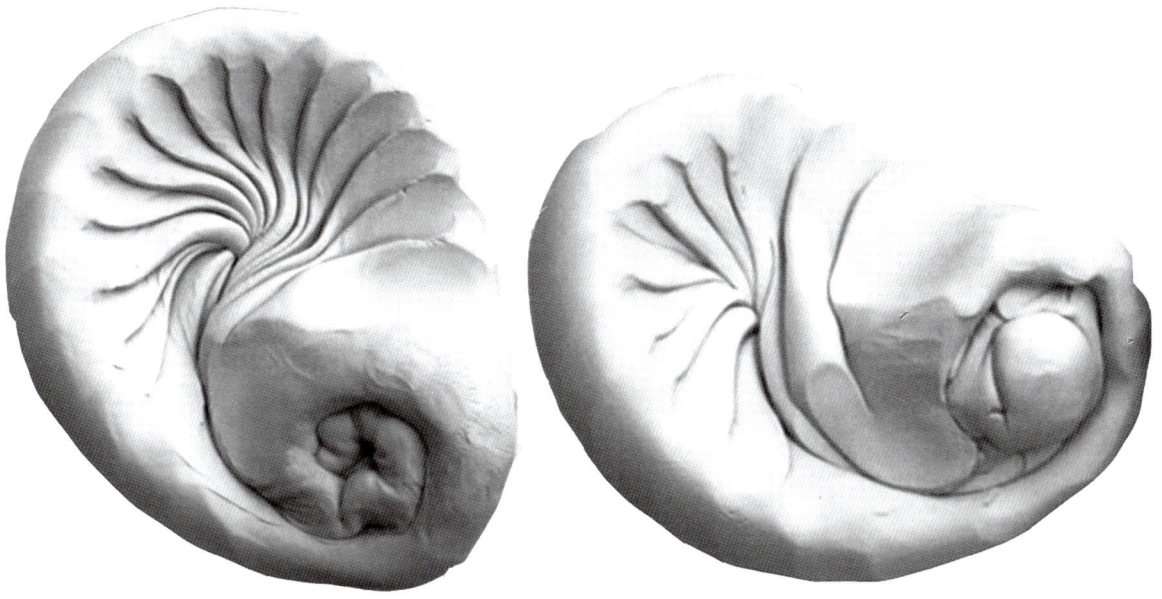

FIGURE 3.15 Kneaded clay, Japanese spiral method

Chapter three

Case study 3.2

Let's now look at a young woman, aged 26, who presented as meek, unimaginably shy and prone to bouts of agoraphobia (fear of being outside of her living environment). In this situation, because of her agoraphobia, there was a certain amount of desensitization required for her to travel to my office/studio space. I had previously reviewed her history form, so after sipping some tea and engaging in small talk, I suggested sitting on a yoga mat and trying coherent breath – breathing into the belly for 4 counts, holding the breath at the top of her lungs for 2 counts and then exhaling for 4–6 counts. After several minutes, this was built to a 6–2–8 ratio. Next, I suggested setting an intention (*sankālpa*) for her practice and sealed this by playing my singing bowl as she meditated on her intention. After she opened her eyes, she decided she wanted to use clay to purge (her *sankālpa*/intention) what she could not voice.

With a bit of prompting, she explained what she could not articulate. Using the clay she represented herself torn asunder, limbs broken in two places, eyes bugged out, no nose for breathing and instead, a hole for her mouth/breathing mechanism (Fig. 3.16). Note the lack of hands and feet, suggesting an inability to defend herself or exit her environment. Her ears were most pronounced, represented as if punched into a cauliflower shape. She explained the image represented her former Self and how she felt after being sexually and physically abused. Then, she collapsed into a sea of tears. Since this was the first admission of this history, omitted from the health forms she had filled out prior to this session, the confession

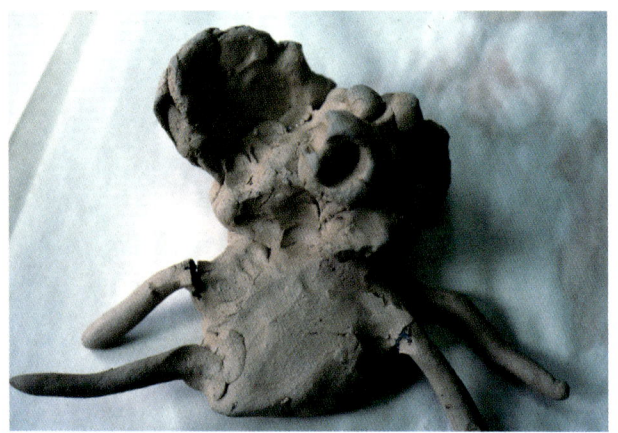

FIGURE 3.16 'The unspoken'

of such a painful and traumatic memory had to be handled delicately.

Oftentimes therapists are too quick to offer tissues to wipe away such painful memories. Welcoming tears (not pooh-poohing them) can be an uncomfortable experience for developing therapists. I just allowed her to sob and after a few minutes I asked her if she wanted me to hold her. To my amazement she sheepishly nodded her head yes. We both moved to the yoga mat and she placed her back onto my chest and then nestled into my arms. I enfolded her and gently held her as she cried and cried. This lasted into the final 10 minutes of the session. Nothing more was said about this incident during this session, but as Swami Kripalu says, 'One who cries knows yoga'. Given that this was our first meeting, it required much trust to allow for this kind of opening. In time, she was able to work through her past trauma.

The experiential component: the yoga and art process

Naturally, in both case studies I texted a recap of the session using my HIPAA-compliant cellphone software (SmartLine). Sometimes, the recap gives highlights of the session and other times it might include homework and/or suggestions for between sessions. If yoga was practiced during the session, I might also email that practice using Sequence Wiz so that there is a written rendition. I also conduct psychological assessments (via the BetterMind app) post-session and before the next meeting, to ascertain the efficacy of the session. Finally, I write up detailed notes for myself. I consider this my homework. Generally, a half-hour before the next session, I re-read these session notes and review the genogram information, so that I am present and prepared.

Basic art materials

Through image, a more common language than words, human beings return to the differentiated state where they work with essence to create healing. During this process of realizing the image and embodying it in the creation of art, we revisit who we are as Self, coming up different, healed, more integrated, recreated.

As you begin to turn your attention toward art materials and their use in the therapy session, it is important to note that when 'formed art' expression (Kramer 1993) occurs, something else happens to the viewer. It is a secondary gain, which I (and my dear, departed friend, Don Jones HLM) coined 'aesthetic arrest'. You may have experienced that feeling when (for example) you were struck by the incredible awe of a sunset, or a painting moved you beyond verbal expression, or a musical piece left you breathless. Such formidable experiences inform your humanity and in turn make you special.

Considerations

Hines (2016) stated, 'In considering the needs and goals of the participant and the setting, the therapist needs to be able to select the appropriate media for a session' (Hines 2016: 231). She also suggested that the therapist 'lead by example' (p.224). This is implicit when donning what Edith Kramer would call the 3-capped process. Kramer (1993) always talked about an art therapist being an artist, teacher, and therapist all at once. And this is exactly what Hines (2016) referred to when suggesting use of media. Hines also recommended involving 'breath awareness and biophysical feedback', to enhance skill-building (p.227). Long known as a Kramerian technique, you can see how Kramer uses breath awareness and the body to warm up the patient for spontaneous art making in her 2011 video (Kramer 2011). As Edith's graduate student in 1977, I witnessed this first-hand; but viewing the 'Mother of Art Therapy' in film should aid the reader's understanding of one way to involve breath awareness and inform biophysical feedback.

You need to start with the person. How does the patient strike you? Given your observation, I always suggest working with dry materials, especially for a first-time meeting. This is for the safety of both the therapist and the patient(s).

Physical parameters to consider

- Always start with dry materials when in doubt.
- Color can lead to affect (even colored pencils can induce affect).
- Wet materials can stimulate regression. While this may be desirable in some situations, when you first meet a patient, it is always best to proceed with dry materials (pencil, crayons, markers, etc.) and then eventually lead up to more regressive materials (pastels, tempera paints, oil pastels, clay, papier mâché and more advanced materials.

Observe important details like:

- motor dexterity, dependency needs
- tenseness, impulsivity, insecurities
- change of tempo, spontaneity of behavior/comments

Chapter three

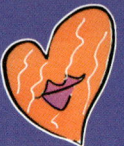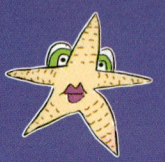

- detail of drawings/paintings or 3-D work.

It is also helpful to know the stages of age progression and normal artistic development in children, whether working with children, pre-pubescent, pubescent, adolescent, and/or adults (see Appendix C). In addition, gauge the following:

- pleasure from producing marks
- imitative and/or reproductive drawings
- learned phase of being able to copy art (not always acquired)
- graphic procedures based on design and balance.

In Horovitz (2017b) I cover all the specifics of studio applications from basic to advanced materials and the use of these materials. I also present these materials in relation to specific populations, with their benefits and contraindications. For a thorough review I refer the reader to that work. However, I will summarize some of the basic materials you might want to consider having in your office.

Basic compendium of art materials for your office

- Pencils of varying hardness (e.g. 6B, 5B, 4B, 3B, 2B, B, HB, F, H, 2H, 4H and 6H).
- Variety of colored pencils, perhaps some which can be used on fabric (e.g. Derwent's Inktense).
- Variety of different-sized paper, including construction paper, watercolor paper and even tissue paper.
- Scissors, blunt and pointed, both left- and right-handed.
- Glue, glue sticks, and a variety of craft supplies.
- Erasers, which can be used not just to remove lines, but create them. There are a variety of erasers on the market (for pencil, ink, charcoal and graphite).
- Crayons, bare minimum is the 8-color set containing red, orange, yellow, blue, green, violet, brown and black. You might also want to include oil crayons.
- Pastels and charcoal are very messy so be prepared for that. Also, they smudge easily, but can be 'set' with cheap hair spray!
- Markers, broad- and fine-tipped. You might also want to have water-soluble markers to protect clothing.
- Gel ink pens in a variety of colors.
- Collage materials are simple: you can recycle magazines, newspaper, even greeting cards for this type of expression. Some art therapists prefer to cut out images and words in advance based on the patients' issues. It is helpful to have pre-cut images of people, places, things and animals at the ready. Dr Rawley Silver (2002) was a great believer in this as she felt that searching for imagery sometimes led to distraction and incompletion of the work at hand.
- Watercolor paints or cake tempera are less messy than acrylic or oil paints.
- Plasticine (oil clay), which is durable and does not dry out if placed in plastic wrap or containers.
- Clay; you can purchase self-hardening clay if you don't have a kiln. After the self-hardening clay dries out, you can coat with a polyurethane finish so that it is durable.
- For both clay and plasticine it is a good idea to have on hand, the following tools: a large pieces of canvas duct-taped to a piece of plywood for the clay, rolling pins, needle tools (which can be made by piercing a wine cork with a needle), plastic knives or clay modeling tools, etc.
- Newspaper to protect table surfaces and allow for easy clean-up.
- Water in a container if you do not have access to a sink. A large empty gallon container can be filled with water and if you need to wash your hands, you can pour the water over your hands into a bucket and discard the dirty water later. I used this method for years before I had access to a sink! It also helps to have soap and moisturizer available.
- Last but not least, make sure you have smocks available to protect your patients' clothing as well as your own.

The experiential component: the yoga and art process

While this suggests the bare minimum of what you can provide, you may choose to only have dry materials in your office.

Digital software programs

Knowing the ABC of art materials should be a given for art therapists but reaching beyond the materials is a commitment to lifelong learning. Think of this as the continuing education credits that one should constantly acquire. It is no different from embracing the DSM-5 or the ICD-10 codes. It all matters. Therefore, I encourage the developing or seasoned art therapist to think of this section as a 'jumping off' point.

In my recent publications (Horovitz 2014, 2017a, 2017b, 2019a, 2019b) I have written about the app Paper53, since I had been presenting on its use for several years. With current technological advancements and ease of access to graphics and photography programs, any individual with a smartphone, tablet or laptop can now create remarkable artwork with the touch of a button. One can take an image created on a tablet using the Paper53 app and then send to a smart phone or computer for further manipulation using a number of other tools available. The final Paper53 image (Fig. 3.17) can be shared and posted to millions of users who can create yet another version of this original sketch. The same thing can be done with any digital image, and if you want to take that same image into software programs as I have done (Horovitz 2011), the possibilities are endless. But, to what end?

While these programs might be appealing for a variety of reasons, such as using such software in restrictive medical environments when conducting medical art therapy, the loss of honing fine and gross motor skills when working with materials such as real pencils, paint, cameras and indeed 3-dimensional materials are lost in this capacity. Still, one needs to add this to the tools that are out there. I have been using the Paper53 app, along with a stylus and my iPad tablet, in order to navigate medical situations that restrict 'traditional' media. Examples of where this technological tool could be employed are chemotherapy units, dialysis units and post-operative units (such as intensive

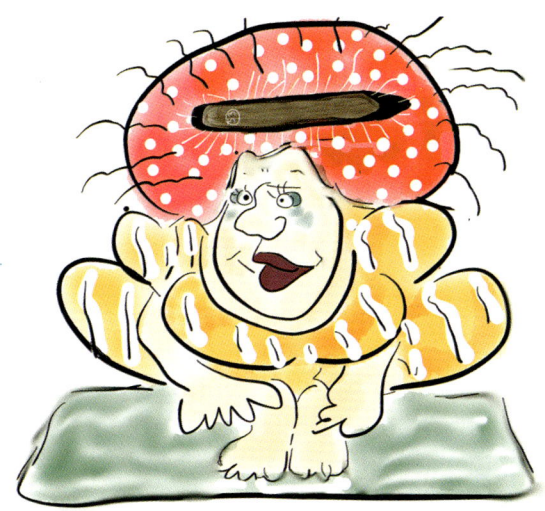

FIGURE 3.17 'Yoga artist', created by author in Paper 53 app

care units). The artwork distilled from such sessions can be output into a journal. Another less expensive option would be to create a screenshot from the image (which yields about 1Mb of information) and print the result onto 2- and 3-dimensional surfaces.

Ultimately such choices lie with the art therapist and I have presented on this at an American Art Therapy Conference (Horovitz 2018). There are good reasons for embracing both old and new technologies, but I urge the reader to be mindful of the reason why art therapy emerged in the first place. One can only imagine how my mentor, the great Edith Kramer, would frown upon such electronic options. Technology both advances and distances us from our roots. And therein lies the rub. Personally, I embrace it all.

I feel the need to be open to digital applications such as Paper53, Genogram Analytics, BetterMind and other such tools since they offer the practitioner a wider base of materials from which to operate. Also, populations more comfortable working with digital platforms need to be accommodated. Rick Garner (2016) also published on the use of digital methods, materials and applications and their use in art therapy. I would highly recommend that the reader peruse his work. If you are not comfortable

Chapter three

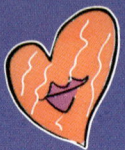 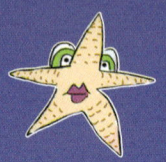

with digital platforms, educate yourself. YouTube abounds with tutorials, and there are many other skill development websites (e.g. https://www.lynda.com) and other venues for learning.

Reflection exercise 3.3

Challenge yourself. Learn a new digital software program or application (app) with which you are unfamiliar. After you have achieved a modicum of success with this, create a few different images and imagine how you might use this process with patients, especially those that (for either emotive and/or medical reasons) do not respond to or cannot use traditional art materials. Compare these two different states, that is the one fabricated in a digital format/program and the one created with actual physical properties. Which did you enjoy more? Was this based on experience and/or the material?

Note how different you felt using a 3-dimensional material (e.g. papier mâché, plasticine or clay) versus a digital app or software program. Observe the differences via fine and gross motor skills, not just physically but also emotionally. Did they engage you the same or differently? Did either offer you a greater 'flow' experience and why do you think that occurred for you? Remember, this may be different for everyone.

Finally, journal about this and contemplate when and how you might operate in a digital format versus physical art materials.

Journaling and the art

Reflective exercise 3.3 brings me to the subject of journaling and art making. Whenever I open a new case, in addition to gathering psychosocial information, at intake I offer the patient a gift of a journal, whether they decide to entertain art therapy, yoga therapy, psychotherapy or all three. The reasons are multifold, and will be explored in the case studies.

Case studies

In a recent family session with a 6-year-old child, I instructed the mother and the child to work on the journal outside of our therapy session. In this instance, I suggested that they bring the journal to the next session. This led to new information regarding the child's willful manipulation and refusal to respond to appropriate parental demands. As a result, we were able to incorporate this into the next session along with yoga therapy. Additionally, the child used the journal to draw images that she could not readily articulate.

I also have used journals and artmaking with adults. In one instance, an identified patient, 'W', was struggling with the issue that her sister's best friend and daughter had moved into her parental home while she had been away at college. While this was part of the urgency that led her into therapy, she had a very complicated medical history (which included kidney reflux from the age of 6 months to 9 years old, resulting in trauma and multiple catheters, eating disorders, recovering addiction and then some). The medical trauma squarely placed her into the category of post-traumatic stress disorder (PTSD) with co-morbid issues. Figure 3.18 gives a fuller picture of the identified patient (IP). (This case is discussed further in Chapter 6, Case study 2.)

This IP decided to bring in a poem (which she transcribed into her journal) from a book that she was reading, *Milk And Honey* (Kaur 2015). As I was unfamiliar with the book, after our session I considered it my homework to familiarize myself with it. I went online and read a large portion. Because of the poem she selected, I texted her the following as part of the recap of our session: 'Try and write your own poem out of these three sentences: Just Bloom; Stay strong through your pain; Grow flowers out of mine. Don't censor anything, just write. Send or bring to your next session.' The lines were from *Milk And Honey*.

The experiential component: the yoga and art process

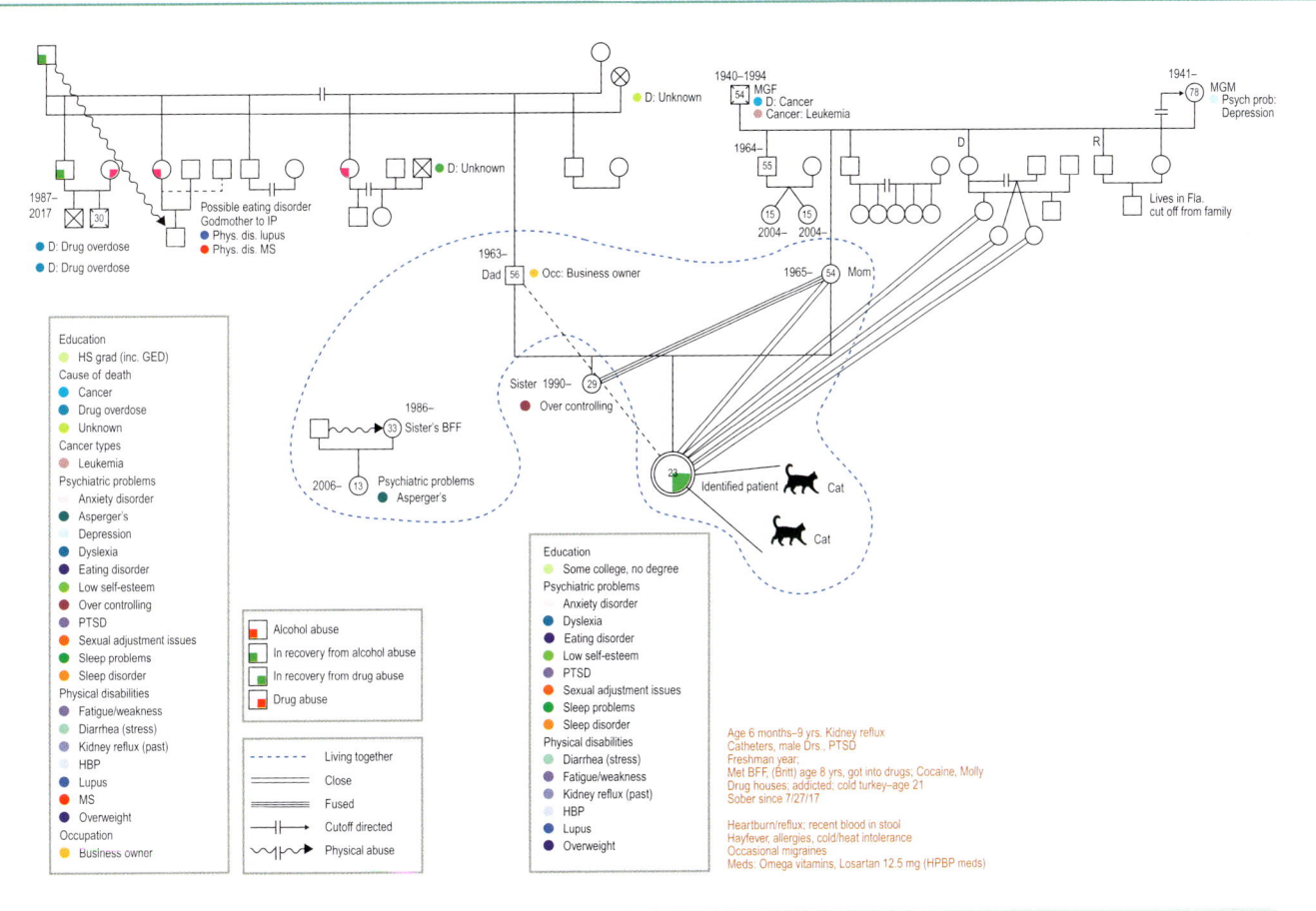

FIGURE 3.18 Identified patient genogram

This is what she wrote and shared at our next session:

Stay strong through your pain. Grow flowers from it. You have helped me grow flowers out of mine, so just bloom beautifully,
dangerously,
loudly, softly bloom.

This led to a written exercise during our next session. After reviewing her homework and her feelings around the journal exercise, I suggested that she pick three random index cards from a pile. I had previously cut up lines from printed matter that I thought might pertain to her issues. The idea presented was to incorporate the three lines into a poem as often (or as little) as she wished. She chose the cards to the right (Fig. 3.19) and to make her more comfortable during the writing process, I chose three index cards at random (mine are on the left). Both of us created a poem from our selected words.

Her poem:

In between mistakes,
I grew
And the results are so encouraging.
I grew,
I grew,
And I grew.
A first failure was too close for me
But I yelled fuck you
Loud from the rooftops
And continued to grow.

Chapter three

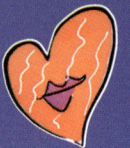 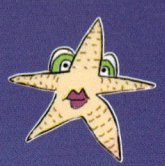

FIGURE 3.19 Index card exercise. The author's selected cards (left) and patient's selected cards (right)

Because she liked my poem, I gave it to her:

Those aren't clouds, God's tongue moves. Over and over it repeats the same message, 'Do you know your own soul?' Those aren't clouds, God's tongue moves. Again, and again, the same refrain repeats, 'But it had the right attitude'. Those aren't clouds, God's tongue moves.

Pre-session her Depression, Anxiety, Stress Scale short-form (DASS-21) results, relative to the sample population, placed her in the moderate range for depression, extremely severe range for anxiety and the severe range for stress. Post-session relative to the sample population, her results were mild range for depression, mild range for anxiety and mild range for stress. This suggests that the journaling exercise led to improved mood. This case is presented in greater depth in Chapter 6.

Importance of recapping/assigning homework to increase emotional and physical regulation

As stated previously, assigning homework, such as journaling, making art, breath (*prāṇayāma*) exercises, meditation, yoga postures (*asāna*) and similar activities (including assigned readings or the like) can lead to emotional and physical regulation. For example, the IP in the previous case study who engaged in the journaling exercise received this following recap based on both the psychotherapy and art therapy (poetry exercise) conducted during a sequential session.

Recap:

1. When you come home from work, try not to feed the negativity between you and your parents: eat, do whatever you need and then retreat to your cave (room) ignoring the 'boarders'. Maybe watch your favorite television show, read, do yoga, or make art!

2. Try and journal more to rid yourself of your anger and frustration with your sister's best friend and her daughter. Remember, harboring this anger gives your power to others. Instead, find creative ways to release your rage other than slamming doors and being negative towards your parents. Take a walk, stroke your cats (animals can be soothing to the soul), watch your favorite shows, clean the shower so you can own the space and have privacy. Wake up earlier so you have the power over that downstairs bathroom as opposed to your sister's BFF who hogs the bathroom.

3. Think about what you want from a session with your parents. Do you want to include your sister? Might that be to your advantage?

4. Finally, try and exercise more; the more you exercise, the less you will ruminate!

5. Hang in there and if it gets tense, TEXT me!

The experiential component: the yoga and art process

For the next session, the IP was finally ready to invite her parents. Her mother had been reticent about therapy since a previous therapist had blamed the mother for all the IP's anxieties, trauma and psycho-emotional issues. During this session, the parents surprised the IP by informing her that her sister's BFF and daughter were moving out that weekend. Joy of joy, the IP no longer had to share her house or her parents' attention – she was thrilled. Still, there were lots of issues that arose during the therapy session.

Both parents agreed they would never repeat offering their home to strangers again. They also mentioned that they did this for the IP and not just her sister. This put a different spin on the issue since the IP's former BFF, who had initiated her into drugs, had previously moved in for a year or so… so the parents had done this twice! 'Never again,' they both refrained.

When the IP became upset and cried during the session, it also became clear that they didn't hug as a family, and apparently that was part of the problem. The IP exhibited anxiety during the session by biting her fingernails. I pointed this out repeatedly during the family session.

The mother admitted that when the IP became angry with her, it 'pushed her buttons', and reminded her of her own mother (MGM) and how she was treated growing up.

As a result, an art therapy assignment was suggested for all to create a door from paper (or cardstock) and on the outside place what feelings they share. On the inside, they were instructed to place what they didn't readily share. All were able to express their feelings through the door assignment. The IP's overarching theme was that she 'didn't feel validated'. Her mother made a cloud inside to represent 'the boarders' and the tension that all three of them had endured. The father's image was just a door with hinges and a lock – nothing was inside because he 'didn't share (his) feelings'. I wanted to address how hard that must have been for him, but I didn't think the time was right to do that, so I just let what he said fill the room. He then began to tear up and said how heartbreaking it was to watch the IP writhe in pain (from age 6 months to 9 years) because he was unable to comfort her and/or prevent that from occurring. I acknowledged how difficult that must have been (not being able to help his child when she was ill and enduring a painful, medical procedure). I also pointed out to the father that he may have bonded with the young boarder (the 13-year-old) perhaps because he identified with her background of past verbal and physical abuse. During the session the IP cried and I suggested that she extract a hug from each of her parents, since no one moved to comfort her.

At the end I suggested that all of them try and hug daily, and in the evening, and/or plant a kiss on top of each other's head (their family modus operandi). It was a very moving session for all. They decided to celebrate by going out for ice cream post-session. This was the recap I sent the IP post session.

Recap:

1. Well the good news is that the boarders are leaving! Wish granted for all concerned. And it seems your parents, too, will be relieved. You heard their words, 'Never again!'.

2. I hope that tonight gave you some perspective on how your family operates: your father doesn't 'share his insides'. Your mother's buttons get pushed when you get angry with her (read: her mother, your grandmother), and you need to feel 'validated'.

3. Is it also possible that some of your anger may be connected to what happened to you as a child? Even though, intellectually, you understand what your parents had to put you through, you may have viewed this (when you were really young) as abandonment, that is before you had WORDS for this. Your medical procedure was traumatizing; but you can heal. We will work on that.

4. Remember your prescription: hug or kiss daily and nightly – ALL THREE OF YOU!

Chapter three

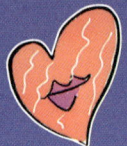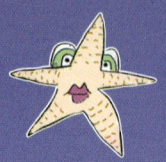

5. Finally, try and share your feelings when you get angry. Your parents really love you. Help them by sharing how *you are feeling* when you become angry.

Additionally, post our sessions, I send my patients psychological tests from the BetterMind app. This allows me to ascertain the efficacy of each session – what has worked and what has not. I also encourage my patients to stay in touch (if they wish) in between our sessions. While some therapists might see this as intrusive and/or an unnecessary burden to their workloads, I consider it part of the therapeutic contract. I do not charge for phone calls (unless they are excessive) and/or texting. I have committed to helping my patients both in and out of the therapeutic time we are in session.

A psychiatrist colleague of mine and I were discussing our caseloads and when she learned how I worked, she exclaimed, 'You must be busy!'. I am, but it is my choice to work this way. While you might not choose to operate in this manner, I am presenting this as my method of working with my patients.

Reflection exercise 3.4

Think of an issue that might be problematic for you. Create a door by either folding the two sides of a piece of paper, cardboard, or cardstock towards the midline. On the outside scribe or draw how you present this issue and your feelings to the outside world. On the inside, place what you don't share with others. Sit with this image and meditate on its significance in your life. Then decide which of the seven chakras this is attached to and meditate on that chakra in order to clear the space. When you are done, journal whatever bubbles up from that place.

Figure 3.20 is a sample created by artist Lyssa Lovejoy (http://www.instapuma.com/drunkinartist) during one of my workshops.

Mandalas and coloring to reduce anxiety

Mandalas have been proven to reduce rumination and anxieties along with adult coloring books, hence the mass profusion of these ideas on the market. By coloring symmetrical and repetitive patterns in a circular shape, the individual focuses on the mandala, allowing for detachment from their negative thoughts and emotions (Chambala 2008, Curry and Kasser 2005, Jung 1972, Sandmire et al 2012). Coloring books provide similar focus and also reduce anxiety in the user (Eaton and Tieber 2017).

In workshops that I have conducted, I have suggested that people create mandalas to reflect how they are feeling.

Nota Bene

Drawing a mandala is also the first step mentioned in the MARI (Mandala Art Research Instrument, Kellogg 1984).

When conducting these yoga and art therapy workshops, creating a mandala is generally part of an opening exercise that might inform the entire day's practice. Generally, I might suggest breathwork/*prāṇayāma*, an *asāna* and/or meditation before beginning the artwork. Then remaining silent, I suggest creating a mandala to reflect that expression through the art.

While multiple platonic solids and sacred geometry coloring books exist that offer prescriptive versions of mandalas, it is always preferable when the artwork comes from within. Figure 3.21 is an example of two participants' response to breathwork/*prāṇayāma* and *aśanā* practice during a 2-day yoga and art therapy workshop that I conducted in New York City. Sometimes, the result can be two or three dimensional as in the case of these two incredible creative art therapists, Yuko Otomo and Yasushi Kenny Iwata.

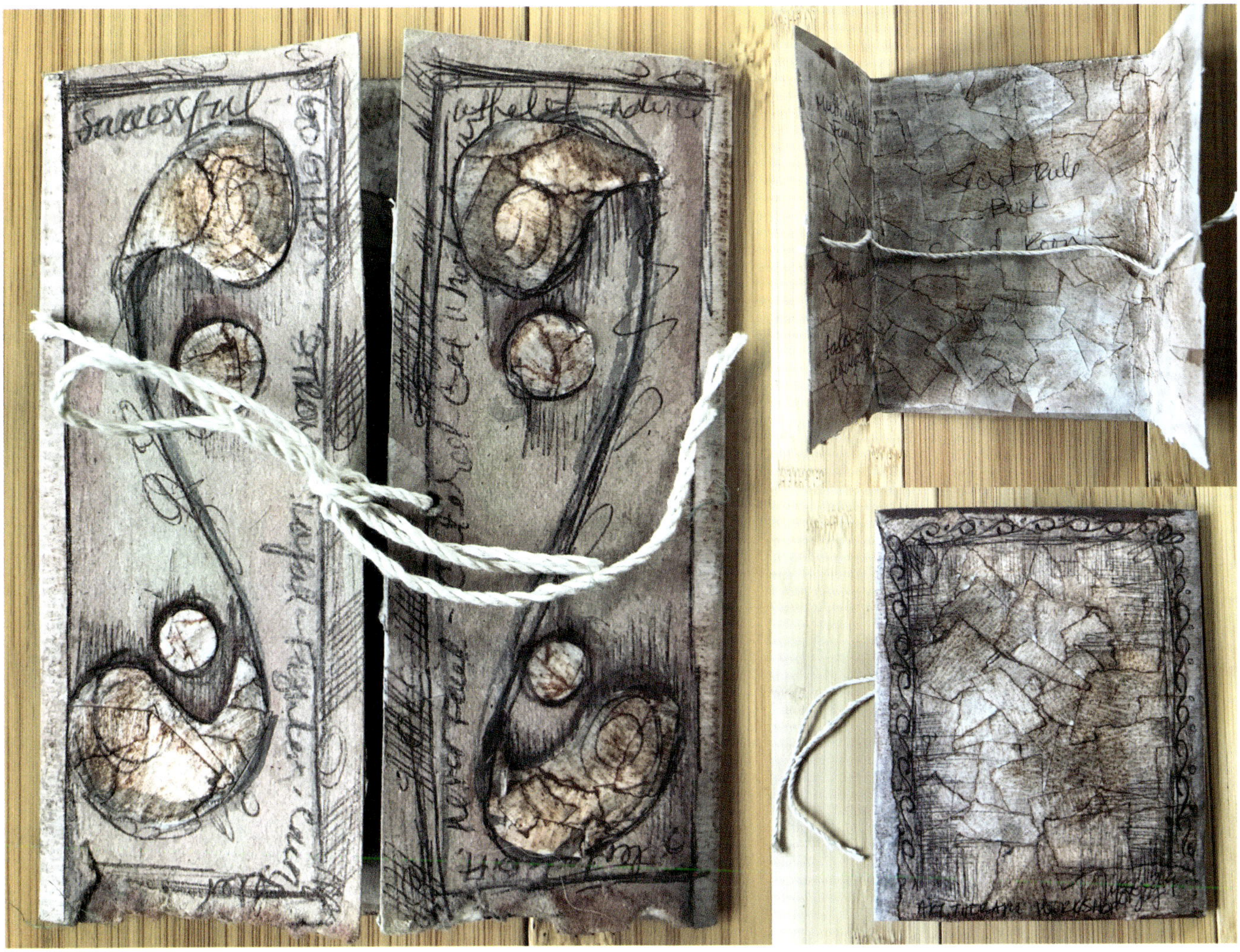

The experiential component: the yoga and art process

FIGURE 3.20 'Sacred Room' by Lyssa Lovejoy (on the left is the front door, upper right is inside, lower right is the back of the door)

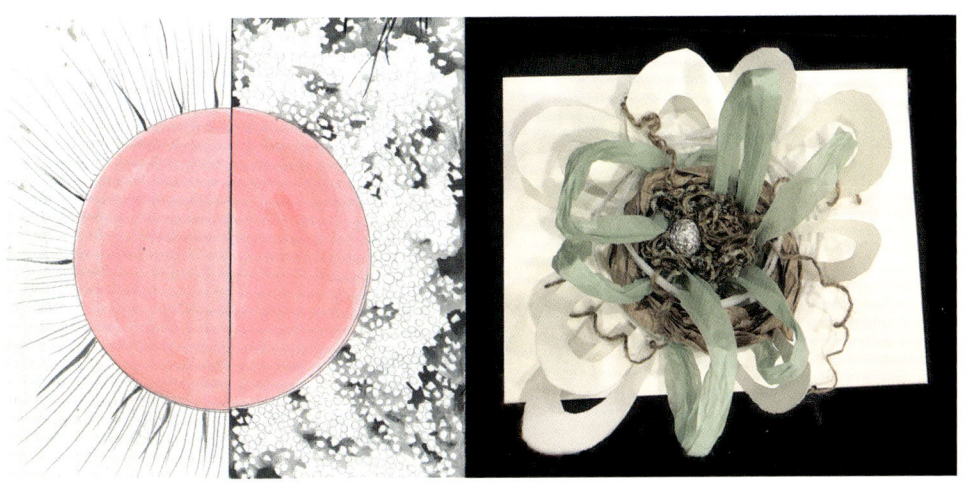

FIGURE 3.21 Mandalas by artists Yuko Otomo and Yasushi Kenny Iwata respectively

Chapter three

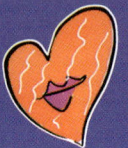
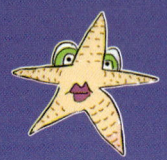

So, try this for yourself by first meditating, conducting some breathwork/*prāṇayāma* and then moving into an *āsanā*. See what bubbles up for you and then you will be prepared to do this with your patients. Remember: the artwork is not product-oriented but process-oriented, so try not to censor the outcome. Welcome it all.

Texting and telehealth: importance of HIPAA-compliant software

All of this brings me to an important subject: using HIPPA-compliant software for texting, telehealth sessions, faxing and similar tasks. As of this writing Dr Amy Wheeler, current President of the International Association of Yoga Therapists, has launched a new software program called Zmaaya, billed as, 'a software solution that helps standardize client documentation, assessment and management' (https://www.iayt.org/page/Zmaaya). This HIPPA-compliant software program currently offers the following features:

- customized electronic intake form that is sent securely to your client
- SOAP notes and outcome measures across all sessions
- detailed assessment
- comprehensive and flexible management plans
- client dashboard
- therapist dashboard
- link to Google calendar to view appointments in one place
- management plan data by Dr Wheeler available only in 'Zmaaya Yoga Therapy'.

There are other HIPPA-compliant software programs available from various vendors that include numerous features at varying prices. My recommendation is to shop around and see what works best for your practice. There are sites that do side-by-side comparisons of different HIPAA-compliant software programs, which is essential when choosing a telehealth site. To date, Capterra is one of the sites that I have visited to make these decisions for myself (https://www.capterra.com/).

I have serviced my patients via telehealth for well over 4 years. This is extremely helpful when patients (and/or family members) are at a distance. In several instances I have used telehealth sites exclusively to conduct therapy and also in between sessions if a patient is ill or traveling for a work-related endeavor.

Nota Bene

Skype and FaceTime are not HIPAA compliant.

I have also conducted yoga therapy at a distance using a telehealth format. While telehealth sessions are certainly not my preference, I offer these services to my patients when they need to travel for business, are recovering from surgery or illness, or have relatives at a distance (see Chapters 4, 5 and 6).

I also use a separate HIPAA-compliant telephone app (SmartLine) through my domain provider (GoDaddy.com). SmartLine operates as a second, completely separate number for patient interaction on my cell phone. SmartLine records voicemails if I miss a call, alerts me if I miss a text, and allows me to text my patients (for recaps, etc.) and send images. Since it is a separate number, if I receive a 'cold call' for my services, the line is identified as, 'Ellen Horovitz, work'. This is a very convenient way to separate your personal cell number from your business cell number. As a sole practitioner, SmartLine is enough for my needs but there are other software programs available for practices that have multiple partners/users. Embodiaapp.com is also recommended.

Finally, I have not had a landline for almost 20 years. The MetroFax app allows me to fax important documents via my computer, iPhone or iPad. Having this software allows me to operate electronically guided by HIPAA-compliant documentation.

The world is ever-changing and given consumer interest, my way of operating as a therapist has continued to evolve and change over time so that I can better serve

The experiential component: the yoga and art process

my patients and their needs. While I still feel that face-to-face is the most optimal method of treating patients, sometimes this is not always possible. Having these kinds of programs (Genogram Analytics, Sequence Wiz, SmartLine, MetroFax, EmbodiaApp, and telehealth sites, etc.) at my disposable is a God-send for me and for my patients.

Next, let's put this altogether by looking at some in-depth clinical cases in Chapter 4.

References

Arora S and Bhattacharjee J (2008) Modulation of immune response in stress by yoga. International Journal of Yoga 1: 45–55.

Brody JE (2018) Preventing muscle loss as we age. New York Times (3 September). Available at: https://www.nytimes.com/2018/09/03/well/live/preventing-muscle-loss-among-the-elderly.html.

Bronfenbrenner U (1994) Ecological model of human development. In: Husen T and Postlethwaite N (eds) International Encyclopedia of Education Vol. 3, 2nd Edn. Oxford, UK: Elsevier.

Brown KD, Koziol JA and Otz M (2008) A yoga-based exercise program to reduce the risk of falls in seniors: a pilot and feasibility study. Journal of Alternative and Complementary Medicine 14(5): 454–457.

Bryant E (2009) The Yoga Sutras of Patañjali: A new edition, translation, and commentary. New York, NY: North Point Press.

Carbonetti J (2001) Making Pearls: Living the Creative Life. New York: Watson-Guptill Publications.

Chambala A (2008) Anxiety and art therapy. Art Therapy 25(4): 187–189.

Colangelo J (2003) Embodied Wisdom: What Our Anatomy Can Teach Us About the Art of Living. Lincoln, NE: iUniverse Inc.

Csikszentmihalyi M (2008) The Flow: The Psychology of Optimal Experience. New York, NY: Harper Collins.

Curry NA and Kasser T (2005) Can coloring mandalas reduce anxiety? Art Therapy 22(2): 81–85.

Desikachar K, Bragdon L, and Bossart C (2005) The yoga of healing: exploring yoga's holistic model for health and well-being. International Journal of Yoga Therapy 15: 17–39.

Eaton J and Tieber C (2017) The effects of coloring on anxiety, mood and perseverance. Art Therapy 34(1): 42–46.

Garner R (2016) Digital Art Therapy: Materials, Methods and Applications. Philadelphia, PA: Jessica Kingsley Publishers.

Garner G (2018) Medical Therapeutic Yoga: Biopsychosocial Rehabilitation and Wellness Care. Edinburgh, UK: Handspring.

Gussak D (1997) Drawing Time: Art Therapy in Prisons and Other Correctional Settings. New York, NY: Magnolia Press.

Held LI (2009) Quirks of Human Anatomy: An Evo-devo Look at the Human Body. Cambridge, UK: Cambridge University Press.

Hines L (2016) Media considerations in art therapy: directions for future research. In: Gussak DE and Rosal ML (eds) The Wiley Handbook of Art Therapy. Malden, MA: John Wiley & Sons, Ltd.

Horovitz EG (1999) A Leap of Faith: The Call to Art. Springfield: IL: Charles C Thomas Ltd.

Horovitz EG (2005) Art Therapy as Witness: A Sacred Guide. Springfield, IL: Charles C Thomas Ltd.

Horovitz EG (2011) Digital Image Transfer: Creating Art With Your Photography. Ashville, NC: Lark Books Inc.

Horovitz EG (ed) (2014) The Art Therapists' Primer: A Clinical Guide to Writing Assessment, diagnosis, and Treatment, 2nd Edn. Springfield, IL: Charles C Thomas Ltd.

Horovitz EG (2017a) Spiritual Art Therapy: An Alternate Path, 3rd Edn. Springfield, IL: Charles C Thomas Ltd.

Horovitz EG (2017b) The Guide to Art Therapy Materials and Methods: A Practical, Step-by-step Approach. New York, NY: Routledge Press.

Horovitz EG (2018) Evidence based practice: legal issues and digital apps. American Art Therapy Association, 49th Annual Conference. Miami, 2 November 2018. Alexandria, VA: American Art Therapy Association.

Horovitz EG (2019a) Efficacy, apps and telehealth: treatment and ethical issues for a digital age. In: Di Maria A (ed) Exploring Ethical Dilemmas in Art Therapy. New York, NY: Routledge.

Horovitz EG (2019b) Foreword. In: Brooke SL (ed) Combining the Creative Therapies with Technology: Using Social Media and Online. Springfield, IL: Charles C Thomas Ltd.

Iyengar BKS (1979) Light On Yoga. New York, NY: Schocken Books.

Iyengar BKS (2005) Light On Life: The Yoga Journey to Ultimate Wholeness, Inner Peace and Ultimate Freedom. Emmaus, PA: Rodale press.

Jung C (1972) Mandala Symbolism. Princeton, NJ: Princeton University Press.

Kaur R (2015) Milk And Honey. Kansas City, MO: Andrews McMeel Publishing.

Chapter three

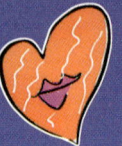
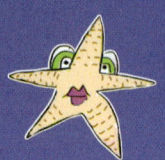

Kellogg J (1984) Mandala: Path of Beauty. Towson, MD: Mandala Assessment and Research Institute.

Kondo M (2014) The Life Changing Magic of Tidying Up: The Japanese Art of Decluttering and Organizing. Berkeley, CA: Ten Speed Press.

Kramer E (1977a) Personal communication.

Kramer E (1977b) Art Therapy in a Children' Community. New York, NY: Schocken Books.

Kramer E (1979) Childhood and Art Therapy: Notes in Theory and Application. New York: Schocken Books.

Kramer E (1993) Art as Therapy with Children, 2nd Edn. New York, NY: Schocken Books.

Kramer E (2011) Edith Kramer: Art tells the truth (video). Available at: https://vimeo.com/33476299.

Laskowski ER (2018) What are the risks of sitting too much? Mayo Clinic FAQs. Available https://www.mayoclinic.org/healthy-lifestyle/adult-health/expert-answers/sitting/faq-20058005.

Life Science Publishing (2018) Essential Oils Desk Reference, 7th Edn. Lehi, UT: Life Science Publishing.

Lin H-C 2010 Learning Spiral Wedging / Kneading Clay, video. Available https://www.youtube.com/watch?v=vj6Kd8RSmVY.

Mason H and Birch K (eds) (2018) Yoga for Mental Health. Edinburgh, UK: Handspring.

McCall T (2018) Foreword. In: Yoga for Mental Health. Edinburgh, UK: Handspring (pp. xi–xii).

McNiff S (1995) Earth Angels: Engaging the Sacred in Everyday Things. Boston, MA: Shambhala Publications Inc.

Raman K (1998). A Matter of Health: Integration of Yoga and Western Medicine for Prevention and Care. Indira Nagar, Chennai, India: EastWest Books Ltd.

Reynolds G (2019, July 24) How weight training changes the brain. New York Times. Available https://www.nytimes.com/2019/07/24/well/move/how-weight-training-changes-the-brain.html.

Sandmire DA, Gorham SR, Rankin NE and Grimm DR (2012) The influence of art making on anxiety: A pilot study. Art Therapy 29(2): 68–73.

Shifroni E (2014) A Chair For Yoga: A Complete Guide to Iyengar Yoga Practice With a Chair, 2nd Edn. Scotts Valley, CA: CreateSpace Independent Publishing.

Silver R (2002) The Three Art Assessments. New York, NY: Routledge.

Streeter C, Gerbarg P, Saper R, Ciraulo D and Brown R (2012) The effects of yoga on the autonomic nervous system, gamma-aminobutyric-acid, and allostasis in epilepsy, depression and post-traumatic stress disorder. Medical Hypotheses 78(5): 571–579.

Ulman R and Dachinger P (eds) (1976). Art Therapy in Theory and Practice. New York, NY: Magnolia Press.

Valnet J (1990) The Practice of Aromatherapy: A Classic Compendium of Plant Medicines and Their Healing Properties. Rochester, VT: Healing Arts Press.

Weintraub A (2012) Yoga Skills for Therapists: Effective Practices for Mood Management. New York, NY: Norton.

Clinical cases: children 4

Grace is how you look, when no one is looking.

Mae Thompson

You just can't make this stuff up. The cases that I will cover herein represent just a smattering of the people that I have worked with over my 40 (plus!) year career. The last 16 years included yoga therapy with individuals, couples, and families. Let's begin to look at some fascinating and challenging cases. Just as I have presented in the previous chapters, in addition to the presented clinical material, I will present suggestions for the reader.

Working with children and family systems

In this first case below, as in all cases where a child is involved, I request an intake appointment with the parental caretaker without the child/children present. There are a number of reasons for this request, some of which are connected to the adult caretaker's ability to attend to the posed questions and respond without the identified child (or children) present. And while this was my request for Case Study 1, the mother arrived with all four children in tow, thus precluding that ability. Also, all four children were interruptive and often wanted to present their information. While there is always time for that, having the parent's rendition to start is paramount, especially if the identified patient has severe mental health issues, as was the case here. While the patient 'T' had not been diagnosed as bipolar by his psychiatrist, in the end, his psychiatrist concurred with my findings.

Case study 1

Bipolar 11-year-old male ('T') and his mother

Background and history

As can be seen by T's genogram (Fig. 4.1), this is a very complicated case. In sum, T and his brother ('A') were the product of a lesbian couple ('R' and 'B') and two different sperm-bank donors. Mom R was the carrier of both T and A. While T presented no abnormal history prior to 5 years of age, it was then that the situation got squirrely.

As a healthcare professional, R was working with the family system of 'D'. D was the biological mother of seven children, including 'C', 'P', and 'S', all from different fathers. D had abandoned all seven children to a homeless shelter. R witnessed the homeless shelter care worker favoring C and purposely starving P, such that P weighed only 12.24 kg. As a result, she and her partner B decided to adopt not just 5-year-old P (when T was also 5 years old) but also P's younger sister S, then 4 months old. While both R and B's motives may have been noble, T witnessed C's mental hygiene arrest (MHA) at the age of 5, while C was visiting his home. That and the recent adoption of P (same age as T) and S (age 4 months) resulted in major complications. T became suicidal, threatened to cut off his testicles with a knife, and was hospitalized for suicidal ideation and this action.

Chapter four

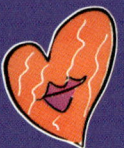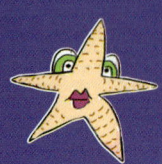

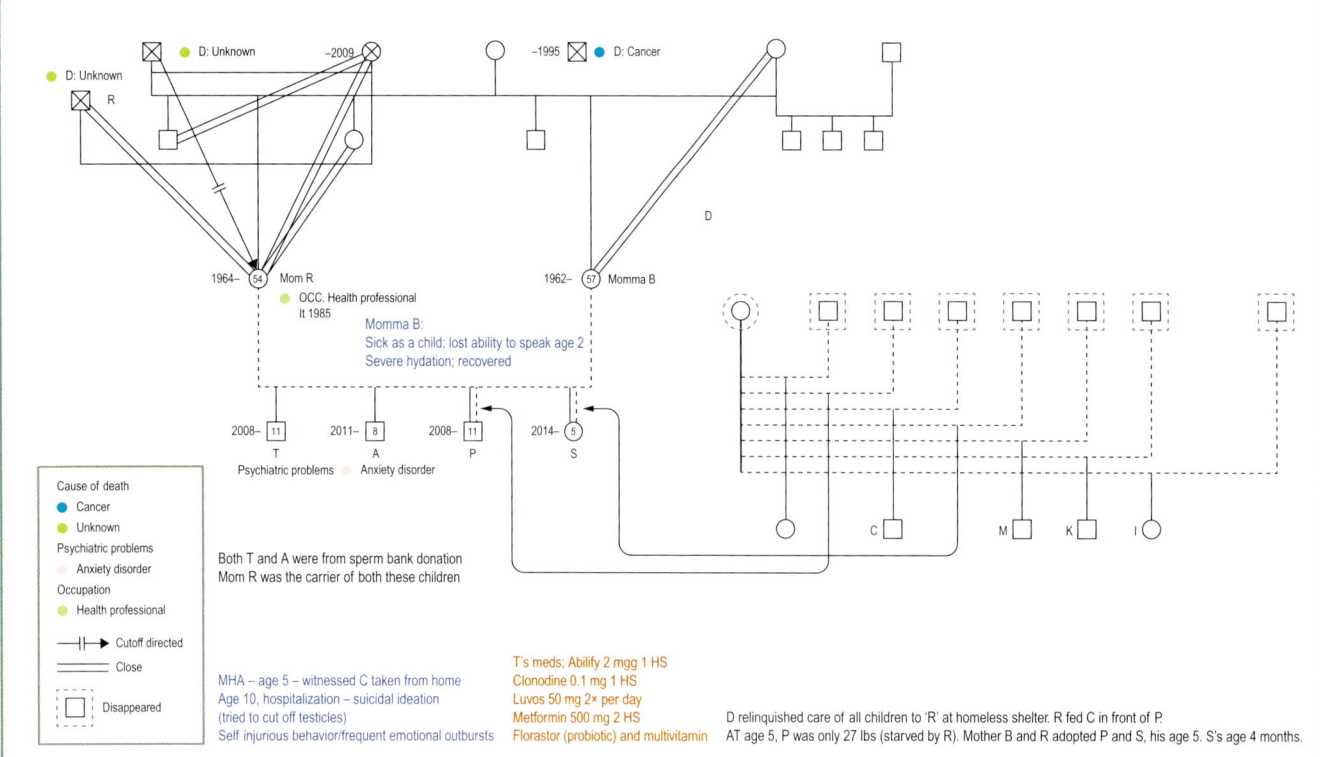

FIGURE 4.1 T's genogram

There were 16 sessions with T, mostly with R, but T's younger adoptive sister S joined for two sessions.

Significant sessions

Session 1 and 2

The first time that T arrived at session with R, he was screaming so loudly that students in the clinic were concerned for my welfare. He arrived in the therapy room (still shrieking) while his mother casually stood outside the office finishing a phone conversation. He seemed volatile and angry. Because of his energy level, I suggested making a hula hoop for him and for Mom to use in future sessions as part of our warm-up. Once the hula hoops were created, we spent the bulk of the time using them, then rolling tennis balls underfoot. That was the extent of the artwork creation (hula hoops) and yoga (tennis balls underfoot). During that session I learned that P and S's sibling C had also been living with them (at his age 5), and that C had been dragged out of T's home by C's biological father. Apparently this traumatized T and led to his MHA, suicidal ideation (threatening to cut off his testicles). Next, R stated (in front of T) that she noticed a difference in him beginning at the age of 18 months. She said, 'Where did my sweet baby go?' This comment forewarned me of R's inappropriate banter to come. I also decided, based on their enmeshment, that conducting dyadic treatment of T and his mother might warrant a paradoxical intervention to address his separation anxiety and their interdependence. I also learned that T was only able to stay in public school

Clinical cases: children

for 2 hours per day. At this juncture, T sobbed face down on the floor, became very histrionic, and began fake crying. But his affect did not match his actions or facial expression. I retrieved a mirror to aid him in seeing this for what it was: pure manipulation. Post the session, I called his psychiatrist to discuss the severity of the case. The psychiatrist begged me to keep the case, which I did, based on the fact that I could consult him when situations warranted this action.

Further progress

The next session, R cancelled due to T having 'a meltdown'. I mailed T a note letting him know that sometimes things get worse before they get better in therapy and I hoped he would return. He was surprised that I had reached out to him in between sessions. When he returned the following week, we repaired his hula hoop, R and T did the cat/cow sequence (*marjaiasāna/bitilasāna*) followed by *supta pādāṅguṣṭhāsana* (hand to toe foot posture), Warrior 1 and 2 (*vīrabhadrasāna* 1 and 2), *Dhi Rhi Ha* (goddess pose) and finally *śavāsana* (Fig. 4.2). During *vīrabhadrasāna* 1 and 2, I suggested that T use Mom like a mirror to improve his pose (paradoxical intervention). He commented, 'ooh, oh that's gross!' This allowed for further independence as he pushed away his mother/self-image. I then reinforced the idea of his taking his own pose and being more himself. During the session, I noticed that he was biting his fingers and later his toes. I addressed his toenail and fingernail biting at the end and learned that this was common for him. I suggested maybe biting a binky or pen top might be less self-injurious and we incorporated this into the homework and their intentions which were:

- R: to have a calm week
- T: to love my mother better and not treat her so harshly

- Myself: for T to love himself more.
- T's homework: substitute a pen at school and binky at home instead of chewing hands and toes. Use hula hoop and the poses that we did in session.

Noticeable during this first yoga session was how dirty T was and his foul body odor. I learned that another problem that R was facing was that T only showered approximately once per month. Thus, the next session, I decided to introduce the eight limbs of yoga, specifically the niyama *śauca* (cleanliness). Because the family was also very religious and attended church weekly, psychologically I tied it to Jesus Christ and the story of Mary Magdalene cleaning Jesus' feet.

Do you recall Reflection exercise 3 in the Introduction, where I asked how you might solve this problem? What I did was purchase two large plastic basins and filled them with warm soapy water before they arrived for session. I had them wash each other's feet as the DASS-21 was conducted pre-session. This became the ritual before we moved to yoga or artwork, and allowed for conversation about what had transpired in between sessions. This became a *sūtra* (sacred ritual/aphorism) for our work together.

In a subsequent session, I met T's *rājasic* move with lion's pose (*simhasāna*), repeated several times and then we moved to *śavāsana*. Post-*śavāsana*, T admitted that he feared that he might kill R (apparently, there had been increased aggression with T pummeling kitchen cupboards, etc.). I suggested that R really be able to hear his concerns, and he screamed at the top of his lungs, directing towards me, that I was, 'NOT helping him'. I comforted him (as did R, by hugging him) and let him know that I heard him, 'loud and clear', and what I heard him saying (repeatedly) was that he was 'afraid' that he would not be able to repress his fear and in fact harm or kill

Chapter four

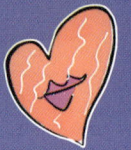
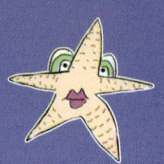

FIGURE 5.2 T's yoga sequence, session 2		
	To stretch the neck and upper back	Warm-up pose
	Supta Pādāṅguṣṭhāsāna	Warm-up pose
	Warrior 1 and 2	This was the pose used to increase autonomy
	Dhi Rhi Ha	Goddess pose with emphasis on clapping at the 'ha' portion
	Savasana	Final relaxation

R. I reiterated to R that she needed to truly hear this and take this seriously. I also directed both of them by suggesting if T got to a place of causing such harm, R would need to act quickly, call 911, and make him safe. While this might be grounds to have T hospitalized, I left that call for his psychiatrist whom I called immediately after our session. It was unknown how much of this was histrionic, true psychosis and/or matricidal tendencies versus attention seeking/manipulative

Clinical cases: children

behavior. Either way, the psychiatrist had to be informed immediately of this situation. I also suggested that R follow up with the psychiatrist as soon as possible.

T became hysterical, crying and stating that he just wanted to leave, which eventually he did. His psychiatrist thanked me for apprising him of this situation. In between sessions and since it was close to Christmas I mailed a card to T (Fig. 4.3), letting him know I was acknowledging his feelings. I wrote:

I know last week was quite difficult for you. Please know your inner 'roar' is safe in yoga therapy. Soon, you will be calmed by your inner strength. Know that expressing your fears, rather than acting on them, is the road to recovery, resilience and inner strength. Remember to breathe and talk about your feelings. Doing so will help you feel safe.

By the seventh session, T's personal hygiene was improving. He was showering more, had a 'movie date' with a girl from school and had increased his school attendance. He was more focused during *aśanā* practice and was able to sustain about 25 minutes of practice (including *śavāsana*).

Session nine was exceptionally important. After the cleansing (feet ritual), T disclosed that he felt closer to his brother A than the other children. I suggested that the bonding might have transpired before P and S moved into the house. We also talked about the genetic bond that A and he shared (with R). At this juncture, T was able to communicate to R that he felt 'unloved', and that he was her 'flesh and blood' and felt more connected to A since it used to be 'just the two' of them. Things escalated and he stated that he should be 'number one' (in essence he was suggesting that he felt displaced). R resented this being raised during session but at the session's end they hugged and T calmed down. He was able to hear from both R and me that no matter how much R tells him that she loves him, these feelings have to emanate from him. It was a powerful session for both of them.

During session 11, T's pre-test scores for the DASS-21 indicated that he was in the extremely severe range for depression, anxiety and stress but by post-session, his scores had dropped considerably (moderate for depression and anxiety and severe for stress).

After the yoga during that session and due to lack of time, T and R used the Paper53 drawing program on the clinic iPad devices. Figure 4.4 shows R's artwork (upper) and T's artwork (lower). In discussing her artwork, R explained that the red lines shooting out from the center were the 'unexpected surprises that occur', and the black snake-like image in the center represents the 'chaos' with which she had to deal.

Meanwhile, T stated that his art was 'all black' save a small corner that Mom talked him into creating since she wished he could be 'happier'. Clearly, he was able to express the dark depressive states that overcome him using this drawing app.

Session 15 was very powerful and videotaped. I suggested that during this session they create masks using papier mâché forms that reflected outside what they shared of themselves to others

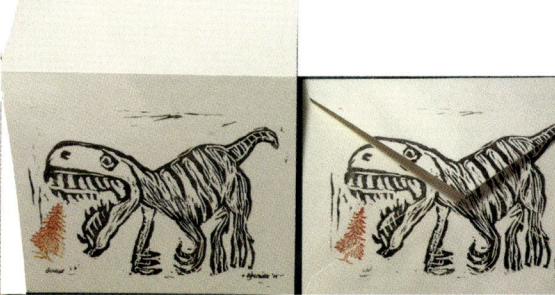

FIGURE 4.3 Card (and back of envelope) made by author for T

Chapter four

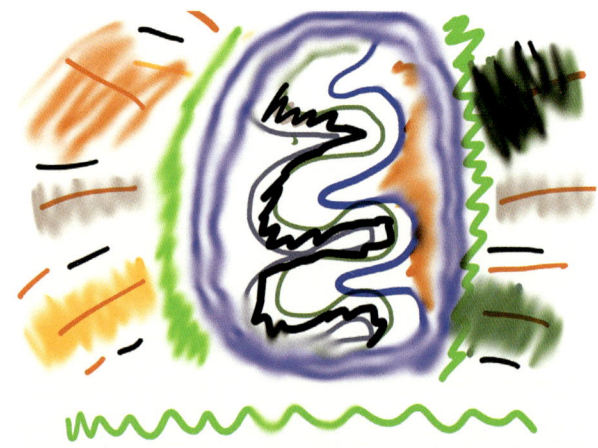

FIGURE 4.4 Paper53 R's artwork (upper), and T's (bottom) created using the Paper53 app during session

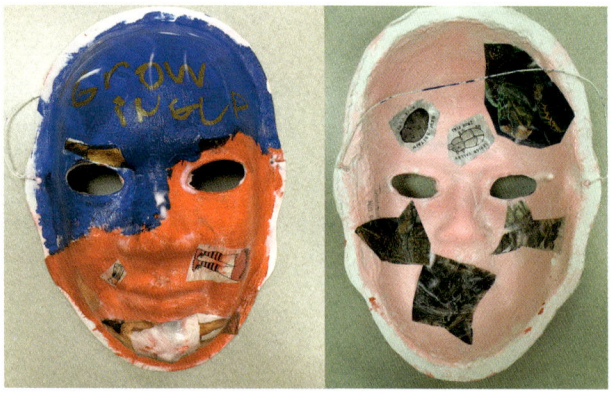

FIGURE 4.5 T's mask (left outside, right inside)

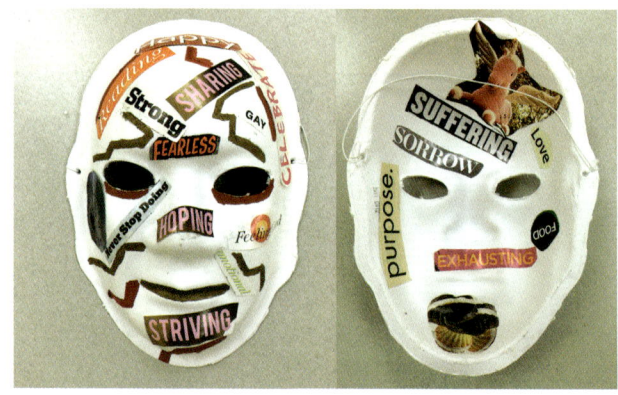

FIGURE 4.6 R's mask (left outside, right inside)

and on the inside, what they kept guarded or secret. A lot came out in this session including T's insight about R and B's recent marital conflicts. (R was frustrated with B's lack of parenting and T sarcastically chimed in, 'I was right', and 'She's a terrible wife'.) Also, T's DASS-21 scores (and R's) were all in the normal range for depression, anxiety and stress, suggesting growth in all areas.

T described the outside of his mask (Fig. 4.5): 'blue is for depression, and red is for my anger', and that he was 'growing up' and in the inside was 'pink' because he was 'cute and cuddly'.

R decorated her mask with magazine clippings, all of which described her struggles and what she wished to project to the outside world (Fig. 4.6). Alas, the inside belied these issues; clippings of suffering, sorrow, food and the like suggested her real struggles. Food was of particular concern as she was obese. Nevertheless, releasing these feelings through the art allowed for healthy discourse during the session.

Of interest is that post this session, T's DASS-21 scores and R's were all in the normal range for depression, anxiety and stress.

I received an email from R a few days after our session. T had written an email to her and stated:

Mommy I'm getting better. I've been working harder than I ever have. I am happier than I have ever been. I feel like a normal, happy child. Wow all the things I've been missing out on. Having fun, enjoying my life. I'm doing things I've always wanted. I'm going out. I am happy. I don't feel the pressure to do bad things. I don't have the thoughts pressuring me to do bad things.

She added in her closing email to me, 'Wow. This really warmed me to the core. Something is going right'.

In fact, things were really improving. Due to the fact that the semester was almost over and this work transpired in a clinic tethered to the school calendar, I attended a Committee on Special Education (CSE) meeting for T and terminated my work with him since I was going on sabbatical the following semester. He was assigned to a new therapist but never returned to the clinic. Six months later, I received an email from R. She reported that T decided not to connect with the new assigned therapist but that he was attending school and that things were going smoothly with him. She wrote that she felt the combined yoga therapy and art therapy had truly helped both of them during this critical juncture in their lives.

Case study 2

6-year-old female: separation anxiety

Background and history

Since I have a profile on the website 'Psychology Today', sometimes I receive referrals from medical doctors that I do not know. This was the case in the mother contacting me to see her 6-year-old daughter ('K'). Presenting symptoms were extreme separation anxiety for both mother and father. Both parents attributed this to the paternal grandfather's death approximately a year earlier and a close neighbor's recent death. K's reaction was restricted to her parents. For example, if mother went upstairs (and was out of K's sight) K frantically screamed for her mother. Surprisingly, K did not experience separation anxiety when she attended school. It was reported that K was very bright, reading book chapters and doing well in school. However, prior to their first appointment, they were also moving to a new home, which may have compounded the issues. K's pull on her parents caused undue stress and anxiety for them, even affecting their marriage (K hampered their 'alone time'). Thus, family treatment was recommended with varied constituents: mother/K; mother/father/K and brother and mother/K.

Of interest was father's background (Fig. 4.7). Raised as a Jehovah's Witness, he grew up without celebrating birthdays, holidays or like activities. Ironically, when the paternal grandfather became ill, he was forced to receive dialysis treatment near his end of life, frowned upon by the religion.

Chapter four

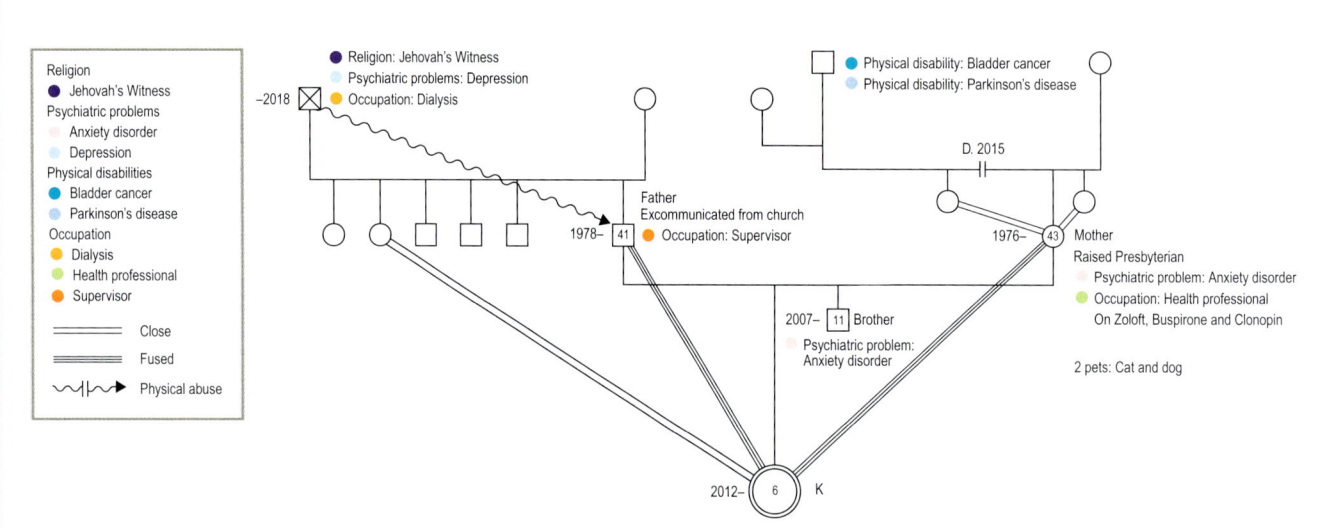

FIGURE 4.7 K's genogram

For Jehovah's witnesses, the decision not to accept blood transfusions is a religious issue rather than a medical one. Both the Old and New Testaments (Genesis 9:4; Leviticus 17:10; Deuteronomy 12:23; Acts 15:28, 15:29) clearly command the Jehovah's witness to abstain from blood. According to Jehovah Witnesses, God views blood as representing life (Leviticus 17:14). Thus, it is commanded that they avoid taking blood not only in obedience to God but also out of respect for Him as the Giver of life (Jehovah's Witnesses 2020).

Father also reported that he had been physically abused by his father and often left in a car for hours while his father went on house calls in the name of church work. Consequently, father's view led to ex-communication from the Jehovah's Witness community.

Significant sessions

During the first session, Mother, Father and K showed up. Lots of discussion ensued around K's inability to separate (specifically from her mother) and her unfounded fear that her parents would die. During the session several things illuminated this discussion: (1) working in clay afforded the opportunity for the parents to express their frustration and sadness, (2) this unleashed a somatic response in K: she broke down in tears when discussing her fear of her parents dying. While both parents were able to express their feelings in clay (Fig. 4.8), K disconnected from the issues at hand, making an image of fireworks (the 4th of July holiday had just passed). The parents were able to delineate their sadness and the father talked about his experiences being raised as a Jehovah's Witness. When I asked K about why she was unable to let her parents out of her sight, she broke down and cried and disclosed her fear that they would abandon her through death. Since neither parent moved to comfort her, I suggested seeking comfort from either. She leapt into father's lap. After she had a good cry, I suggested alternative ways of dealing with her rumination/fear. I suggested she get up and perform 20 jumping jacks with me (counting as we jumped). I suggested turning to exercise (and like activities) since the physicality and counting precluded rumination. She uses this activity to date when rumination overtakes her.

Clinical cases: children

Exercise staves off rumination; thus, performing yoga *asānas*, which require mental and physical concentration, counters anxiety.

Because there was still more time left, I suggested that K sit between her parents since she was still in her father's lap and that all three of them do a drawing together. This revealed more information. Father's work revealed his drawing of his wife, son, and daughter in protective bubbles (Fig. 4.9). But as he explained the drawing, he added that he gave them air vents, which made sense, but I wanted to know why. He detailed a story about having been left for hours in a car when his father went into people's homes spreading the word of Jehovah's Witness. He became very teary at this point and further elaborated on stories of such abandonment by his father during his childhood. Thus, I was able to weave this information into the 'homework' for K.

Homework

1. K will draw, exercise, write, etc., when she has these unfounded fears; parents to remind her of 'the string' between you and that she is in charge of not thinking these thoughts, not Mom or Dad. Also, when she feels left out of brother's play dates, remind her she can offer to help either of you with chores (unpacking, cleaning, etc.).

2. K will remind Dad to enjoy his future birthdays and to celebrate life in general since he was not raised to do so.

3. Mother will exercise more and when she feels sad or despondent, she will take a walk alone or with someone from the family.

Session 2 (mother and K)

The focus was on yoga and the journal that K had been drawing in. To start, I taught K both some breathwork such as coherent breath (Elliot 2005) and *nadi śodhana* to reduce her anxiety (Fig. 4.10).

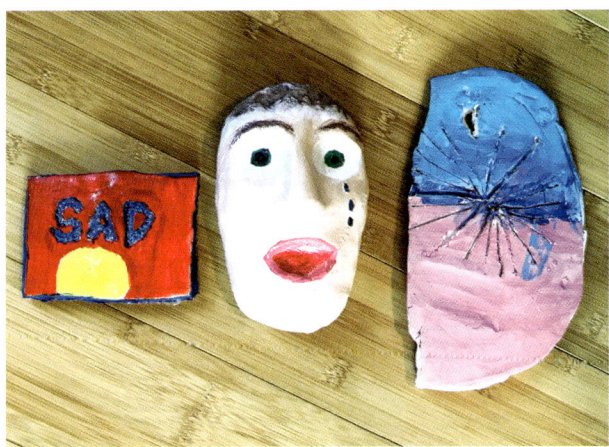

FIGURE 4.8 Clay work by family at session 1 (left to right: Mother's work, Father's work and K's 'firecracker.')

FIGURE 4.9 Father's work (left); K's (middle) and Mother's (right)

Chapter four

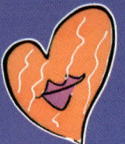 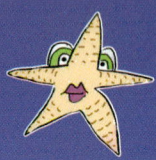

FIGURE 4.10 Mom and K: yoga session

	Krama inhale (segmented inhalation) Energizing effect, useful for increasing breathing capacity.	Begin to inhale expanding the top of the chest, pause for a moment; continue to inhale expanding the rib cage, pause for a moment; complete your inhale expanding the abdomen. Exhale slowly and smoothly.
	Krama exhale (segmented exhalation) Calming effect, useful for increasing breathing capacity.	Inhale slowly and smoothly. Begin to exhale, contracting your abdomen above the pubic bone, pause for a moment; continue to exhale, contracting the abdomen around the navel, pause for a moment; finish your exhale contracting the muscles between the navel and sternum.
	Belly breath and coherent breath	Bring hands to belly and heart if easier; inhale into belly for 4 counts; hold your breath for 2 counts and then exhale for 4 counts; try to increase to 6:2:6 and repeat at least 10× to calm your feelings.
	Nadi śodhana (alternate nostril breathing) Balancing effect.	Inhale through the left nostril; exhale through the right nostril; Inhale through the right nostril; exhale through the left nostril. 1 cycle.

Clinical cases: children

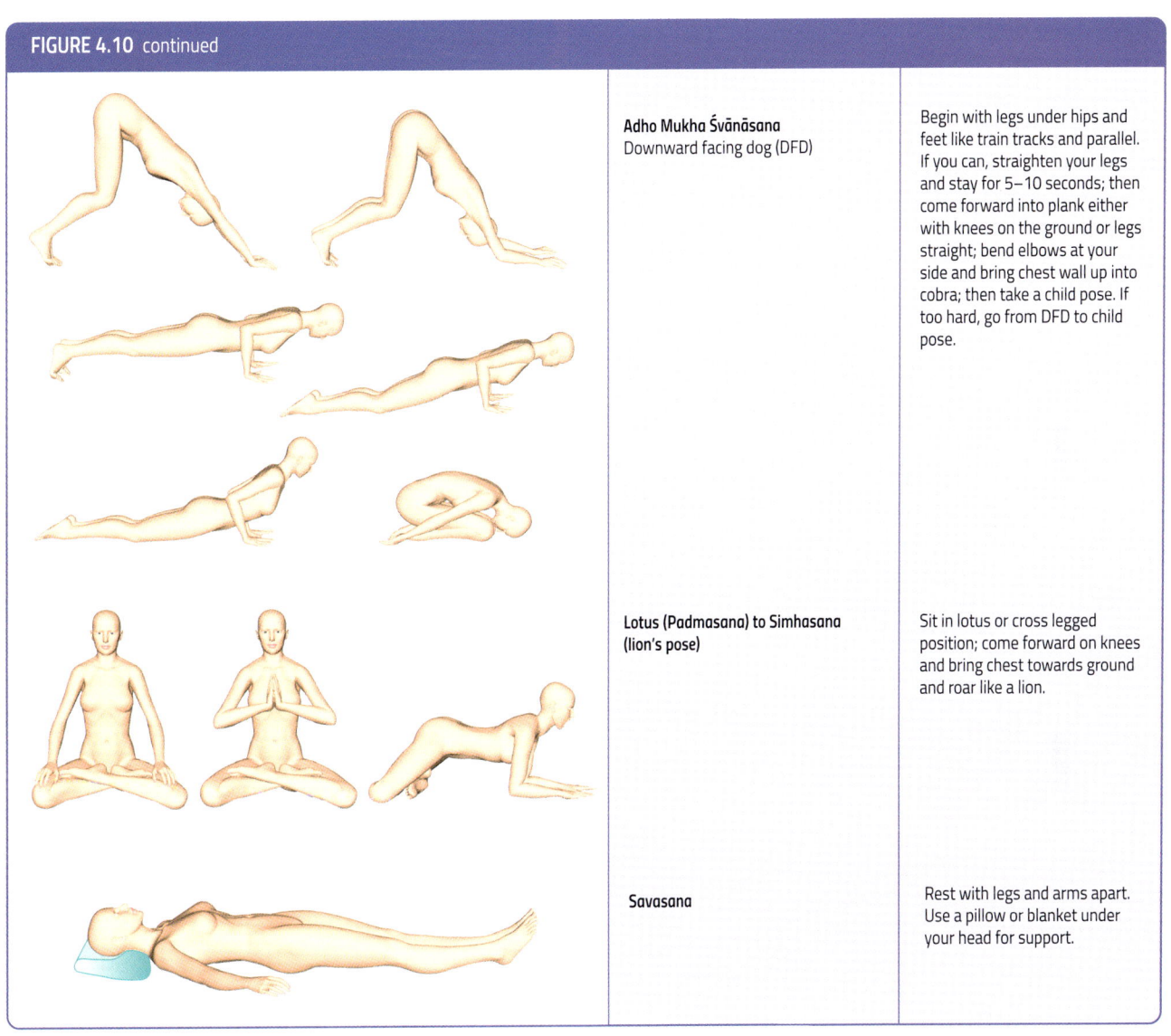

FIGURE 4.10 continued

During the discussion of K's journal, mother brought up the children's book, *The Invisible String*, with which I was unfamiliar (I now own the book, Kearst 2000). The concept behind it addresses separation anxiety and so K's schoolteacher thought it would be a good book for them to read.

The premise behind *The Invisible String* is that no matter what separates the children from their mother, they are always connected by this invisible string that binds their love and their hearts. My mentor/yoga teacher, Sri François Raoult commented (after reading the book) that it was 'a *sūtra*'.

Chapter four

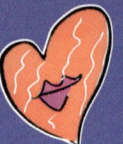 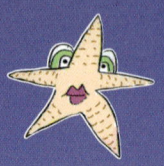

After the breathwork, we moved into the yoga *asānas*, but the mother became almost aggressive with K, attempting to force her legs into lotus during *simhasāna*, lion's pose. I had to warn her several times not to force K's legs into lotus and explained that K could obtain similar results cross-legged. It was almost as if mother felt this was akin to competitive athletics and gave me a hint of what she might be like when K attended dance classes and like outside activities.

What remained a steadfast issue throughout the therapy sessions was that K watched television and movie programming that heightened her anxiety. For example, in this first session she disclosed that she watched the *Batman* movie and talked about the scene where Batman's parents died in a car crash. Of all the things she could have gleaned from the movie (forget that he was a crime fighter), this is what she clung to. In a later session, K arrived wearing costumes that led to discussion of more cartoon characters, specifically *Miraculous* and the *Descendants*. So (reader) you already know that if I am unfamiliar with a book, character, movie, etc., I make it my homework to educate myself. Ten minutes of both *Miraculous* and the *Descendants* made it abundantly clear to me that these cartoons/shows were wildly inappropriate for this 6-year-old and served to fuel her anxiety about losing her parents. Naturally this was recapped to the parents in later sessions, but unfortunately my warning/suggestion did not deter them from allowing K to watch these disturbing narratives.

In clinical speak, the vernacular for the parents' rejection of change (veering from such activities) is referred to as one step forward and one step backward (or approach and avoidance). While this may be discouraging for the therapist, it is part of the therapeutic dance: homeostasis is always preferable to change, which is hard and requires real work.

Session 4

The session started off by discussing how things had been going. Keeping a calendar marked with stars when K's behavior improved worked extremely well, so I suggested that they continue to use the calendar to monitor and reinforce desired behavior.

At the beginning of the session, when discussing progress, K was practically on top of her mother when the mother mentioned her inability to go grocery shopping without her. I talked about barnacles, how they adhered to boats and pointed out K's clinging behavior during session. We used the co-operative blankets and the elastaband to point out that she was still connected to her parents even when they were slow dancing. That cemented the idea, and then we moved to art therapy. We put everything in perspective (Mom's work, which she loves, Dad's work, which he loves, and Ks schoolwork, which she loves). Mimicking *The Invisible String* book, I suggested that each of them choose a colored marker and make a dot on the page to represent themselves. I sat next to K, and Mom and Dad sat opposite K and next to each other. K was the pink dot connected to Mom's purple and Dad's red dots, respectively (Fig. 4.11).

I suggested K use words to connect her pink dot to Mom (she repeatedly wrote the word 'love'). This was repeated first between Mom to Dad. Mother wrote 'always' (as in, 'you are my always'), and Dad wrote 'life' (as in, 'you are the love of my life'). Then Dad wrote to K, 'heart' (as in, 'you are my heart'), and Mother wrote to K, 'everything' (as in, 'you (and your brother) are my everything'). Looking at the paper, I had an 'aha' moment: I turned the paper upside down and pointed out that Mom and Dad were the foundation from which K sprung. I suggested that they create that mountain, its foundation and the sky above.

Clinical cases: children

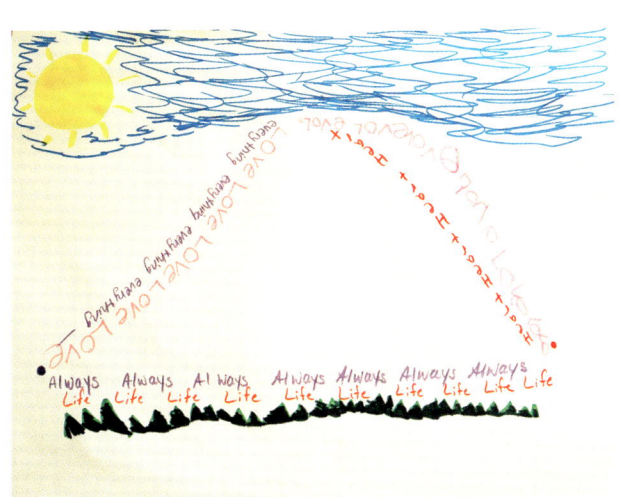

FIGURE 4.11 Family Mountain

K detailed the grass, Mom colored the blue sky and Dad drew the sun. Next, I had K take *tādāsana* (mountain pose) and state, 'I am strong, stable, and secure, I am the mountain, *tādāsana*'. I also pointed out that school (for K) was like Mom and Dad's work and there she excelled and was strong, independent, and need not be a barnacle. I reiterated that when she was feeling needy that she take the pose, *tādāsana*, and repeat to herself, 'I am strong, stable and secure, I am the mountain, *tādāsana*' (Fig. 4.12). I also suggested taking the artwork home so that her parents could use this drawing to reinforce independent behavior.

Striking the mountain pose, *tādāsana*, enhances confidence, grounding, stability and strength (Gibbons 2015: 96). This *āsana* can be used with numerous patients and can incorporate a number of intentions and *mudras*. While people have varying etiologies, almost everyone who comes to my door is in need of bolstering their self-esteem, strength and stability. This seems to be fairly universal.

In a later session, once again, we discussed *The Invisible String*. I shared a story with K and

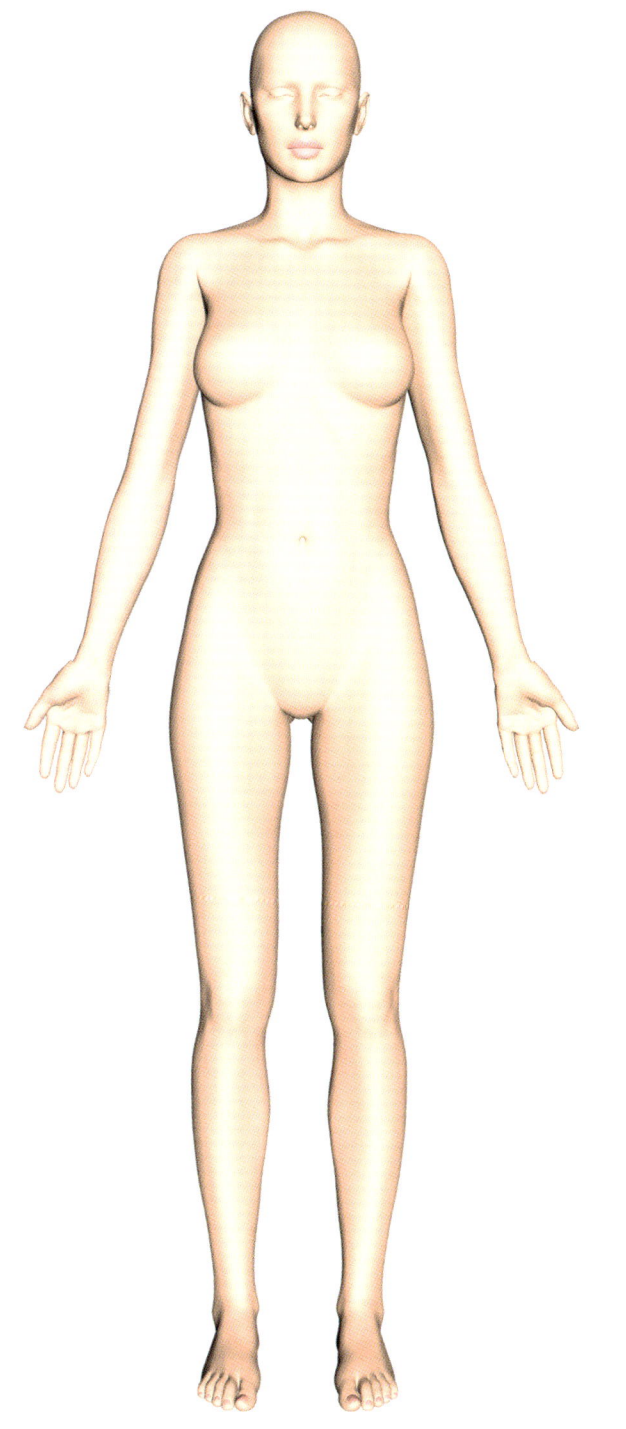

FIGURE 4.12 *Tadaśanā*, I am the mountain.

Chapter four

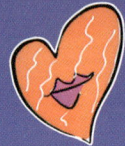
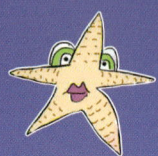

her mother about my graduation from my yoga advanced teacher training (ATT) with Sri François Raoult and how we tied strings around our wrists as both a remembrance and also to mark the importance of the occasion, while psychologically binding us together as our 'yoganaut' group (Raoult 2019). My thin string, now faded from its original bright yellow, still adorns my wrist and will continue to until it falls off. I suggested that they make an invisible string bracelet for each other, which they commemorated with attached buttons (Fig. 4.13).

Update

The case has terminated since all were doing so well. K no longer has separation issues, pronounced as they were. She responded to limit-setting, adjusted to her new school placement and has become increasingly independent. As a result, the parents have increased couple time and everyone seems happier and more well-adjusted. Of course, my door is always open to K and her family should they need my counsel in the future.

Addendum: The family returned during the coronavirus pandemic; individual sessions with K's brother and then the entire family aided him during the isolation of COVID-19 times.

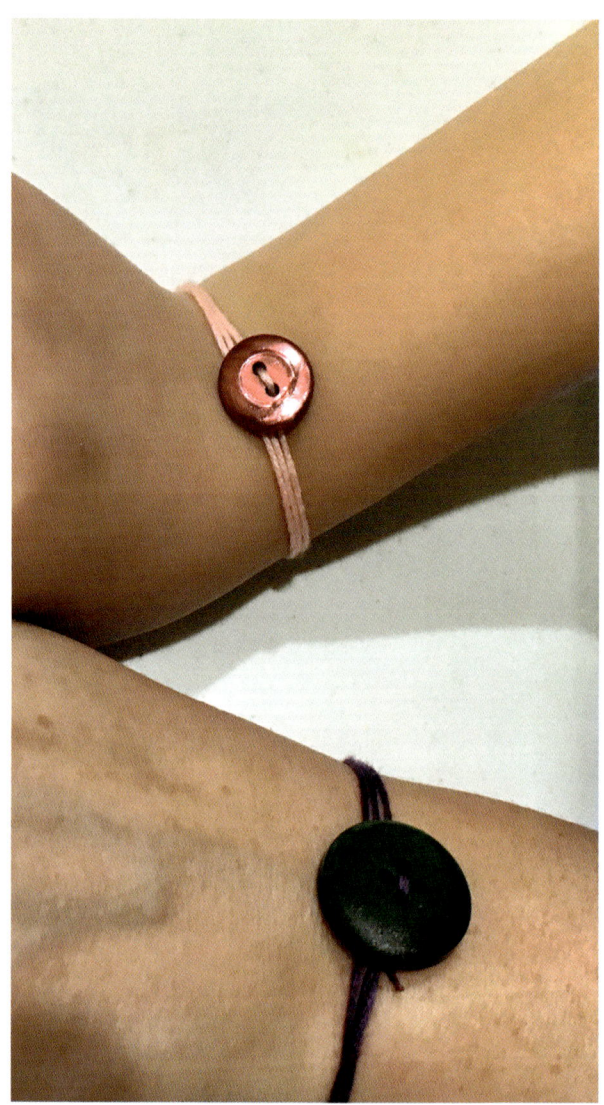

FIGURE 4.13 K's invisible string bracelet (top, K's; bottom, Mother's)

Clinical cases: children

Somatic integration and yoga therapy

When looking at K's case in terms of somatic principles and education, one is concerned with the living body (or soma) – how the body learns, functions, becomes aware and moves in space. Hanna (1991: 31) clarifies this as follows: 'The soma, being internally perceived, is categorically distinct from a body, not because the subject is different but because the mode of viewpoint is different: it is immediate proprioception – a sensory mode that provides unique data'.

Because it is impossible to separate the body from the mind when proprioception is at work, I incorporate both as learning agents within the confines of therapy. Historically, one can trace somatic thinking (and the elusive Self) all the way back to William James (1890). Antonio Damasio, a present-day scientist, wholeheartedly agrees with James' account of the body/mind generating emotions capable of separating the contents that belong to the Self and those that do not. Damasio (2010) called these feelings 'somatic markers'. He explained that when these contents occur in the mind stream, they generate an appearance of a marker and thus accomplish a distinct feeling between the Self and the non-Self: 'in a nutshell, feelings of knowing' (Damasio 2010: 9). According to the field of somatics education, a body can be dead or alive, but soma refers to a living body, or according to Joly (2001), the sum total of the body's subjective (first person) lived experience.

Hanna (1986) defined somatics as: 'the art and science of the inter-relational process between awareness, biological function and the environment, all three factors being understood as a synergetic whole'. Eleanor Criswell (1989) explains soma in terms of the psychophysiology of yoga and its workings in the brain. She discussed the 'neural' inputs achieved through yoga as 'providing input to your brain' (e.g. central and peripheral nervous systems). These 'neural inputs' are achieved through skin senses, eyes, ears, nose and visceral senses, while humoral inputs (plasma constituents and their characteristics) are received via oxygen, carbon dioxide, temperature, glucose, etc. (Criswell 1989: 110).

Going even further, Bessel van der Kolk (2014) talks about trauma leaving an imprint on the mind, brain and the body. Healing depends on 'experiential knowledge… you can be fully in charge of your life only if you can acknowledge the reality of your body, in all its visceral dimensions' (pp. 21–27). He has gone on to say (van der Kolk 2019):

Our studies show that yoga is equally as beneficial as – or more beneficial than – the best possible medications in alleviating traumatic stress symptoms. In the studies we did involving neuroimaging of the brain before and after regular yoga practice, we were able to show that the areas of the brain involving self-awareness get activated by doing yoga, and those are the areas that get locked out by trauma and that are needed in order to heal.

Mirror neurons, empathy and relations

Tronick (1989), Sravish et al (2013) and van der Kolk (2014) have demonstrated that when infants and caregivers are 'in sync' on an emotional level, they are also in sync physically. Heart rate variability (HRV), hormone levels, and the nervous system are entirely affected by this 'invisible string' or empathic relatability.

In terms of mirror neurons, the same can be true for the yoga therapist and their patients. If you are out of sync with yourself and not attuned to your patient, a secure attachment will not be forged. Thus, the 'invisible string' between therapist and patient is what Wampold (2001) was suggesting (as previously discussed in Chapter 1) being the greatest predictor of efficacy in patient

Chapter four

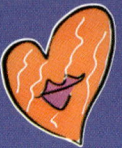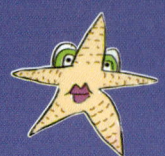

outcomes: it is not necessarily the therapeutic modality used, but the relationship between the therapist and patient.

According to Criswell (1989: 111), there are three levels of the brain: (1) the reptilian brain, including the brain stem and thalamus, (2) the old brain (or limbic system), which we have in common with other animals, and (3) the neocortex or new brain, the primary function of which is inhibitory or to be eased/quieted. In yoga practice, the task is to quiet the neocortex allowing the lower brain to function more freely.

> ### Reflection exercise 4.1
>
> Distinguishing the importance of soma and authenticity in mirror neurons between yourself and your patients, ponder a time when you worked with someone that was like 'K' (adorable but sycophantic and suffocating in nature). How would you remain connected to that patient, yet paradoxically cause an intervention that allowed for individuation (much like I suggested in *tadāsana*) using art, journaling, assigned readings, and/or therapeutic yoga? Also, what would you do for yourself to navigate this situation and remain connected to yourself in a truly compassionate and caring way?

Recent research on attention deficit disorder (ADD) and attention deficit–hyperactivity disorder (ADHD)

A secondary gain occurs every time I practice yoga – I enter what Csikszentmihalyi (1996) coined a 'flow' state and I literally transform. The more I become in touch with this part of myself, the sharper my interoceptive (gut feeling) becomes. Sommer Anderson (2008) interviewed countless analysts who relayed stories about this 'sub-symbolic and nonverbal symbolic mode' of processing information. Truly, this is the language of art therapy and yoga therapy – it is the interoceptive, proprioceptive and kinesthetic experience; it is that 'felt' experience when you 'know' something immediately in your body, even if you cannot verbally articulate it in the speech center of your brain. I have come to rely on this second brain, this visceral patch, housed in the stomach organ. This has served me well and as a clinician I often 'thin slice' (Gladwell 2005) accurately when analyzing client facial and body language. Thin slicing is accepting our first impressions seriously. According to Gladwell (2005), 'sometimes we can know more about someone in a blink of the eye than we can after months of study' (p.76). Yoga heightens that awareness for me both personally and as a practitioner. Exercising my body also exercises my brain.

Years ago, a report in the *New York Times* (Reynolds 2012) confirmed this need to incorporate movement into therapy: 'Exercise, the latest neuroscience suggests, does more to bolster thinking than thinking does'. In a laboratory setting, Justin S. Rhodes, a psychology professor at the Beckman Institute for Advanced Science and Technology at the University of Illinois, gathered four groups of mice and set them into four distinct living arrangements. The animals completed a series of cognitive tests at the start of the study and were injected with a substance that allowed the scientists to track changes in their brain structures. Then they ran, played, or if their environment was unenriched, lolled about in their cages for several months. It turned out that the toys and tastes, no matter how stimulating, had not improved the animals' brains. Only one thing mattered, and that was whether they had a running wheel. Animals that exercised (whether or not they had any other enrichment in their cages) had healthier brains and performed significantly better on cognitive tests than the other mice. Animals that didn't

Clinical cases: children

run, no matter how enriched their world was otherwise, did not improve their brainpower in the complex, lasting ways that Rhodes's team was studying (Reynolds 2012). Since then, there have been numerous publications on exercise and its ability to maintain the brain in its plastic, ever-evolving development. Somehow, my interoceptive, proprioceptive, kinesthetic self knew this for a very long time. Forget Sudoku, this was the mother lode.

Daniel Goleman wrote a piece for *The New York Times* entitled 'Exercising the mind to treat attention disorders' (Goleman 2014). According to the article, experts claimed that, 'there are no long-term, lasting benefits' from taking medications to alter attention disorders. Furthermore, it was suggested that, 'mindfulness seems to be training the same areas in the brain that have reduced activity' in attention disorders. According to this latest research, the singular mental ability of mindfulness training predicted success in school and in work life: 'specialists are now suggesting this might be particularly beneficial in treating ADHD and ADD'. Indeed, a recent report in *Clinical Neurophysiology* on mindfulness-based cognitive therapy suggested improved inhibitory regulation (Schoenberg et al 2013). Pag and Ruiz (2017) reported that children with ADD may be inattentive, have difficulty following directions, may exhibit impulse control issues, can display excessive motor activity in many (but not all) cases and may demonstrate difficulty conforming to social norms.

Today, more healthcare professionals recommend a multidisciplinary, multimodal approach to the treatment of ADD, which includes medication but also may include therapy and dietary changes as well as a host of mind-body approaches, such as biofeedback, neurofeedback, and yoga. Integrated Movement Therapy™ was one such approach suggested by Kenny (2002). It had consistent results with children diagnosed with autism spectrum disorders.

Case study 3

11-year-old female and mother: attention deficit disorder (ADD)

Background and history

Initially, I met with the mother in order to obtain a detailed three-generation genogram and medical history on 'E', then aged 9 (Fig. 4.14). However, what became clear during both the intake and the first session was that treating as much of the nuclear family system as possible would be the optimal course of action. After the initial yoga session with E, I decided to conduct the Kinetic Family Drawing (KFD) assessment in order to ascertain psychosocial familial issues, cognitive and developmental functioning, and analyze the artwork in terms of the Formal Element Art Therapy Scale (FEATS) (Gannt and Tabone 1998). Because E was only 9 years old when treatment began, I ascertained after her initial yoga therapy assessment that E might be more comfortable if her mother were present for some of the sessions. After the mother joined the combined yoga/art therapy sessions during session 2, occasionally I checked in with E to determine whether or not she was interested in individual, weekly sessions, but she continued on from session 2 with her mother joining all sessions for the next 2 years. Occasionally her brother joined sessions but mostly the focus was on the mother/daughter dyad. The brother and father attended a few sessions towards the end of treatment. E was seen for approximately 40 sessions over an academic 2-year span.

Chapter four

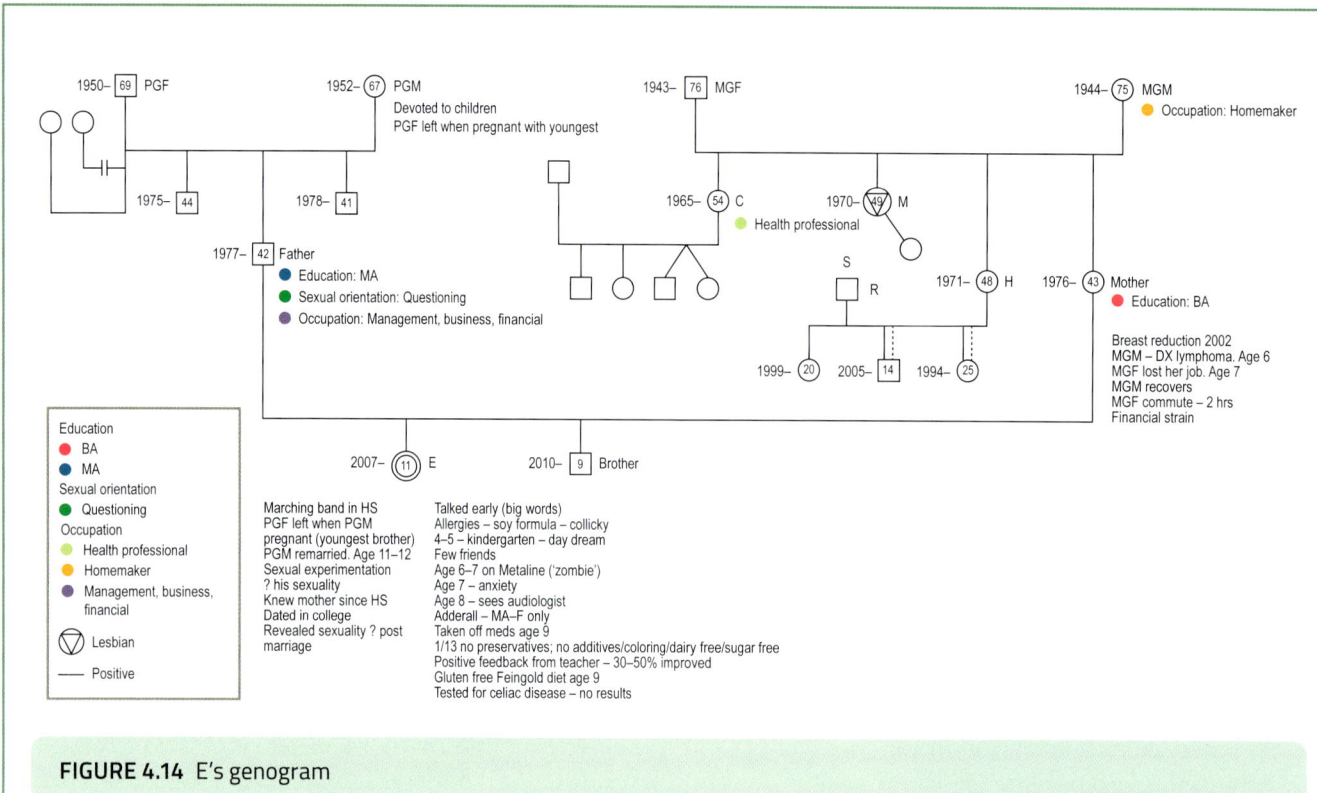

FIGURE 4.14 E's genogram

Yoga therapy and KFD assessment

I wanted to gauge E's breathing and pranayama capacity. I demonstrated how to hold one hand to the stomach area and the other to the chest in order to inform her of the differences in breathing and teach her coherent breath (Elliot 2005). She admitted difficulty sitting still. And while yoga was new for her, she persevered. Her ability to make eye contact and conversation increased as the session wore on with statements like, 'I don't like my brother, he is annoying, he is always repeating others' jokes'. Nevertheless, her mood was depressed, her balance was off (even though she was proficient at ice-skating, winning competitions), and her energy level was clearly low. All of this was palpable during the yoga therapy assessment and caused me to conduct a preliminary art therapy assessment to corroborate what I was witnessing in the yoga therapy session.

When I conducted the KFD (the instruction is to 'draw yourself and your family doing something'), while E was able to engage and seemingly relax, her drawing (Fig. 4.15) was surprisingly disconnected and reflected her diagnosis of ADD Inattentive type, and general dissociation from her body. All family members were depicted as floating heads. Mother was drawn first, then father and finally her brother between them. Brothers placement in and of itself (between the parents) was revealing regarding E's perception of the parental system.

Clinical cases: children

Next, she inquired whether or not she should add herself, clearly suggesting feelings of displacement within the family system. While E eventually drew her head larger than the other family members, this may reflect her escape into fantasy and dissociation (yet none of the family members sported bodies). When I asked what they were doing, she explained that they 'watch(ed) movies together', but that is the extent to which they 'did things together'. Also, the fact that mother, father and brother are on one plane may suggest that she views them as aligned, yet herself (detailed below them) as not on the same playing field.

First family session: mother and E

Because the sessions were limited to a full hour of treatment, generally the first 30 minutes was dedicated to yoga therapy. This often consisted of:

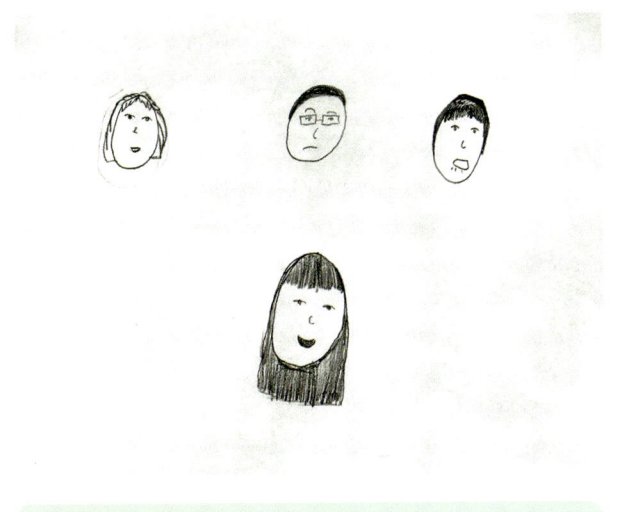

FIGURE 4.15 Kinetic family drawing

- coherent breath regulation/ meditation
- warm-ups using hula hoops
- warm-ups, *bhāvanās*, specific *āsanas* (often with mantras) depending on physiological/ emotive factors that influenced which postures to employ; *śavāsana* and setting intentions.

I was surprised that the mother did not let me know that she intended to join but instead made that decision for E. This gave me some clue into the family dynamics and my need to 'challenge unproductive assumptions' (Boscolo and Bertrando 1992, Horovitz 2017). Since it was the first family session, we focused on stretches and warm-ups. We did several exercises and mother joined in. I joined them using hula hoops, which was great fun for both of them (Nichols 2007). Here, E soared with skill. Next, several yoga exercises were implemented to aid E's complaint of possible plantar fasciitis, one in which they partnered together. During the ending stretches (*supta pādāṅgusthāsana*), where they were supine on the floor with one leg stretched over the other as their arms were out at the shoulders (T-shaped), mother jokingly tipped me off to her underlying passive–aggression by kicking E.

It became clearer during the art therapy component just how much anger mother harbored towards E. I realized then that tiptoeing around mother's passive–aggressive actions would be crucial to the treatment in order to realign the family system and challenge unproductive assumptions (Boscolo and Bertrando 1992); otherwise the case would be lost.

Chapter four

The mother became increasingly tuckered during some of the poses and so *savāsana* (corpse pose – where the body relaxes and restores itself) was welcomed by mother following the yoga session. On the other hand, E, ever unable to relax, twitched and opened her eyes, while her mother was completely calmed by the restorative and healing qualities of the 5–10-minute *śavāsana*. After *śavāsana*, I asked them to silently head to the art table and make a drawing together that communicated something to the other taken from their yogic practice and intention set during *śavāsana*. Had the yoga therapy component been absent from the dynamics of the family session, the mother's passive–aggressive behavior might have been overlooked (when she jokingly kicked E during *supta pādāṅgusthāsana*). But having that replicated in the same session through the artwork (*vis a vis* the mother colonizing the space and creating a self-revealing tornado) triggered my need to be vigilant.

Mother worked on the left side of the page and took up approximately 66% of the space, a clear reflection of her need to dominate. Colonized, E worked in the upper right corner. Like E's KFD (see Fig. 4.15), no bodies were present (save E's thought-bubble of a princess and a castle, clearly suggesting continual dissociation and retreat into fantasy, a factor that annoyed her mother). Yet, cognitive improvement was evident since E's initial KFD drawing (Fig. 4.16). Here, E was able to create an entire princess (complete with body) in her thought bubble. Yet, interestingly enough, the princess lacked feet, suggesting her immobility to make change in her own life. Mother's upper component was described as representing the calm feeling that resulted from the yoga and the area below represented the chaos. E aptly pointed out that the image below looked like a tornado. Mother explained that it was a tornado, but it was 'dying out'. Nevertheless, E's ability to aptly point out the

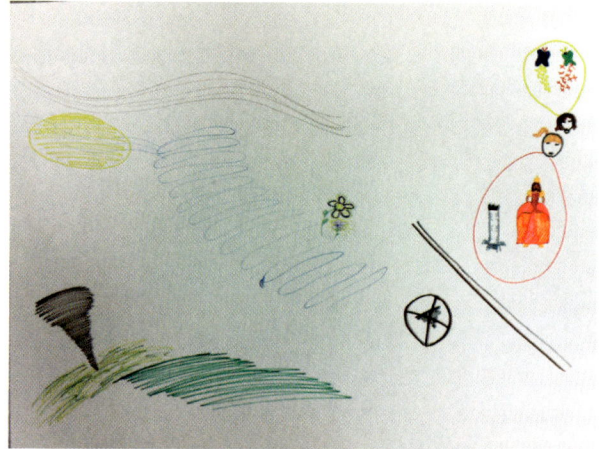

FIGURE 4.16 Family session artwork post yoga

brewing storm reflected her ability to 'thin-slice' (e.g. using our instincts and first impressions, Gladwell 2005) her mother's emotive state.

E drew her mother's head (elevated) above hers with butterflies coming out of the thought-bubble. Her own head sported a princess and tower, suggesting an increased desire to retreat into fantasy. She remarked that the princess in the tower reflected her desire to escape from her brother, who 'annoyed' her on a 'daily' basis. Once again, sibling rivalry rose to the surface and I was presented with a need to remap the family system. While the mother talked about the tornado, E separated out their two respective spaces by drawing two black angled lines below her princess/tower in her head; she then created a tornado enclosed by a circle and placed a cross over it, as if to excise it from both mother and its effect on the family system (and possibly create a boundary for herself). This theme of setting boundaries with her mother became a precursor to the therapy ahead and spoke boatloads about E's need to recast the homeostasis and realign the family system (Boscolo and Bertrando 1992, Horovitz 2011, 2013, 2017).

Clinical cases: children

That was my window into their dyadic dance. Changing that tempo (Boscolo and Bertrando 1992, Horovitz 2011, 2013, 2017, Nichols 2007), while not unseating mother's parental control, was a dance of two steps forward and two backward. In all therapy, but always when working with family systems, one has to be mindful of this progression/regression.

Homeostasis always rules the day. The adage is that it's easier to remain the same than walk towards a trajectory of wellness. One of my past family therapy supervisors, Sybil Baldwin, once told me, 'it's easier to love a bad mother than none at all'. Not that this mother was bad – on the contrary. She was committed to getting her daughter the help she needed and recognized (in the process) that she too needed help with her own issues. When I coupled the mother and E through yoga therapy postures, this enabled me to challenge unproductive assumptions and co-create a new reality system for the family (Boscolo and Bertrando 1992).

Significant family sessions

Let's dance ahead into treatment, since sessions ranged over a 2-year period. My yoga therapy direction in treating this family system was organized around coherent breathing and what I learned from my yoga therapy teacher Amy Weintraub: setting intention through regulated coherent breathing, *prāṇayāma*, *bhāvana* (Sanskrit for the development or cultivation of the heart/mind through a suggested story idea), meditation, sharing intentions and making art. I always started with the body first: warm-ups (hula hooping and the like) was the direction and then I progressed to whatever seemed most pertinent at the time I checked in (meditation, coherent breathing, *prāṇayāma*, *bhāvana*, *āsana*, etc.).

Sri François Raoult taught me the importance of honestly answering formulaic requests from others with his stock answer, 'it depends'. He is so right. You see, there really is no yogic recipe, no magic formula. However, I insist on one ingredient – the patient always sets an intention. The intention is what threads the yoga and weaves it into the art. Clues are always offered to me by 'thin-slicing' a family's facial and body gestures and verbal associates to the yoga therapy/body work, but it is their intention that enables the body to chart its course through the art.

Several times post yoga therapy, mother and E chose to work in clay. Clay, being a most malleable medium, is extremely forgiving. Undoing and redoing rules the day, since this is the nature of clay. Even if 'mistakes' are made, they can easily be 'erased' and reshaped and molded anew.

In terms of media, clay is unquestionably the ultimate mirror for forgiveness (Horovitz 1999, Henley 2002). The medium itself can be used to reflect ambivalence in acts and word. For example in one dyadic session, which I videotaped, mother created a 'straight and narrow path', and talked easily about how it was 'okay to fall off the path', but likened this passage to be lined with the possibility for growth, change and acceptance of things that were not necessarily an exact recipe. Here, mother may have been self-projecting, yet this verbal translation allowed E to view herself as fallible yet accepted, while simultaneously offering mother a platform to air grievances about her daughter's 'differences'. Being authentically accepted despite her differences and limitations was liberating.

In later sessions, the mother and E continued to focus on forgiveness and self-acceptance by making mosaic clay mirrors (Fig. 4.17). This project required several weeks to complete: the clay

Chapter four

had to go through both a bisque and glaze firing, the mosaic clay pieces then had to be adhered to a plywood backing, and finally, the mirrors had to be attached. Of interest is E's piece, which housed a small pinch pot (lower left of her mirror frame). Her utilitarian pinch pot (meant to hold earrings) was fastened with a screw joint and compound. While the mother's mirror (Fig. 4.17, left) sports a more sophisticated design element, E's abstract mirror (Fig. 4.17, right) required much forethought and planning, thus dovetailing with her objective of increased focus and attention.

By the second year of treatment, E complained of 'no longer wanting to be sick' (thus rejecting the IP (identified patient) notion and realigning the subsystems (Nichols 2007)). Much of the artwork post yoga flowed around those issues. While E was struggling with flu-like symptoms, the meta-message was clear: she was also tired of being identified as the 'patient' in the family system and was struggling to be viewed as healthy and thus challenged unproductive assumptions (Bertrando 2007, Horovitz 2017, Nichols 2007).

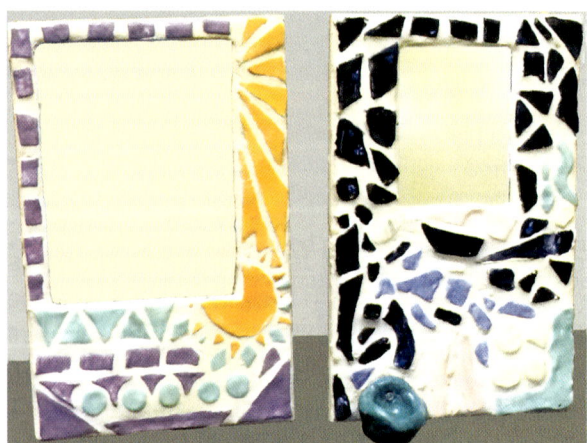

FIGURE 4.17 Clay mirrors (left, mother's; right, E's)

Another 3 weeks elapsed due to E's illness, the family's vacation, and my own. But all family members were present during the next session. As a result, I started with warm-ups (hula hoops, etc.) and then we moved to cat–cow and balance poses with all of them doing tree, which was fun and challenging for all. Next, I partnered them in *navāsana* (boat pose), using two belts per partner for support (Fig. 4.18). Mother and E climbed the wall in modified handstand for about 15 seconds, showing off their prowess. Father took to the yoga, and while E and her brother were difficult to keep focused, when *śavāsana* occurred, they all melted to the ground. It was very interesting to watch this dynamic, where suddenly E focused more than others and was the star during yoga.

Before the art therapy, the following intentions post *savāsana* were:

- Mother: togetherness
- E: for everything to just get better (which led to explanation about the upcoming New York State regent exams)
- Brother: to get a good grade on the state test (regent exams)
- Father: togetherness.

Surprisingly, after the clay artwork was created around the upcoming regent exams, the father suggested making a clay Berenstain bear family (based on the children's Berenstain Bear literature books) (Fig. 4.19). While the father had been absent for almost all of the family sessions, he took the lead with the clay materials and aided both E and her brother towards fruition. This required another session to complete. Our sessions ended shortly after these family sessions since I was leaving for a sabbatical.

Clinical cases: children

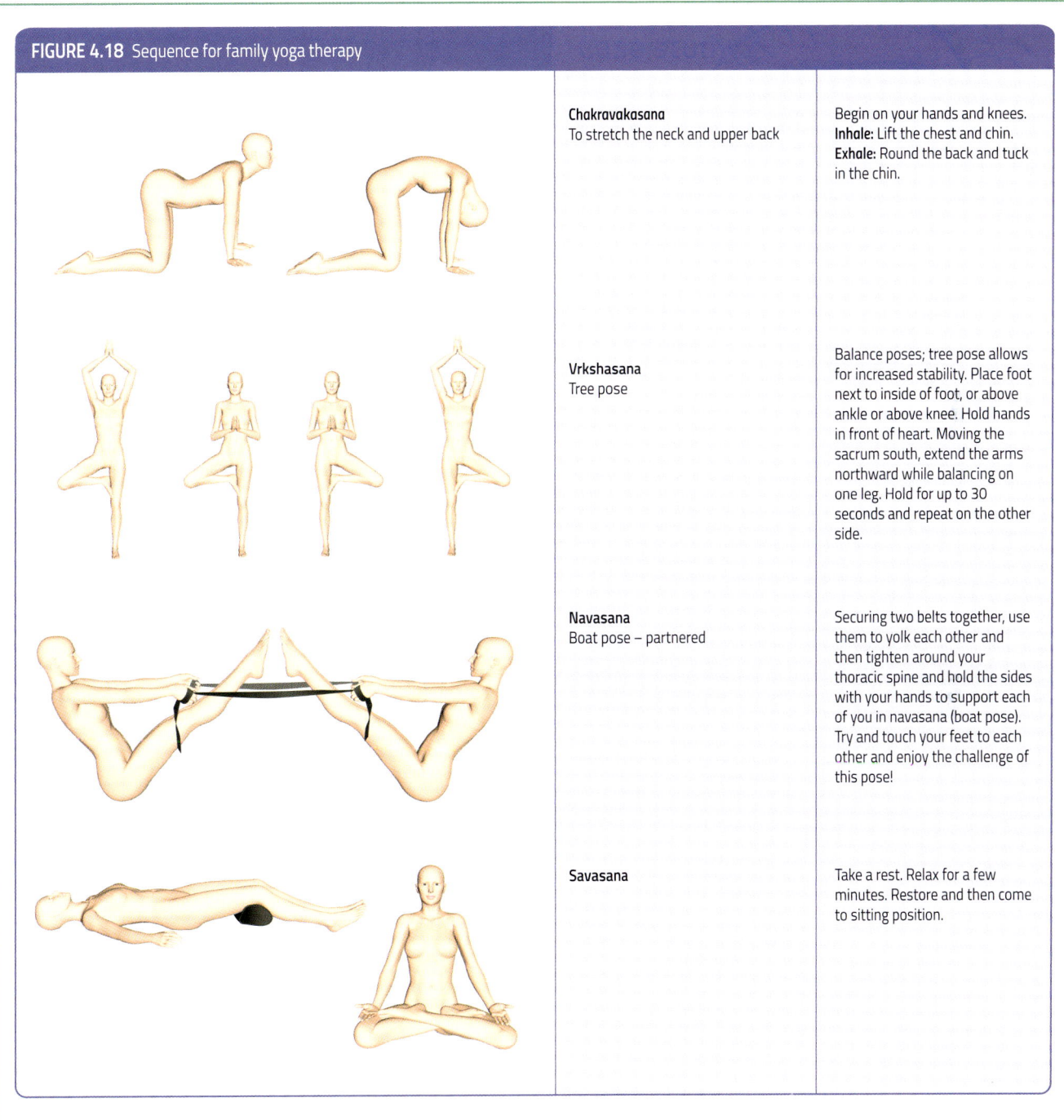

FIGURE 4.18 Sequence for family yoga therapy

	Chakravakasana To stretch the neck and upper back	Begin on your hands and knees. **Inhale:** Lift the chest and chin. **Exhale:** Round the back and tuck in the chin.
	Vrkshasana Tree pose	Balance poses; tree pose allows for increased stability. Place foot next to inside of foot, or above ankle or above knee. Hold hands in front of heart. Moving the sacrum south, extend the arms northward while balancing on one leg. Hold for up to 30 seconds and repeat on the other side.
	Navasana Boat pose – partnered	Securing two belts together, use them to yolk each other and then tighten around your thoracic spine and hold the sides with your hands to support each of you in navasana (boat pose). Try and touch your feet to each other and enjoy the challenge of this pose!
	Savasana	Take a rest. Relax for a few minutes. Restore and then come to sitting position.

Chapter four

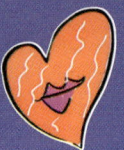 

Discussion

In sum, there had been a cognitive, emotional and developmental shift in E as well as in her relationship with her mother, brother and father. After approximately 2 years of treatment, the mother had come to accept E's differences and in fact had embraced those variances as can be seen in Figure 4.20 and Figure 4.21. During the final session, E and mother coupled in yoga: trust was involved to support each other's weight. Here E was most comfortable, since the bodily activity allowed for the interaction and connection for which she so hungered. E's attention was improving in all areas of her life: home, school, and her competition ice-skating. While much work remained, there had been enormous progress. And while E often complained about their 'hectic schedule' (mother's choir practice, ice-skating practice/competitions, brother's hockey and then some), she verbalized on more than one occasion both in and out of the therapeutic sessions that she did not want to 'give up' the yoga/art therapy. Clearly the yoga/art therapy had 'yoked' this family into a healthier form of attachment.

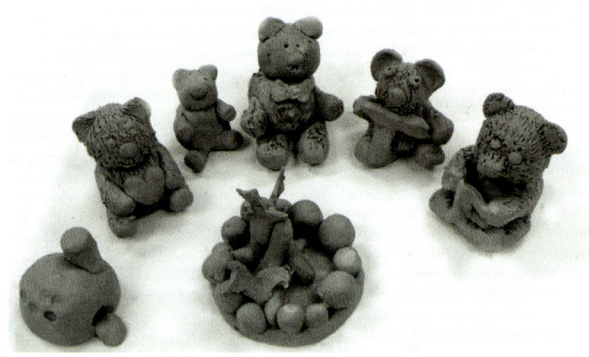

FIGURE 4.19 The 'Berenstain Bear family' with tent and campfire (foreground). Back left to right: mother's bear and extra baby bear, Father's bear (sporting a bowtie), Brother's bear (holding a T for terrific) and E's bear (holding her initial E)

FIGURE 4.20 Mother and E's yoga sequence

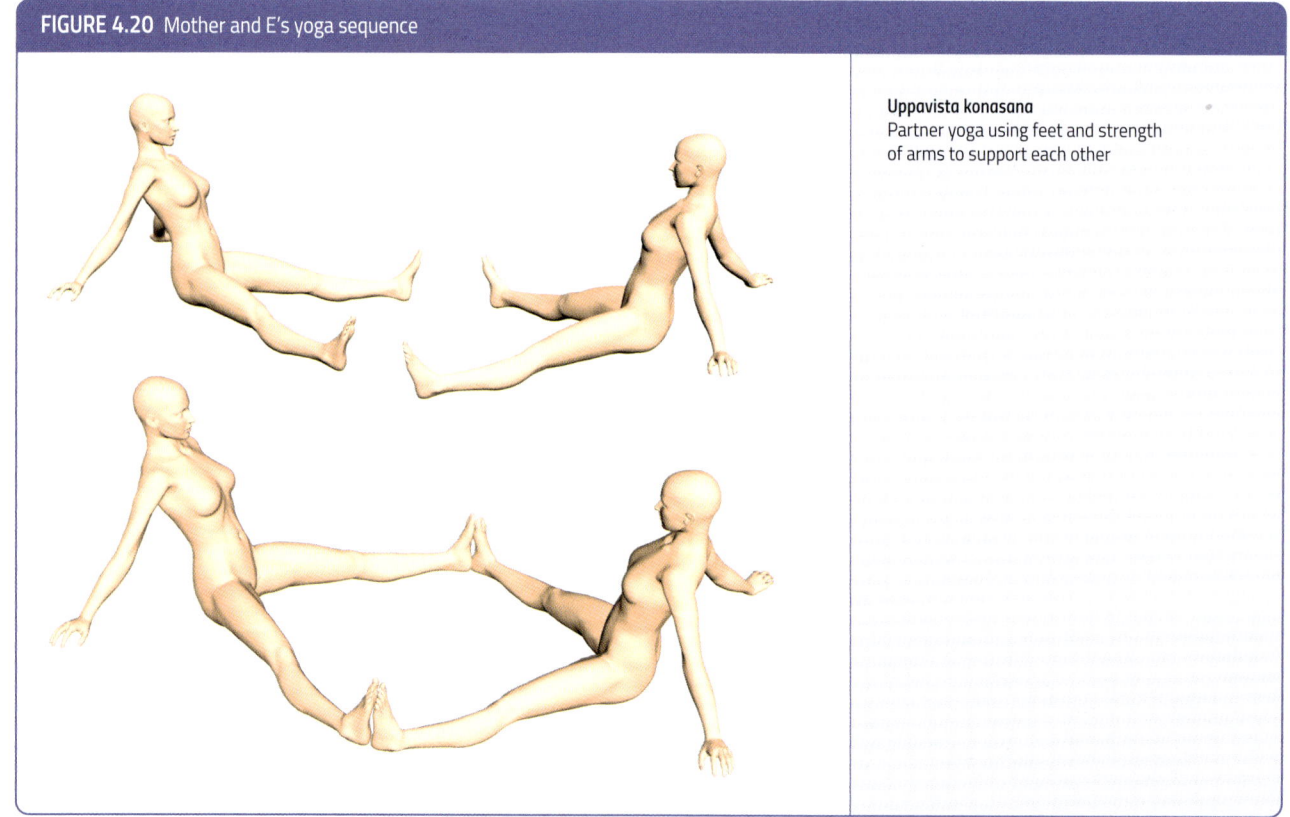

Uppavista konasana
Partner yoga using feet and strength of arms to support each other

Clinical cases: children

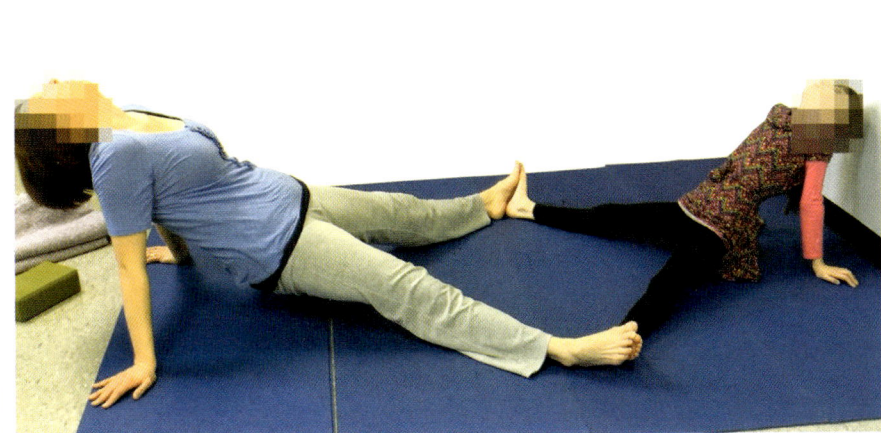

FIGURE 4.21 Mother and E with faces redacted

Reflection exercise 4.2

- In this case, save the final few sessions, there was a notable absence of the father. How would you have addressed this in the family yoga therapy/art therapy sessions?
- Given the family issues, E's diagnosis and health issues, how do you feel this case might have been affected if E and the family embraced an Ayurvedic lifestyle, which they did not explore?
- Imagine yourself combining yoga therapy with expressive arts (art, dance, music, narrative, play or similar expressive art therapies). What expressive art would you use to aid this family into co-creation and healthy functioning?

Case study 4

10-year-old with ADHD (child custody case) and telehealth

Background and history

This case of 'A' will be discussed from several vantages: ethical, legal, psychological and supervisory. Only I was actually involved in seeing the child and his family. However, as the case moved towards the court system and I was asked to be an 'expert witness' in the case, I sought out the supervision of my friend and colleague, Dr Marcia Sue Cohen-Liebman, a forensic art therapy expert in testifying for the legal system.

It is important to note that part of the therapy I conducted involved telehealth with the child's (estranged) biological mother. Additionally, I discussed the complexity of the case via both telephone and email with Dr Cohen-Liebman. I had signed consent forms allowing me to communicate with A's educational members, all lawyers involved in the case, the child's law guardian, the judge, A's primary care physician and Dr Cohen-Liebman.

Chapter four

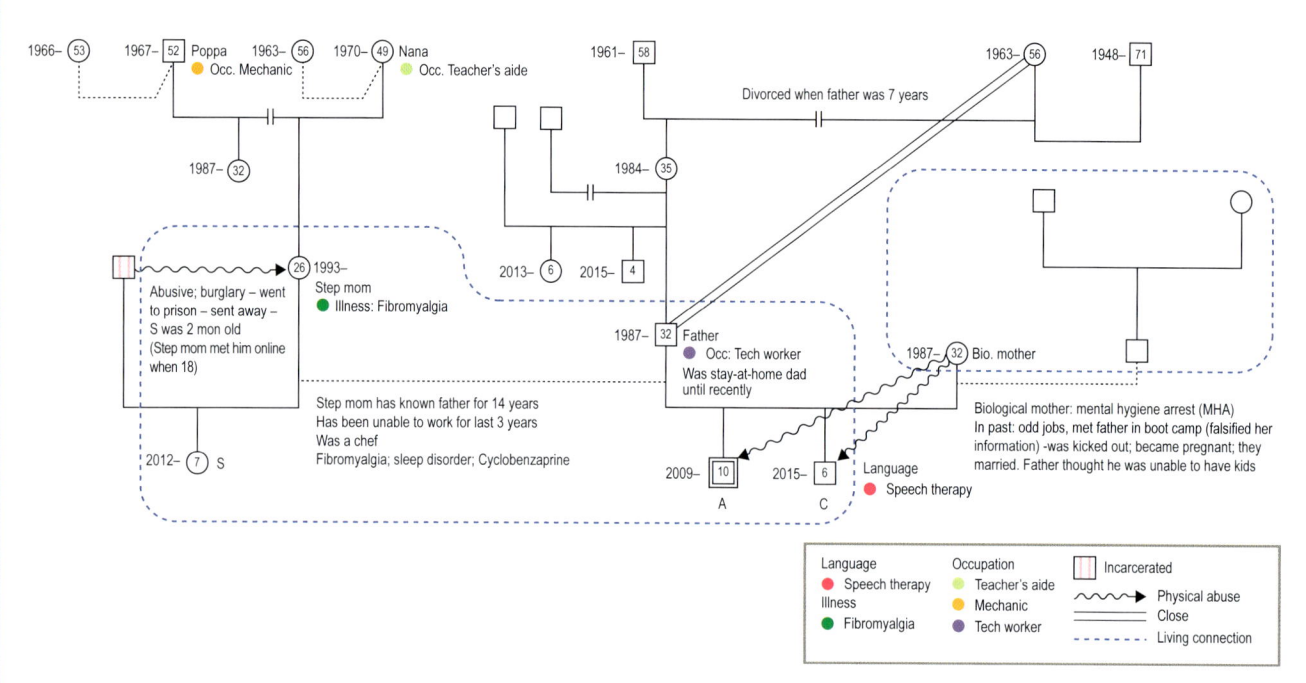

FIGURE 4.22 A's genogram

Because the biological father's insurance company did not cover my services, I accepted this case at a reduced rate due to the adverse conditions which affected A. As can be seen in the genogram (Butler 2008, McGoldrick et al 2008) (Fig. 4.22) this complicated case included severe neglect and abuse by the biological mother and her fiancé.

Based on Child Protective Service reports, at the age of 6, A had been malnourished, was not toilet trained, was left in urine-soaked diapers and was living in squalor with his 3-year-old brother (C) and biological mother. The caseworker's report included allegations of 'inadequate guardianship, food, clothing and shelter,' citing that the mother's trailer was in 'deplorable condition and there was no food in the kitchen and the floors were covered with garbage and other debris'. Fortunately, due to C's age he had little memory of this time.

> **Nota Bene**
>
> It is important to note that I did not receive this information until just before the case went to court, approximately 4 months after the initial intake.

Technology employed

Beyond the use of telehealth with the biological mother, I employed the BetterMind app (a suite of psychological assessments) to ascertain efficacy of sessions and to track changes over time.

Clinical cases: children

Specifically, the psychological assessments I conducted on A were the Spence's Children Anxiety Scale (self-report) and the DASS-21 (Depression Anxiety Stress Scale–Short Form).

It is important to note that the BetterMind app allows a practitioner to conduct the assessments remotely between sessions. This acts as a barometer between sessions should the clinician wish to use the app in this format. Patients can take the assessments on their computers, smart phones and/or tablets.

When the mother handed the care of her children to the father, she left for the midwest and had intermittent Skype contact with the children for approximately 4 years. Then, after 4 years of absence, she arrived in town and demanded an unsupervised, 2-week visitation with both children.

Intake with father and stepmother

At intake, A was 10 years old and in an educational environment with a 6:1 ratio (children: staff). Many of the children in his educational setting had severe developmental lags and emotional issues. While A had initially been referred to this educational setting because of aggressive outbursts, his educational functioning was at a 6th grade level for both reading and math. At the time of intake, A's biological father and stepmother were unsuccessful in getting A moved from his special educational level into a mainstream classroom. Additionally, the biological mother and father were involved in a legal dispute in which the biological father was seeking full custody of his sons and was attempting to block visitation by the biological mother.

Updates prior to court date

Using the Spence's Children Anxiety Scale (SCAS) self-report, A scored in the clinically significant range for:

- Social phobia
- Physical injury fears
- Generalized anxiety disorder
- (Raw Score = 38, percentile = 81.3)

A's total scores indicated greater severity of anxiety symptoms. These scores are also converted into percentiles based on age and gender from normative samples reported on the SCAS website (www.scaswebsite.com). Percentile scores of more than 84 for any subscale score or the total SCAS score indicates clinically significant anxiety symptoms.

During the initial session, I asked A if he knew why he was seeing his biological mother. He blurted out that she made him look at pictures on the internet (e.g. he stated that he was forced to look at images of 'vaginas' which he found 'disgusting'). He also admitted that he became so anxious in school over possibly disappointing his father and stepmother that he considered 'hurting (himself) with a knife'. It was later explained to A that suicidal ideation, self-harm or harm towards others had to be reported to his parents. This was done via a HIPAA-compliant telehealth therapy session with both his biological father and stepmother present. I also urged A to share these thoughts with his biological father and stepmother should they arise again.

During this same session, the kinetic family drawing was conducted (Burns and Kaufmann

Chapter four

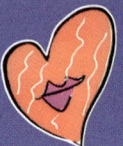 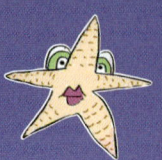

1972) (Fig. 4.23). A's response indicated developmental delays that seemed to be emotionally based since he read at the 6th grade level (Lowenfeld and Brittain 1987). The drawing was created from a bird's eye perspective. A close-up of how he drew his family is 'seen from the top'. A explained that all family members were 'hanging onto the outside of the car', and that he was inside visible from the moon roof in the van. His separation of himself contained by the family van suggests a

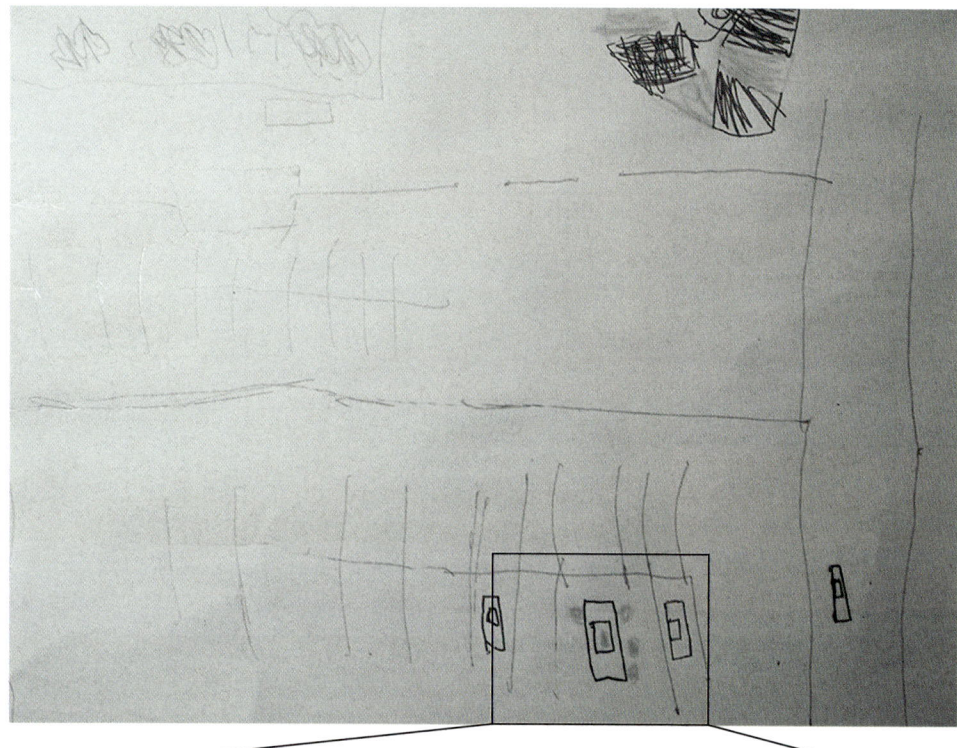

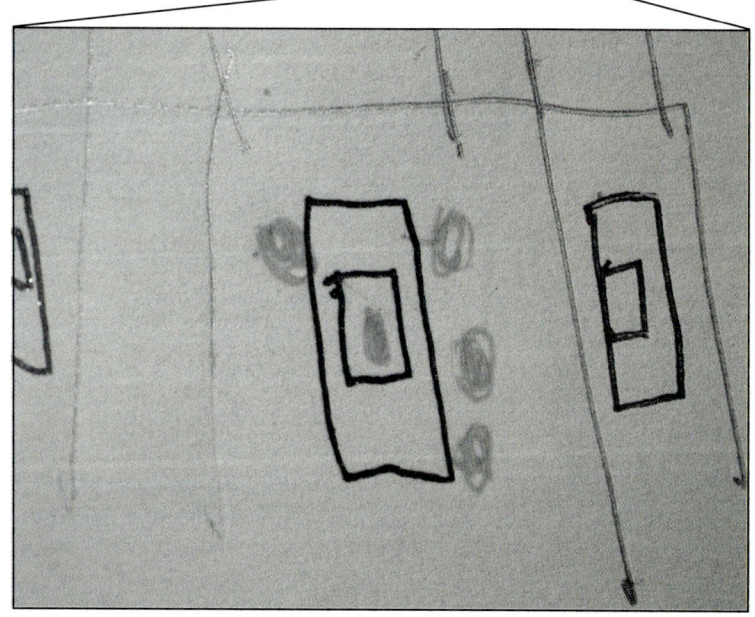

FIGURE 4.23 A's kinetic family drawing (top) and close-up (bottom)

Clinical cases: children

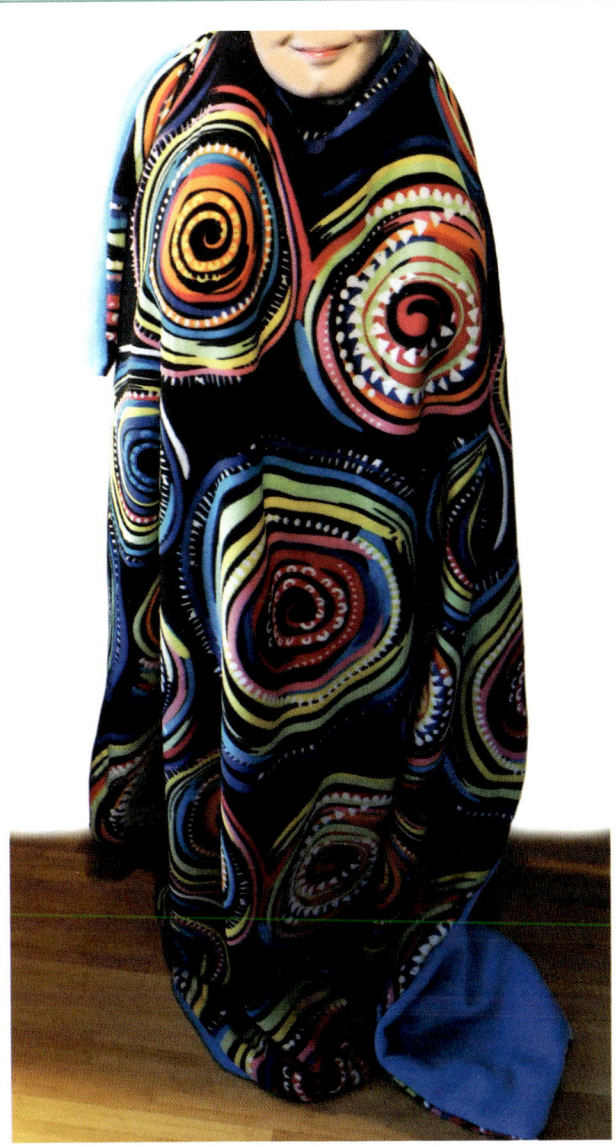

FIGURE 4.24 A inside his blanket

Developmental and psychological assessments

A summation of all psychological testing (the Bender Gestalt Visual Motor Integration Test II, the Spence Children's Anxiety Scale and the DASS-21 will be reported in three components: (1) developmental and psychological updates, (2) significant session summations, and (3) recommendations.

Results for A's Bender Gestalt Visual Motor Integration Test II:

- Raw score 27
- Standard score 126
- T-score conversion 67

This placed A at the high end of children his age with a percentile rank of 95.22%. On the motor test and perception test, A had perfect scores of 12 and 10 respectively, placing him in the top 1% for children his age. Due to time constraints, the recall subtest of the copy phase of the test was not administered. Nonetheless, frequent erasures and poor planning (the last two designs were executed on the back) suggested impulsivity and aggressive tendencies.

Results for the Spence Children's Anxiety Scale – Child (SCAS-Child) (Fig. 4.25) were that:

- A scored as being in the clinically significant range for separation anxiety and social phobia
- A scored as being below the clinical range for: total anxiety; obsessive compulsive; panic attack and agoraphobia; physical injury fears; generalized anxiety disorder.

heightened need for protection and containment. After he created this, he asked me if I could help him make a 'blanket', again suggesting a need for containment and comfort (Burns and Kaufmann 1972, Cohen-Liebman 1997, 2002, 2003, Gussak and Cohen-Liebman 2001, Horovitz 2014, Hulse 1951, 1952, Oster and Crone 2004). It took a few weeks to complete his reversible blanket, shown in Figure 4.24, where A is cloaked inside.

A's social phobia scores, separation anxiety and physical injury scores increased – this may have been reflective of excess bullying in the classroom. On the other hand, panic/agoraphobia and generalized anxiety scores decreased since the last testing date and may be the result of feeling safer in his home and the family support he was receiving in the care of his biological father and stepmother.

Chapter four

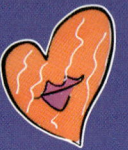

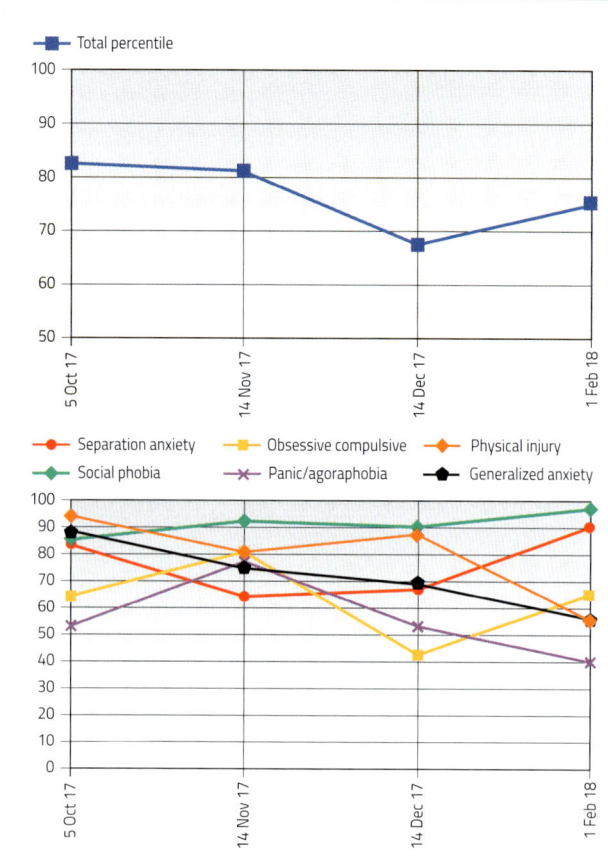

FIGURE 4.25 SCAS-Child results for A

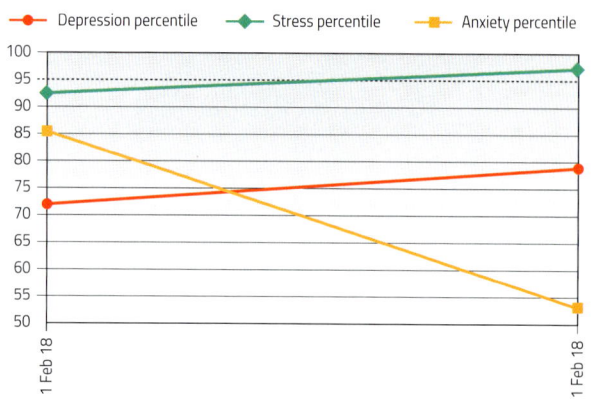

FIGURE 4.26 DASS-21 score results for A

Looking at A's DASS-21 results relative to the sample population (Fig. 4.26), A was in the:

- Mild range for depression
- Normal range for anxiety
- Severe range for stress.

When A took this test prior to the looming court date he may have been experiencing depression and stress as a result of the impending decisions, which were discussed during the session. He also seemed very stressed by his educational environment and badgering by other children in his class.

Artistic level of development

Artistically, A was functioning at the high end of the Gang Age of Development (except for his KFD, which is generally regressed for most since familial issues cause emotional and generally cognitive arrestment (Burns and Kaufmann 1972, Horovitz 2014)).

Significant session summations

There were a total of 12 sessions: five family sessions with the father, stepmother and A; one telehealth session with the biological mother and A; two sessions with the stepmother and A; and four individual sessions with A. There was also one telehealth individual session with the biological mother. When it became clear that the biological mother was fighting for custody and visitation, her lawyer suggested that we meet for an individual telehealth appointment. What was clear from that meeting was that she seemed unfit to take care of her children, yet she intended to go to court to ascertain visitation and custody rights. The previous agreement had stipulated no out-of-state visitation and supervised visitation. But she had hired a lawyer to contest that decision.

Having both the father and stepmother present for family sessions allowed me to observe their parenting skills (as well as A) in a more natural environment. Based on my observations, my findings were presented to all the respective lawyers and the child's law guardian. Based on my observation of the father, I unequivocally stated

Clinical cases: children

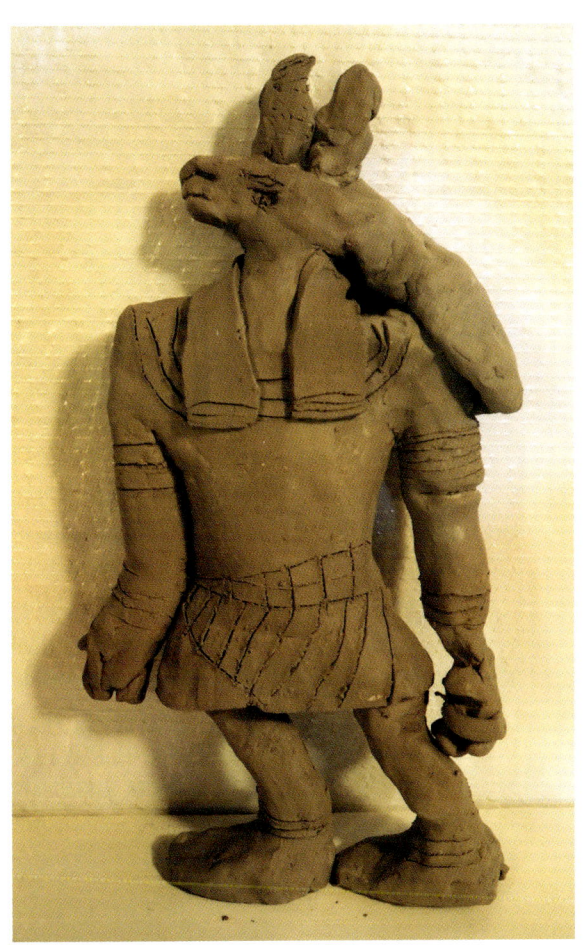

FIGURE 4.27 Anubis clay sculpture, approximately 11" high, conducted during several family sessions with A, father and stepmother interacting

that he was not in need of parenting classes and the stepmother presented as a model parent. But I could not make this same recommendation for the biological mother.

Prior to the telehealth session with A's biological mother, in a family session, A insisted that he was not ready for another telehealth session with the biological mother. Indeed, he reiterated his position that his father, stepmother, brother, and stepsister were whom he considered to be his 'family'. The sculpture of Anubis (Fig. 4.27) took over three family sessions to complete. He had

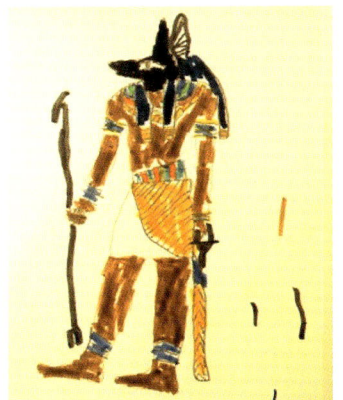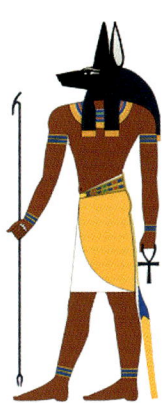

FIGURE 4.28 Anubis sketch (and Wikipedia image) completed during telehealth session with biological mother

created the sketch for Anubis (Fig. 4.28) during his telehealth session with his biological mother.

Partner yoga therapy session with stepmother and A

Intermittent yoga sessions occurred with A and his stepmother but the most powerful was a partner yoga session. A arrived exceptionally anxious about the upcoming court date and so I suggested some coherent breathing (Elliot 2005) as well as some preliminary meditation. Then we did some partner yoga as indicated in Figure 4.29. Immediately after this session, A had visibly calmed down and relaxed.

At the end of the sequence, I placed essential oils on both A's and his stepmother's temples, massaged the back of their necks and then played the song, *An Ending, A Beginning*, by artist Dustin O'Halloran (2013). *Nada*, or yoga for sound, has a way of cutting through emotions, especially after yoga. The right song chosen for *savāsana* can often unleash a flood of emotions. In this case, when A sat up post *savāsana* and I asked him how he felt, it was clear from his demeanor and affect that a shift had occurred. His eyes welled with tears. His comment, 'relieved', said it all. Yoga was the new maxim: rinse and repeat.

Chapter four

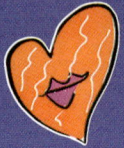
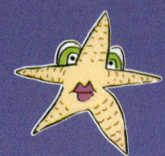

FIGURE 4.29 Partner yoga sequence with A and stepmother

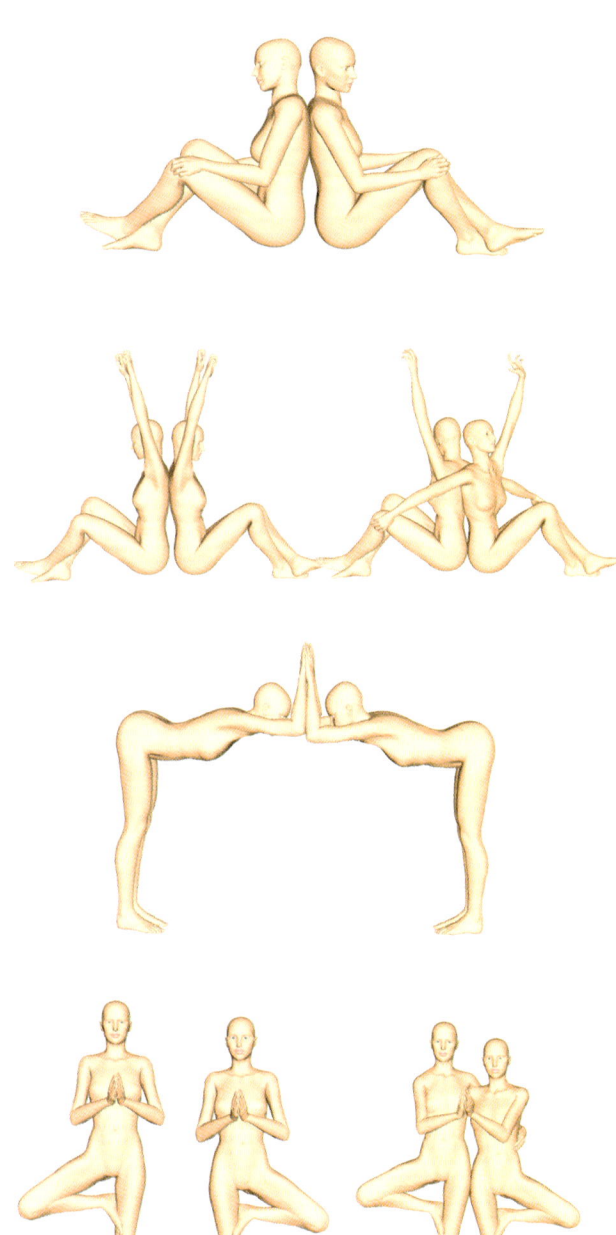

Partner breathing
Start in a seated position with legs crossed at the ankles or shins, with your backs resting against each other.
Rest hands on thighs or knees and allow yourself to feel and connect with your partner.
Begin to notice how the breath feels as you inhale and exhale; especially notice how the back of your ribcage feels against your partner's. Begin to 'breath alternate' with your partner, so as you inhale, they exhale. Practise for 3–5 minutes. This is a gentle way to connect with your partner, helps open the heart and is an easy way to connect with your breath.

Partner twist
Sit back-to-back with your partner in a cross-legged position. As you both inhale, reach your arms up by your ears. Exhale as you both twist to the right, resting your right hand on your partner's left knee or thigh. Lengthen your spine up on each exhale. Stay in the twist for a minute then switch to the other side.
Benefits: Increases spinal flexibility, stretches and strengthens external and internal oblique muscles.

Temple pose
Start by facing each other in a standing position. Set feet under hips, then inhale, extend arms overhead and begin to hinge forward at the hips until you meet hands with your partner. Slowly begin to fold forward, bringing elbows, forearms and hands together so they rest against each other and release chest and belly toward the floor.
Hold for 5–7 breaths, then slowly walk towards each other, bringing torso upright and release arms down. This helps open the shoulders and chest, which is the seat of our energetic heart.

Partner Vrikasana (tree pose)
Start by standing next to each other facing in the same direction. Standing a few feet apart, bring palms towards each other with the arms in a 'T' shape, or draw the elbows together in a cactus shape. Begin to shift onto right foot and have your partner shift weight onto their left foot. Draw the opposite leg into tree pose by bending the knee and bringing foot to the ankle, calf or inner thigh of the standing leg. Balance for 5–7 breaths, then release and turn around to face in the opposite direction and repeat on the opposite side.
Benefits: Balance poses encourage focus, and this specific pose invites playful focus while being a gentle hip opener.

Clinical cases: children

Recommendations

Severe neglect issues (such as A's) take a long time to resolve. A continued to reject the idea of visitation with his biological mother. Without resolve of his anger, A might experience emotional and developmental arrestment. Therefore, I advised that supervised family therapy sessions with his biological mother be added to his treatment when A was ready. Based on my telehealth appointment with the biological mother, she was attempting to improve her lifestyle and choices that affected her children, but nonetheless her presenting behavior was emotionally fragile. She appeared psychologically unprepared to see either of her children despite her verbalization of intent to do so, and she was visibly shaken and upset during the telehealth appointment with A. Upon meeting her at court, it was clear that she suffered from trichotillomania – she had no eyebrows and almost no eyelashes (this was not visible via telehealth as there were no close-ups with the computer camera).

Because of A's emphatic protestations, I recommended that any visitation granted to the mother be supervised in order to provide him the emotional buffer that he needed. Forcing unsupervised visitation could prove deleterious to A's psychological and developmental well-being, and in fact reverse his current progress and adaptation to his present home environment.

I also suggested a psychological evaluation of the mother by her psychiatrist (and/or the medical doctor who was dispensing her medication) to ascertain her readiness for unsupervised visitation. Should that examiner deem her prepared for unsupervised visitation, I recommended several telehealth sessions occur with both A and the mother to ascertain readiness for such visits by both.

Conclusion and discussion

What is abundantly clear is that any therapist needs to be aware of the legal issues surrounding child abuse and neglect. My dear friend and colleague Dr Marcia Sue Cohen-Liebman (2018) suggested being abreast of any of John EB Myers writings (specifically Myers 1998), since knowing the legal information if placed in a position of being called either as a lay or expert witness requires ample preparation and, in some instances, separate counsel. While I was surprised that the prosecutor refused to accept my status as an expert witness, the judge trumped the situation: he agreed to my augmentation and suggestions for visitation by the biological mother as agreed upon by all parties. By doing this, in some sense A's rights were minimally protected.

Nevertheless, what is regrettably clear is that the law often does not protect the interests of the child, and in this case the child's legal guardian not only sided with the biological mother but also did not represent the child nor his testimony during court. Indeed, the father's actions (obtaining custody of his children once he learned of the abuse at the hands of the biological mother) seemed to be lost in the decision of this case. Because the case was being decided '*De Novo*' (or devoid of the facts behind the case), these actions never came up. In this respect, the outcome was a tragedy. Had this gone to trial, and had the facts been heard, the outcome may have been different and indeed the children's rights might have been more amply protected.

Chapter four

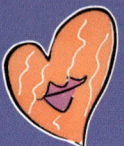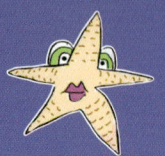

Combining art therapy, yoga therapy and specific apps (Genogram Analytics and BetterMind Healthcare) to track the efficacy of the sessions (which included cognitive behavioral therapy, art therapy and yoga therapy) allowed me to ascertain best practices when working with this child and his family.

To quote Mae Thompson, 'Grace is how you look, when no one is looking'. May I continue to be guided by those words, and those of my teachers.

> ### Reflection exercise 4.3
>
> This case (like so many I have experienced) rocked my world. I felt so defenseless after talking to my colleague (Dr Cohen-Liebman). It made me wish my graduate studies had armed me with legal expertise. I recall admitting to Dr Cohen-Liebman that had I been younger I would have returned to law school just to be educated. The system seemed so twisted. The last time I felt this way was over 20 years ago and I wrote about it subsequently (Horovitz 2005). I contemplated leaving the clinical field. But Dr Irene Rosner-David reminded me in a recent phone call that I have touched so many lives and for the greater good. I knew what she meant but it still left me with this gnawing feeling: is it enough? Are we ever enough? So, ask yourself, how can you be enough to those damaged souls that come before you for help? Write about it, create around it – may it offer you some solace.

References

Bertrando P (2007) The Dialogical Therapist: Dialogue in Systemic Practice. New York, NY: Routledge.

Boscolo L and Bertrando P (1992) The reflexive loop of past, present and future in systemic therapy and consultation. Family Process 31(2): 119–130.

Burns RC and Kaufman S H (1972) Actions, Styles and Symbols in Kinetic Family Drawings (K-F-D): An Interpretive Manual. New York, NY: Brunner/Mazel.

Butler J (2008) The family diagram and genogram: comparison and contrasts. American Journal of Family Therapy 36(3): 169–180.

Cohen-Liebman MS (1997) Forensic Art Therapy. Preconference course presented at the Annual Conference of the American Art Therapy Association. Milwaukee, WI: American Art Therapy Association.

Cohen-Liebman MS (2002) Intro to art therapy. In: Giardino AP and Giardino ER (eds) Recognition of Child Abuse for the Mandated Reporter, 3rd edn. St. Louis, MO: GW Medical Publishing.

Cohen-Liebman MS (2003) Using drawings in forensic investigations of child sexual abuse. In: Malchiodi C (ed) Handbook of Clinical Art Therapy. New York, NY: Guilford Press.

Cohen-Liebman MS (2018) Personal communication.

Criswell E (1989) How Yoga Works: An Introduction to Somatic Yoga. Novato, CA: Freeperson Press.

Csikszentmihalyi M (1996) Creativity: Flow and the Psychology of Discovery and Invention. New York, NY: Harper Perennial.

Damasio A (2010) Self Comes to Mind: Constructing the Conscious Brain. New York, NY: Pantheon Books.

Elliot S (2005) The New Science of Breath: Coherent Breathing for Autonomic Nervous System Balance, Health and Well-being. Allen, TX: Coherence Press, LLC.

Gantt L and Tabone C (1998) The Formal Elements of Art Therapy: The Rating Manual. Morgantown, WV: Gargoyle Press.

Gibbons K (2015) Integrating Art Therapy and Yoga Therapy. Philadelphia, PA: Jessica Kingsley Publishers.

Gladwell M (2005) Blink, the Power of Thinking Without Thinking. New York, NY: Little Brown.

Goleman D (2014) Exercising the mind to treat attention deficits. New York Times, 12 May. Available at: http://well.blogs.nytimes.com/2014/05/12/exercising-the-mind-to-treat-attention-deficits

Gussak D and Cohen-Liebman MS (2001) Investigation vs. intervention: Forensic art therapy and art therapy in forensic settings. The American Journal of Art Therapy 40(2): 123–135.

Hanna T (1986) What is somatics (Pt.2). Somatics VI(1): 39.

Hanna T (1991) What is somatics? Journal of Behavioral Optometry 2(2): 31–35.

Henley D (2002) Clayworks in Art Therapy: Plying the Sacred Circle. London, UK: Jessica Kingsley Publishers, Ltd.

Horovitz EG (1999) A Leap of Faith: the Call to Art. Springfield, IL: Charles C Thomas Ltd.

Clinical cases: children

Horovitz EG (2005) Art Therapy as Witness: A Sacred Guide. Springfield, IL: Charles C Thomas Ltd.

Horovitz EG (2011) Advanced Practice Half-Day Workshop: Healing Mind and Body: The Integration of Art Therapy and Yoga Therapy. American Art Therapy Association 42nd Annual Conference, Washington DC, 10 July.

Horovitz E G (2013) Embracing the Mind, Body and Spirit: Integrating Art Therapy and Yoga Therapy. Georgia Art Therapy Association, 5–6 April.

Horovitz EG (2014) The Art Therapists' Primer: A Clinical Guide to Writing Assessment, Diagnosis and Treatment, 2nd Edn. Springfield, IL: Charles C Thomas Ltd.

Horovitz EG (2017) Spiritual Art Therapy: An Alternate Path, 3rd Edn. Springfield, IL: Charles C Thomas Ltd.

Hulse WC (1951) The emotionally disturbed child draws his family. Family, Quarterly Journal of Child Behavior 3: 152–174.

Hulse WC (1952) Child conflict expressed through drawings. Journal of Project Technology 16: 66–79.

James W (1890) The Principles of Psychology. New York, NY: Dover Press.

Jehovah's Witnesses (2020) Why Don't Jehovah's Witnesses Accept Blood Transfusions? Available at: https://www.jw.org/en/jehovahs-witnesses/faq/jehovahs-witnesses-why-no-blood-transfusions/

Joly Y (2001) The Feldenkrais method of somatic education. International Feldenkrais Newsletter, January: 17–20.

Kearst P (2000) The invisible string. Camarillo, CA: DeVorss & Company, Publishers.

Kenny M (2002) Integrated Movement Therapy™: yoga based therapy as a viable and effective intervention for autism spectrum and related disorders. International Journal of Yoga Therapy: Vol. 12(1): 71-79.

Lowenfeld V and Brittain WL (1987) Creative and Mental Growth, 8th Edn. New Work, NY: MacMillan.

McGoldrick M, Gerson R and Petry S (2008) Genograms: Assessment and Intervention, 3rd Edn. New York, NY: WW Norton.

Myers JEB (1998) Legal Issues in Child Abuse and Neglect Practice (Interpersonal Violence: The Practice Series). Thousand Oaks, CA: Sage Publications.

Nichols MP (2007) The Essentials of Family Therapy, 3rd Edn. Boston, MA: Pearson, Allyn & Bacon.

O'Halloran D (2013) An Ending, A Beginning. Late Night Tales: Bonobo. Available at: https://nighttimestories.co.uk/

Oster GD and Crone PG (2004) Using Drawings in Assessment and Therapy: A guide for Mental Health Professionals, 2nd Edn. New York, NY: Routledge.

Pag F and Ruiz E (2017) Focusing on ADD. Yoga Journal, 5 April. Available at: https://www.yogajournal.com/lifestyle/focusing-on-a-d-d

Raoult F (2019) Personal communication.

Reynolds G (2012) How exercise could lead to a better brain, 22 April. Available at: http://www.nytimes.com/2012/04/22/magazine/how-exercise-could-lead-to-a-better-brain.html?_r=1&emc=

Schoenberg PLA, Hepark S, Can C, Berendregt HP, Buitelarr J and Speckens AEM (2013) Effects of mindfulness-based cognitive therapy on neurophysiological correlates of performance monitoring in adult attention-deficit/hyperactivity disorder. Clinical Neurophysiology 125(7): 1407–1416

Sommer Anderson F (2008) Bodies in Treatment, the Unspoken Dimension. New York, NY: Routledge Press.

Sravish AV, Tronick E, Hollenstein T and Beeghly M (2013) Dyadic flexibility during the face-to-face still-face paradigm: a dynamic systems analysis of its temporal organization. Infant Behavior and Development 36(3): 432–437.

Tronick EZ (1989) Emotions and emotional communications in infants. American Psychologist 44(2): 112.

van der Kolk B (2014) The Body Keeps the Score: Brain, Mind and Body in the Healing of Trauma. New York, NY: Penguin.

van der Kolk B (2019) Befriending your body. Available at: https://kripalu.org/resources/befriending-your-body-how-yoga-helps-heal-trauma

Wampold BE (2001) The Great Psychotherapy Debate: Models, Methods and Findings. Hillsdale, NJ: Lawrence Erlbaum.

Clinical cases: adolescents 5

It's easier to floss with barbed wire than admit you like someone in middle school.

Laurie Halse Anderson (1999)

Today's culture and adolescence

Chances are, if you are reading this, you are no longer an adolescent. Navigating in-crowds, cool kids, jocks and the have-nots was just a small part of the mayhem I encountered growing up, and when and where you grew up tinted your adolescent spectacles. But growing up now is a smorgasbord of social media ills that makes my experiences pale in comparison. Sure, there were tales about outcasts that might have been bandied about by the rumor mills, but nothing compares to the speed and velocity of today's internet and social media platforms for discharging heinous barbs and cruel comments.

When the Internet first became available to the public (in August of 1991), I doubt anyone would have predicted how nefarious it would become, yet here we are. Parents are accused of posting about their children without permission (otherwise known as 'oversharenting') (Durlofsky 2018) and some adolescents have taken them to task for doing so. According to industry statistics (Statista 2019), from the spring of 2019, the most popular social networks used by adolescents were Snapchat (41%), Instagram (35%), Twitter (6%), Facebook (6%) and Pinterest (1%). There are more obscure social media sites popping up all the time, perhaps to keep adult users out and adolescents in control. One of which mentioned in this next case is Houseparty, a group video chat that is closed to a specific circle of friends that the user establishes. What is also important to understand is not only the 'cancel culture' (when one is rejected by a group of people, generally through social media) (Yar and Bromwich 2019) and how that impacts individual sense of Self, but also the stigma of 'aloneliness' (Ratner and Hamilton 2015), as discussed by Higgs (2019), which is different from 'FOMO' (fear of missing out) and 'JOMO' (joy of missing out).

According to Higgs (2019), the concept of 'aloneliness' or choosing to spend time alone can have mental, emotional and social benefits. Alas, reaping those rewards is dependent on electing to spend time alone. In a culture that confuses being alone with loneliness, the ability to appreciate time by yourself is often negatively processed. On the contrary, identifying your need for solitude and recharging by yourself, can improve your ability to handle stress and burnout.

Case study 1

13-year-old female with type 1 diabetes (T1DM) and her family

If the aforementioned issues weren't enough of a challenge for the average adolescent, along with the pressures of drugs, sex and gender identity, in this first case the co-morbid influences of type 1 diabetes mellitus (T1DM) (onset aged 4 years) and hidradenitis suppurativa (HS) compounded and fed into 'R's depression and ongoing anxiety (Lerner and Steinberg 2009). And as will be seen, the familial background also greatly influenced the parameters of this case.

Background and history

I have been seeing R and her family for about 2 years. Due to the nature of R's medical history and ongoing issues (anxiety, depression and co-morbidity of T1DM and HS), there are constant challenges. Compounding that is the familial background (Fig. 5.1) and several emotional and physical challenges resulting from her upbringing and recent life events.

Let's start with a little historical background at intake. R was born around her mother's age 19 years. R's father had dual citizenship and so her mother didn't want him involved in the relationship for fear that he might take R to another country. The father's parents remained distant (until recently) and wanted nothing to do with the mother or R. It is important to note how close in age R and her mother are – more sessions than

Chapter five

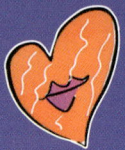
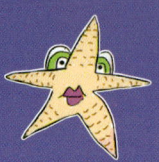

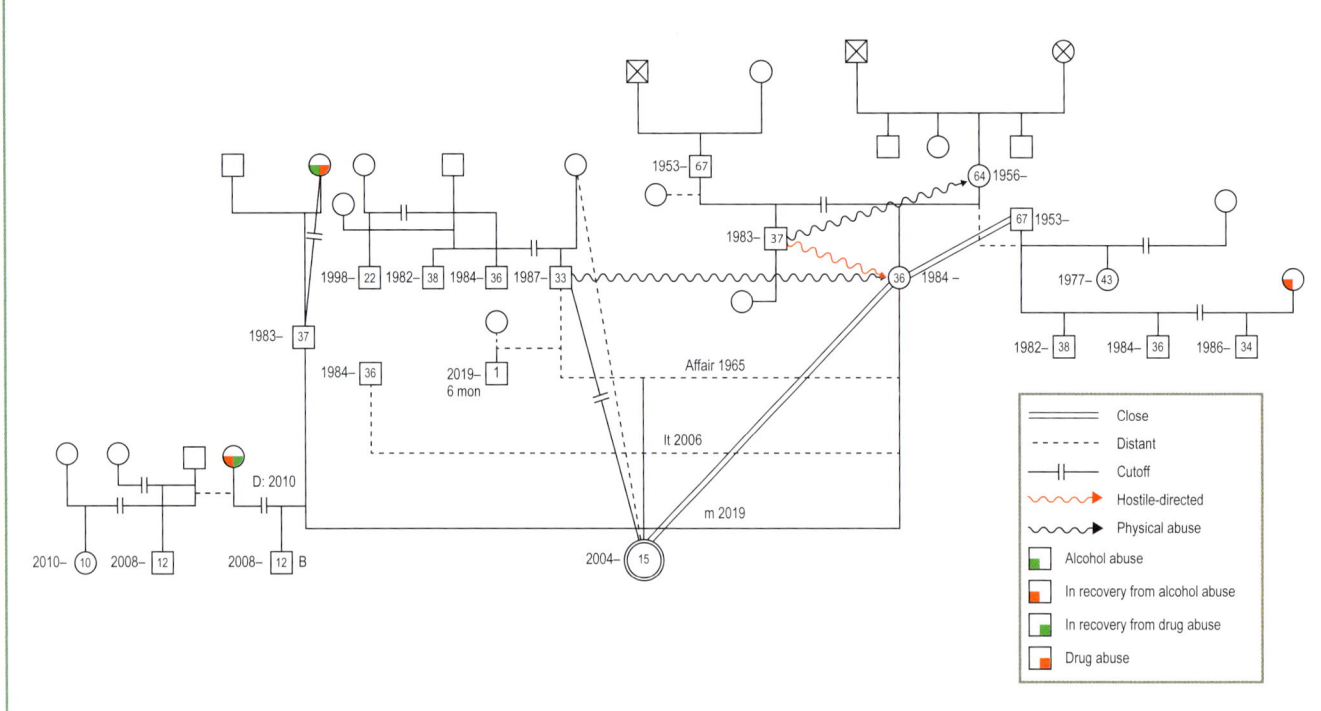

FIGURE 5.1 R's genogram

not have included the mother, since sometimes she felt more like a 'sister'. The father had nothing to do with R until R's age 9 years. He became overly involved for about 2 weeks and then dropped out of her life completely until recently, when she started therapy with me (aged 13). His involvement was intermittent at best and caused R to be confused and feel rejected by his overtures. Her relationship (or lack thereof) with her father became part of our treatment objectives, however R has remained unwilling to have him directly involved in family sessions, as detailed below in the significant sessions section. Recently, R's mother took her father to court when he had a baby with his girlfriend (who apparently looks and acts like R's mother). He now pays child support for R.

Before mother's marriage to R's stepfather, she had been living with an ex-fiancé, LT, from R's birth to her age of 6.5 years. Mother claimed she loved him but when he had an affair with her best friend that severed the relationship.

At intake, R was residing with her mother, her mother's fiancé (now stepfather – they married in 2019) and stepfather's son, B. Of import is stepfather's background. He had been in the armed services and was deployed 2 months after B's birth. For 8 months, the stepfather did not know the whereabouts of his ex-wife, who had been toting B to drug houses and exchanging sex for drugs. When the stepfather learned of this, he urged his parents to intercede and assume care of B until he returned from duty.

Skipping ahead about a year: R's mother was waitressing and met the stepfather and B at the restaurant where she worked. They dated for about 6 months, during which B was described as

Clinical cases: adolescents

'defiant'. R was 7 years old when she was introduced to her stepfather and B. Mother and stepfather moved in together shortly after that and although mother had been 'engaged' to the stepfather, she stated her resistance to getting married (they had been together for about 6 years at intake). Part of her hesitation seemed linked to her ex-fiancé, boyfriend LT, who still had an amicable connection with R. Having never parked her feelings regarding the betrayal, R's mother hesitated to fully commit to the stepfather. Her reasoning for finally committing will become clear in the significant session descriptions. Currently, mother is employed as a primary schoolteacher and has a master's degree, and stepfather is employed as a mechanic at a local firm.

Regarding R's medical background (see Fig. 5.1), it is important to note that when her T1DM was discovered at 4 years of age it was traumatic for all, since her mother had to chase R around to get her to take her injections and test her glucose levels. R is presently overweight. Reportedly, she 'steals' or sneaks food, especially if she is home 'sick' and tending to herself. So, her eating disorder has also been addressed in the sessions.

According to Lotstein et al (2013), transferring from pediatric to adult care is associated with an increased risk of poor glycemic control at follow-up. Their findings suggest that young adults need additional support when moving to adult care. However, R's mother did a bit too much of the caretaking (e.g. waking R up in the middle of the night to check her glucose levels) and her inability to offer the reins to her daughter cemented their enmeshment/co-dependent behavior. At a time when rebellion and individuation (Mahler 1968) is the natural order of adolescence, mother's behavior negated this. R therefore rebelled in her own ways: getting 'sick' on a regular basis, lying about completion of her homework and hiding aspects of her social life from mother.

Yoga and diabetes

Since I wanted to incorporate yoga into this case, I researched and scoured the literature. I looked for books that were fairly accessible so I could loan them to R and her mother. Thinking that American Diabetes Association publications would be a good place to start, I purchased Kay and Nelson's (2015) book. While this book was easy to digest and break into manageable sequences, I was left feeling underwhelmed by it. Nevertheless, I gave the book to R and her mother to take home after the second session so that they could browse through and hopefully develop an interest in yoga management for diabetes. Simultaneously, I had been using this and other books with an adult case with T1DM, so it seemed a likely place to start.

An older study by Sahay (1986) seemed fairly restrictive in its particular recommended asanas, but reported significant control of T1DM and T2DM: 'fasting and postprandial blood glucose levels came down significantly and good glycemic status was maintained for long periods of time' (e.g. infection and ketosis were significantly reduced). Sahay's protocol included the following asanas: *dhanurāsana* (bow pose), *ardha matsayendrāsana* (half-spiral twisted pose), *bhujangāsana* (cobra pose), *naukasana* (boat pose), *halāsana* (plow pose), *vajrāsana* (thunderbolt/kneeling pose) and *pachimotanāsana* (forward folding pose) along with *prāṇayāma* (breath control practices) (Sahay 1986:123). In the article it stated that the subjects practiced four different types of *prāṇayāma*, but it did not detail which exercises were employed.

In a more generic study by Kahley-Isley et al (2010), the authors reviewed yoga as complementary therapy for children and adolescents, including those with medical disorders. However, this review covered only T2DM in children and adolescents in need of lowering their body mass index (BMI). The protocol used was an Ashtanga yoga

Chapter five

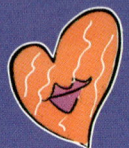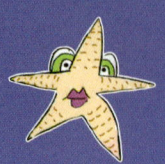

class (modified to decrease the physical intensity so the children/adolescents did not fatigue). The duration was 75 minutes, three times a week for 12 weeks. Participants 'displayed positive outcomes of weight loss, improved self-concept, and improved anxiety symptoms'. The authors suggested that the findings should be considered preliminary as the small sample sizes and interventions lacked appropriate controls, but nevertheless, the case studies seemed promising.

In a more recent study by Innes et al (2016), yoga was reviewed for T2DM. Results indicated that yoga might reduce stress (specifically on metabolic function, neuroendocrine status and inflammatory response). It was also postulated that yoga might modulate the autonomic nervous system (ANS) by stimulating the vagal system and target areas of the brain associated with cognition and mood. However, according to Jeter and McCall (2017), while evidence supported improvements, there were methodological problems with the studies and, 'clear reporting standards were needed to confirm and elucidate the potential therapeutic benefits of yoga programs for adults with T2DM'.

And so, the research continues. Suggested is that improved BMI, self-concepts, lowered anxiety and modulation of the ANS (via vagal system stimulation) may result from yoga in T2DM, but clearly more standardized studies are needed.

Zinman's (2017) book is graphically appealing, personally relatable (recounting the author's T1DM diagnosis aged 42 and her search for alternative therapies) and informative (detailing yoga sequences, diet and medication to manage T1DM and T2DM). For the layperson, she accessibly outlines the Ayurvedic approach of personalities and body types (*vata*, *pitta* and *kapha*). At the book's end, yoga sequences designed to relieve specific symptoms of diabetes are connected to these Ayurvedic principles. While the author was not an adolescent, both R and her mother benefited greatly from this read.

Finally, Iyengar (1979) suggests additional *asanas* (p.494) to those already described. He also recommended *nādi sodhana prāṇāyāma* (alternate nostril breathing) and *uddīyāna* and *nauli* (both *bandhas* (binds) and purifications). He explained that in *uddīyāna* the *prāṇa* 'moves from the abdomen to the head... increases gastric fire and eliminates toxins in the digestive tract' (p.425) and in *nauli* (a *kriya*/purification) the 'abdominal recti are strengthened' (p.428). Because these are fairly advanced practices and R's physical system had not been fully developed, I chose not to teach her the *uddīyāna* and *nauli* practices, although they could certainly be added to a seasoned adult's yoga practice.

In R's case, I used patient self-report on psychological instruments before and after yoga therapy, art therapy and psychotherapy modalities. Because I kept very detailed notes on all my sessions, I could target best practices with this specific adolescent. It is important to note that in Year 2 of our work together, R found great solace by attending a summer camp for diabetic children and adolescents. All the camp counselors had either T1DM or T2DM (and were thus role models). R served as a counselor the second week for the children's camp after having attended the camp for adolescents. She made strong connections at this camp and still connects with her peers through the app 'Houseparty'. While R had been directed to various online support groups (e.g. Taking Control of Your Diabetes, www.tcoyd.org; Everyday Health, www.everydayhealth.com: Juvenile

Clinical cases: adolescents

Diabetes Research Fund, www.jdrf.org and similar organizations), she fared better in a face-to-face environment (McCoy 2009). This was the beginning of R's 'aloneliness' stage, rejecting unhealthy relationships and reducing online communication as a primary source of functioning (Statista 2019).

When people ask me for specific how-to recipes for working with this or any population, my stock answer is, 'it depends'. According to the Wellcome Trust Sanger Institute (2017), researchers anticipate being able to use technologies derived from stem-cell research to treat cancer, spinal cord injuries and muscle damage among a number of other diseases and impairments, so perhaps someday individualized treatment might, in fact, be the right approach to treatment of T1DM or any disease. I choose to operate via a case-to-case (heuristic, phenomenological) method, tailoring treatments for each individual, rather than rigidly following prescribed regimens. While this is perhaps considered out of step with data-driven methods, I find this methodology satisfying; and while the primary gain is the patient's, I obtain a secondary gain as clinician. By this, I am not disabling patient change but in fact walking the path alongside my patient, and this transformation is affecting me as well. These are the reasons that I write, to share these stories with you. Should you come across like patients in your journey, I hope these cases will aid you in your trajectory towards wellness.

Significant sessions: year one

To date, R and I have met for 36 sessions over a 2-year period. There have been numerous interruptions and R generally comes (with or without a family member) every other week. In the second session, R arrived greatly upset with one of her schoolmates. Practicing how she could verbally address this, we worked on some letter writing. Then to lessen her anxiety, we practiced belly breath and coherent breath. We leafed through the Kay and Nelson (2015) book and practiced a variation of the first sequence (belly breath, Elliot's coherent breath (Elliot 2005) (not in the book), tāḍasāna (mountain pose), vṛkṣasāna (tree pose), ardha matsyendrāsana 1 (seated twisted pose), modified setu bandha sarvāṇgāsana (bridge pose) and śavāsana (rest or corpse pose). This was quite a bit for our first yoga/art therapy session. R was anxious and depressed upon entrance, but after she completed the yoga sequence (Fig. 5.2) followed by her artwork (Fig. 5.3), her depression, anxiety and stress scores (DASS-21) dropped significantly by session's end (Fig. 5.4). I suggested that her mother purchase the book for her.

The next session, R's mother joined for yoga and we started with coherent breath, ujjayi (ocean breath) and then moved onto nādi sodhana prāṇāyāma (alternate nostril breathing). The yoga sequence is detailed in Figure 5.5.

Involving the mother in the therapy was dicey: R clearly needed her own therapy and while mother tried to focus on R's issues, her own issues inevitably spilled out. The psychotherapeutic aspects of the session were almost symbiotic in nature, as they were dually directed, aimed at mother's issues and R's. Mother was frustrated with: (1) R's behavior (lying, sneaking food, lack of control regarding her T1DM), (2) R's bouts with HS – debilitating sores common in T1DM patients, which resulted in R's frequent hospitalizations, (3) her own commitment phobia (with fiancé, now stepfather), (4) anxiety, and (5) enmeshment with R.

R's issues, beyond the management of her T1DM and HS, were: (1) her eating disorder (specifically bingeing) and lying, (2) depression and

Chapter five

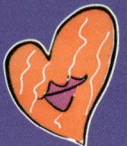
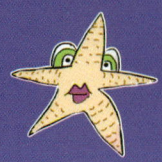

FIGURE 5.2 Yoga sequence 1

	Krama inhale (segmented inhalation) Energizing effect, useful for increasing breathing capacity.	Begin to inhale expanding the top of the chest, pause for a moment; continue to inhale expanding the rib cage, pause for a moment, complete your inhale expanding the abdomen. Exhale slowly and smoothly.
	Krama exhale (segmented exhalation) Calming effect, useful for increasing breathing capacity.	Inhale slowly and smoothly. Begin to exhale, contracting your abdomen above the pubic bone, pause for a moment; continue to exhale, contracting the abdomen around the navel, pause for a moment; finish your exhale contracting the muscles between the navel and sternum.
	Tadasana (mountain pose) and **Vṛkṣāsana** (tree pose).	Tree pose was first modified (using a chair) until R felt steady. Then it was repeated without the chair.
	Ardha matsyendrāsana and **Setu bandha sarvāṅgāsana**	Simple seated twisted pose, followed by bridge pose.
	Śavāsana (rest or corpse pose)	Final relaxation pose with blanket or pillow under head for support.

Clinical cases: adolescents

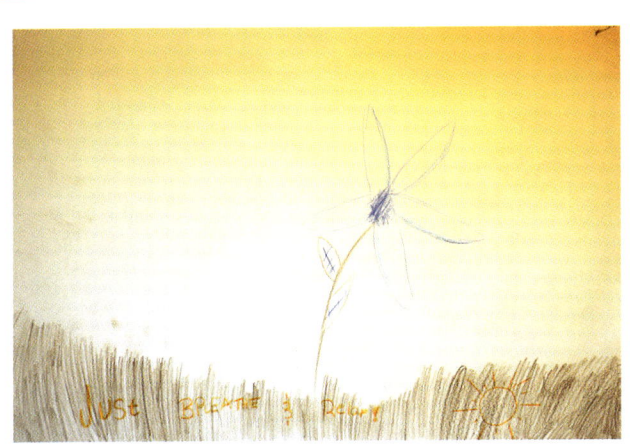

FIGURE 5.3 R's artwork post yoga, 'just breathe and relax'

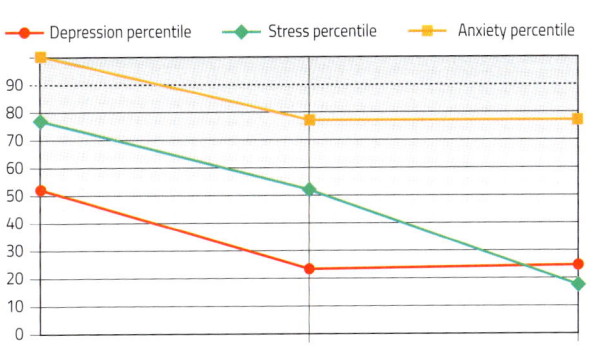

FIGURE 5.4 R's DASS results pre- and post-yoga and art therapy

anxiety, (3) low self-esteem, (4) obesity (her 5' 4" frame (152.67 cm) sported close to 200 lb (90.16 kg), (5) familial struggles with her brother, B (diagnosed Asperger's syndrome with concomitant symptoms of oppositional defiant disorder (ODD), although undiagnosed), (6) abandonment issues regarding her biological father, and (7) unhealthy face-to-face (F2F) friendships in person and online.

It is important to note that all family members (mother, stepfather, R and B) joined in for four sessions. These family sessions explored B's aggressive and assaultive behavior towards all family members. Post the second family session, it became clear that B needed his own treatment, so that R's therapy was not usurped. Creating this separation allowed R to invest in her treatment and success.

The house fire

Due to R's comorbidities, sessions vacillated between the above issues, ping-ponging between psychotherapy, yoga therapy and/or art therapy, depending on what came up. And then life really threw this family a curve ball: they had moved into a new home and on a July 4th weekend their home caught on fire. It was suggested that B had not been careful putting out sparklers and might have inadvertently been responsible for the fire. Later, a family session ensued in order to aid B with his feelings of guilt around this terrible accident. Because they lived in the countryside with no access to a nearby fire hydrant, the home burnt to the ground. They and their pets were safe, but all of their belongings were destroyed. For about a month, they moved in with the maternal grandmother, including their animals – quarters were tight, to say the least. Eventually, they moved into temporary housing, which they all described as 'awful' and 'lacking privacy and space'. Another 8 months elapsed before their home had been rebuilt.

In my own home we had unused furniture stored in our basement that was earmarked for our adult children (dressers, bedframes, a dining room table with chairs, etc). We discussed it with our adult children and all agreed that this family should take whatever could be of use to them for their temporary and eventual new home. We cleaned up the furnishings/household items and offered them to R and her family. Now, I know

Chapter five

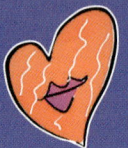
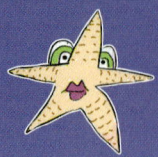

FIGURE 5.5 Yoga sequence with mother

		Balance on your toes for up to 1 minute. Reach up skyward. Arms overhead, come up on toes and stretch your calves. Benefits: Strengthens arches, ankles, knees and thighs – especially if you scissor the mat, adducting your legs. Lengthens spine and opens up pectoralis major and minor. Opens the shoulder girdle, especially the anterior deltoid. Hold for 10 seconds 5–10×.
	Warrior 1 to Triangle pose	Benefits: Improves digestion and circulation, relieves menstrual discomfort, relieves sciatica. Stretches arches, hamstrings, calves and groin. Opens throat, chest, shoulders and hips. Stabilizes and strengthens the torso. Increases muscular endurance.
	Paschimottanasana (seated forward bend)	Stretches spine, hamstrings and calves. Stimulates lymphatic and reproductive systems. Relieves menstrual discomfort. Improves liver, kidney and colon function. Alleviates high blood pressure (HBP). Reduces fatigue and insomnia. Soothes nervous system. Relieves stress, anxiety and mild depression. Hold for 25–60 seconds or more if you like it.
	Sphinx pose	Place arms directly under shoulders. Bring diaphragm to spine to strengthen core. Keep knees and lower legs on the ground. Improves posture, stimulates circulatory, digestive and diaphragmatic systems. Opens chest, shoulders and throat. Strengthens the spine.
	Savasana (rest or corpse pose)	Final relaxation pose with a pillow or blanket under head for support.

Clinical cases: adolescents

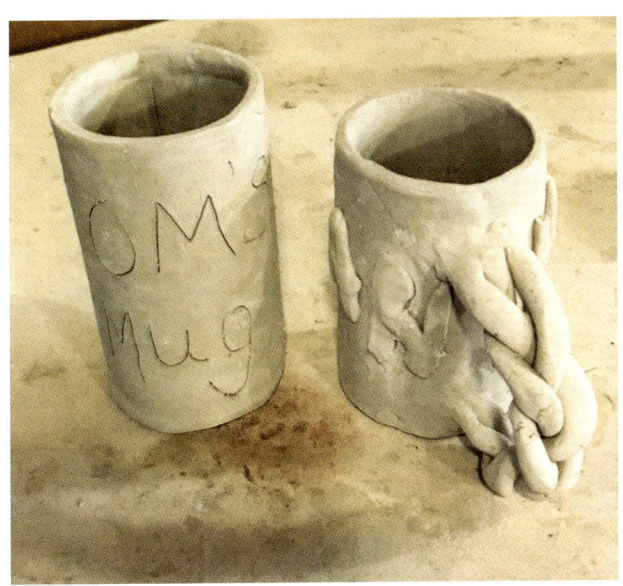

FIGURE 5.6 Mother and R's ceramic mugs

that some therapists might disagree with my decision, but it meant boatloads to this family (and our adult children) to extend this simple act of kindness. Having worked with burn survivors for years (Horovitz 2005), I knew from experience just how devastating and traumatizing a house fire could be.

In a family session following the fire, mother and R made themselves new ceramic drinking mugs (Fig. 5.6). Making new drinking vessels, containers for the future, also spoke to their resilience to contain themselves in light of these devastating circumstances.

Further significant sessions

A few months later, B joined a session with R and mother. The focus was mostly on B's inability to focus on his homework, and his defiant assaultive behavior towards all family members. He stated that he had four personalities and had little control over which personality came out. He named them: the 'Good Boy', his named Self 'B', the 'Evil Boy' and the 'Funny Boy'. He claimed that these different personalities were always within him. This allowed me to talk about his past situation when he had been abandoned and neglected by his biological mother. I lightly suggested that these different personalities might have served as a coping mechanism for him and were still active. We talked about his desire to be the 'Good Boy' and how crippled he felt when the other personalities took over. I also explained that these visceral feelings might be embedded in him from the time when he was not receiving adequate care from his biological mother. The family (specifically B's father) had been tip-toeing around these past events. I suggested that B needed some clarity around what had actually occurred. His father had explained that his biological mother and he had 'differences' and they split up because she preferred a 'party mode'. This doctored story was a disservice to B: he knew what he felt but didn't know why. Having truth to attach to his feelings and subsequent coping mechanism was preferable to skirting over his past experience. So, I explained this as best as I could while also explaining the disconnect between his father and mother.

During the session, it seemed more important to concretize B's actions with his past abandonment issues and explain to him that his visceral reactions were connected to a preverbal experience of fear and abandonment. He was clearly traumatized, beyond splitting off into what could be diagnosed as a dissociative identity disorder (Mayo Clinic 2020).

The DSM-5 classification of diagnoses describes 'dissociative personality disorder' thus:

A disorder characterized by the presence of two or more identities with distinct patterns of perception and personality which recurrently take control of the person's behavior; this is accompanied by a retrospective gap in memory of important personal

Chapter five

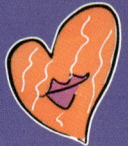 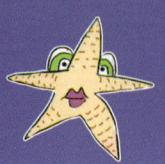

information that far exceeds ordinary forgetfulness. The changes in identity are not due to substance use or to a general medical condition… Each personality is a fully integrated and complex unit with memories, behavior patterns and social friendships. Transition from one personality to another is sudden.
APA 2013

Van der Kolk (2014) talked about the reptilian brain being the 'ultimate emergency system'. He suggested that this system is most likely to engage when we are 'physically immobilized…when a child has no escape from a terrifying caregiver'. In these situations, the dorsal vagal complex collapses and disengages into an 'ancient part of the parasympathetic nervous system'. According to van der Kolk, once this system takes over, 'we cease to matter… awareness is shut down and we may no longer register physical pain' (van der Kolk 2014:83). Clearly, this described what B experienced at the hands of his mother, during her time as an addict in crack houses – but explaining this to a child takes quite a bit of finesse.

At aged 10, B seemed capable of understanding what had occurred, and even though his biological mother was now a recovered addict, had remarried and had a new baby, it was especially difficult for B to grasp why he wasn't living with her and instead only 'visited'. His father had full custody. B also stated his fear of his mother's new husband, who 'yelled' at him if his homework was not completed. Next, he talked about his own father who 'yelled (at him) every day since (he) was born'. Naturally, this might have been an exaggeration, but it defined some of the polarities in his world, how he viewed his interactions with his caregivers and why he might have relied on these multiple personalities. As I have seen time and time again, while R had been the 'identified patient' in this family, all were multiple players in getting this family into treatment.

In this same session, B talked about his fear of fires (since their house had burned down, perhaps at the hands of the 'Evil Boy' persona). This came up because I had mentioned the kiln firing that would take place after their clay works dried. This allowed for some closure around B's guilt that he might have caused the house fire. We discussed this at length (as he worked with the art materials) and I suggested that his father might join us for a future session. Figure 5.7 shows the work that was created. I assisted B in completing his finished penguin. B had seen the 2005 movie, 'The March of the Penguins', and while this may have influenced his creation, penguins are known to live in extreme conditions that most others could not survive. Because of his background, I thought that his choice to create this indomitable animal (which was quite large, about nine inches tall) may have been reflective of his need to overcome his adversities.

While I attended to B during the session, R and mother's behavior felt very adolescent: they bonded like schoolgirls and seemingly left B out of their interactions. Rather than address this

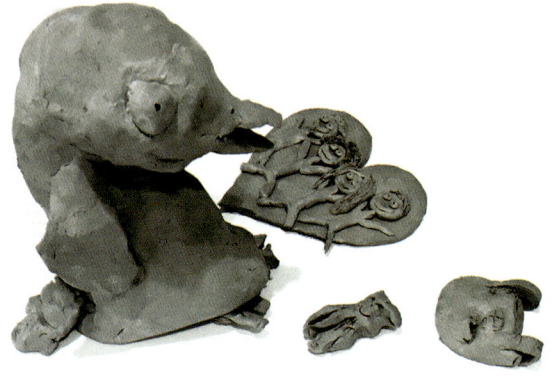

FIGURE 5.7 B's penguin (left), mother's family plaque (upper right), squid made by R for B (lower-right, center) and ceramic pocket vase made by R (lower right)

Clinical cases: adolescents

directly, I decided to leave that for my recap to both. They may also have felt the need to extract themselves from B given his persistent level of aggression. Still, it reflected a dynamic that I might not have witnessed had B not attended the therapy sessions.

R's DASS-21 scores also went down, suggesting the therapy had calmed her stress, anxiety and depression. Nonetheless, after the session I texted the following recap of our session to both R and her mother. Sending recaps has been instrumental in my summarizing the sessions for my patients and leaves the door open for them to connect with me in between sessions.

1. B will complete his homework 7/10 days so he can return to art therapy. You will help him complete his work (if he asks); but he will also allow you to complete your homework. Then B will 'teach' you how to play his video games for every day that he finishes his homework in a timely manner.

2. You will push yourself to go to school and perhaps draw in your journal or write about what is really going on and making you feel the need to be absent. Feel free to send to me via text.

3. Meanwhile, you need to know that on some level, when B becomes the focus (either through bad behavior or you get less focus because you are attending school), that this may constitute self-defeating behavior, so be aware of where this is coming from. Write about it, draw about it, invite all that bubbles up.

4. And remember this is your therapy: today it was important to focus a bit on B in order to draw him in and make him feel comfortable, but clearly you and your mother could see that he wanted your attention. He wasn't sure how to break in between the two of you. Your closeness is obvious and to him: he may feel left out, and thus acts out. So perhaps you and your Mom need to look at your interactions (or lack thereof) with B.

A few weeks later, the entire family attended and together they made a clay house (Fig. 5.8). Mother and R created the furnishings for the inside and stepfather and B created the exterior. This required another family session to complete. Once it was fired, it was taken home to be painted and displayed in a place of honor. During this time, and because his father was present, we again focused on B's visceral feelings and his admission that he wanted 'to be hugged' by all. Paramount was getting B to recognize that when he had these feelings, he could ask for what he needed (love, hugs) rather than act out to receive attention.

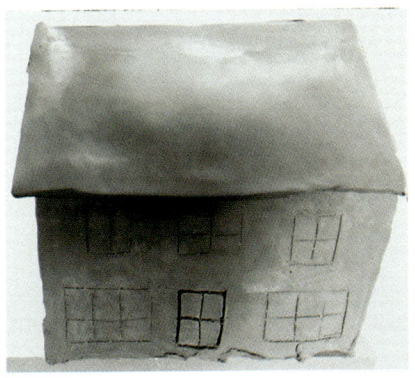 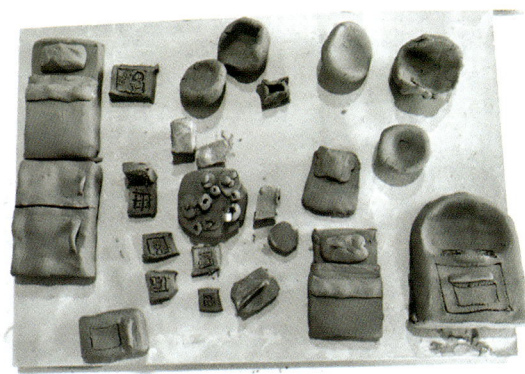

FIGURE 5.8 Exterior house created by B and stepfather (left), insides for house created by mother and R (right)

Chapter five

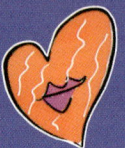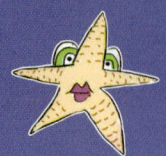

According to Hong and Park (2012), securely attached children are more resilient and develop into competent adults. On the contrary, 'those who do not experience a secure attachment with their caregivers may be unable to develop a sense of confidence or trust in others' (p.449). B missed this step and thus had no locus of control. Developing both secure attachments and a locus of control would be B's lifework. According to van der Kolk (2014), 'our maps of the world are encoded in the emotional brain'. Changing that requires a 'reorganization of the central nervous system' (p.129). Not an easy fix. It was for these reasons that I recommended that B begin his own therapy. Since that point, he has also been diagnosed with ADHD regarding his inability to succeed in school. He has been placed on medication, which has helped with his frequent outbursts, aggression and untoward behavior. However, due to his abusive childhood and lack of locus of control, he has a long road ahead of him.

In the following individual session with R, we discussed her frustration with B. What helped was paralleling his behavior with her own: I discussed that last year (due to hospitalizations and illness around her T1DM and HS) she missed a lot of school. Her illness and subsequent hospitalizations became a secondary gain: she received a lot of attention. I suggested that B's failing and concomitant desire to stay out of school might be his way of getting the focus that she had received. I also explained that it might be very hard for him to break into the repartee between herself and mother. She understood.

Next we talked about typical adolescent frustrations with her classmates and friends and her admission to being 'fluid'. Many of her friends had identified as cisgender, bisexual and transgender. Much to my surprise, she identified as pansexual. That sparked the beginning of more typical adolescent conversations and forecast things to come.

The next session revealed more about typical adolescent behavior and how this upended R. Because R's mother wakes her nightly to check her glucose levels, she was awake when one of her friends ('Q') shot out several group texts that she had overdosed in her attempt to suicide. R panicked, ran into her mother's bedroom and told her what had occurred. Mother immediately tried to reach Q's parents. Several phone calls were made and finally Q's mother picked up, angry for the late-night intrusion. Fortunately, Q was hospitalized and then stayed a minimum week in the psychiatric ward.

This was handled very badly at school: all of the friends who were part of the 'group chat' were required to hand in their cell phones to the school counselor so that the data could be extracted. Next, the entire group was forced to sit down with the school counselor, and then required to meet individually. For R, this seemed little short of interrogation. Also, instead of dealing with how traumatizing this was for her (she kept thinking, 'what if I hadn't been awake?'), R felt awash with guilt for saving her friend's life. Q's parents never called to thank her mother or R. Instead, the school counselor instructed R and her friends not to talk about the incident once Q returned to school. R couldn't park her feelings.

In the following session, I suggested that she write a letter to Q explaining how she felt. In the letter, R stated that she felt like she was 'walking on eggshells', and didn't want to push her over the edge but wrote, 'Are you safe at home? Are you compelled to do it again? Why didn't you come to us? I get it's hard, but why?'

In this same session, R was also able to admit how hard it was to see her father all over Facebook talking about his girlfriend's pregnancy and how much this compounded her feelings of rejection. This sparked the beginning of social media ills and spiraling into depression.

Clinical cases: adolescents

Significant sessions: year two

Sometimes, it gets worse before it gets better. R's mother called to address the fact that once again, R had been failing in school and cloaking how badly she had been doing. R had been getting up late or refusing to get up on time for the bus, and sometimes was so depressed that she would fall asleep on the school bus on the way home. I turned to art therapy so both mother and R could express their feelings. Figure 5.9 is reflective of this period.

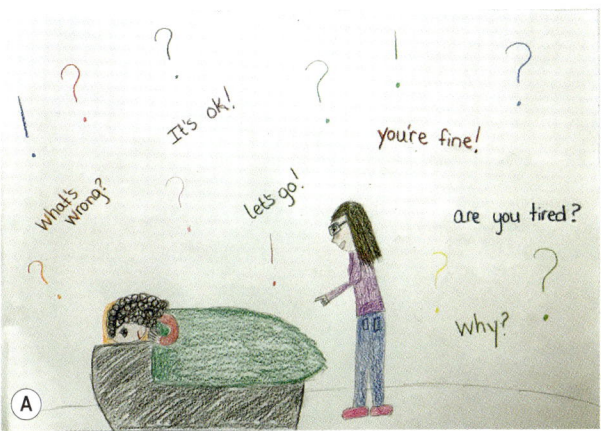

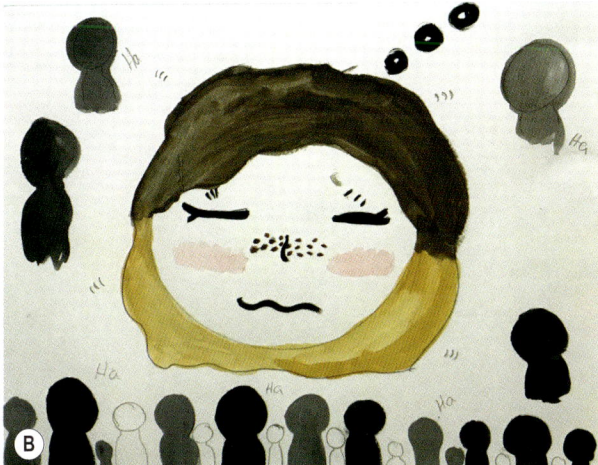

FIGURE 5.9 Mother's artwork (top) and R's artwork (bottom)

Mother's artwork is pretty self-explanatory: she is trying to rationalize what she is witnessing – R not getting out of bed and not communicating what is wrong. The questions that surround the scene vacillate between confusion and probing (What's wrong? Why?) to denial (You're fine! Let's go!). One can sense mother's urgency to eradicate the problem and her frustration with her inability to resolve the situation.

R's work was a bit more cryptic. Her explanation pinpointed the root of her depression. She explained that no matter where she went, she felt people were, 'staring at her because of her weight'. Her recent Eating Attitudes Test-26 (EAT-26) results highlighted the following three subscale areas of concern: dieting, bulimia, food preoccupation and oral control.

The discussion revolved around talking about her eating disorder, her paranoia that everyone was talking about her or staring at her, and her admission of anger towards her father for, 'not being there for her', even though he will be there for his girlfriend and the new baby.

Since there had not been enough time to fit in the yoga, I taught R stair-step breath. The technique is part breath/part visualization. The steps are fairly straightforward. Sit in easy pose or *sukhāsana*. Draw the breath through the chakras from the root chakra to the crown chakra in small increments, as if sipping through a straw. Then once at the top, pause for a moment and then release your breath like you would an elevator going down. Repeat for several minutes until calm.

Post-session I mentioned the book *Speak* (aimed at adolescents) to R's mother (Anderson 1999). The book discusses the issues of not talking, holding these secrets inside and being an 'outcast', especially from classmates. This is similar to today's culture of being 'canceled'. I suggested that she have R read it and if she couldn't locate it, I would give her my copy.

Chapter five

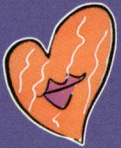
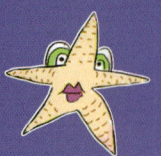

In the next session, mother stated that R had a habit of taking care of others (like her friend Q) before administering to herself. I likened her lack of self-care to being on an airplane and not giving herself oxygen first if the masks fall down. I mentioned a local diabetic support group that I located and possibly taking a friend who was also T1DM. Both R and mother were encouraged by this new information.

Next I conducted yoga with both of them for 20 minutes (Fig. 5.10). Both seemed noticeably relieved post session and R's DASS-21 results yielded these positive results:

- normal range for depression
- mild range for anxiety
- normal range for stress.

I hadn't seen R's scores this low since before the fire occurred.

Compounding R's T1DM and HS issues were her depression, stress and anxiety. Placing her on psychotropics was certainly an option but one which she and her mother wanted to avoid. I knew that pumping up her exercise regime would help regulate her moods (van der Kolk 2014, Stearns 2018, Weintraub 2012), reduce exogenous insulin requirement and improve her metabolic control (Admon et al 2005). However, getting R and mother to buy into increased exercise was hit or miss. With encouragement, I finally convinced mother and R to join a local YMCA (a nonprofit organization for youth development, healthy living and social responsibility). This was a start, as was R's decision to join the school softball team. Beyond exercising, this increased her camaraderie and widened her circle of friends.

After a few months, R once again spiraled into negative behavior. She kept getting sucked into bad relationships via online communications with people and lying about her homework. On Easter Sunday she fell apart. Apparently, one of her 'friends' had fabricated a character online (a bogus albino cancer patient) with whom R had been 'communicating'. It took some time before R realized that the scenario was faked. This allowed me and mother to talk about the dangers of the internet. We encouraged her to invest in face-to-face relationships. I also talked to her about JOMO versus FOMO.

This was a turning point for R. She had lost weight since starting softball and forged friendships with her teammates, but stacking up the issues and talking about how she been contending with them really helped:

- the house fire
- displacement into a home with little to no privacy
- B taking center-stage and being abusive to all family members
- her friend Q, who attempted suicide
- her own health issues, hospitalizations and setbacks.

It was a lot for one person to bear in a year. I suggested that perhaps she needed to 'fail' at school to get the much-needed attention that had been going to B. Because she complained of her inability to 'focus', I showed her the open-focus method (Fehmi 2014, Fehmi and Robbins 2008) and suggested that she continue to use her desk as an 'office' for schoolwork. As a result, her DASS-21 scores were better than in past months: all normal in the range for depression, anxiety and stress, which was very affirming for R, mother and me.

The method of open focus that I taught her is akin to visualization and meditation, but the aim is to let go and become immersed in the four states of narrow, diffuse, immersion and objective focusing (Fehmi 2014). I showed R how to do this by using a sample of reading from a book and becoming aware of those four states. As a result, once R practiced and understood how to achieve this open-focused state, she truly understood how to tap into her own state of awareness and ground herself.

Clinical cases: adolescents

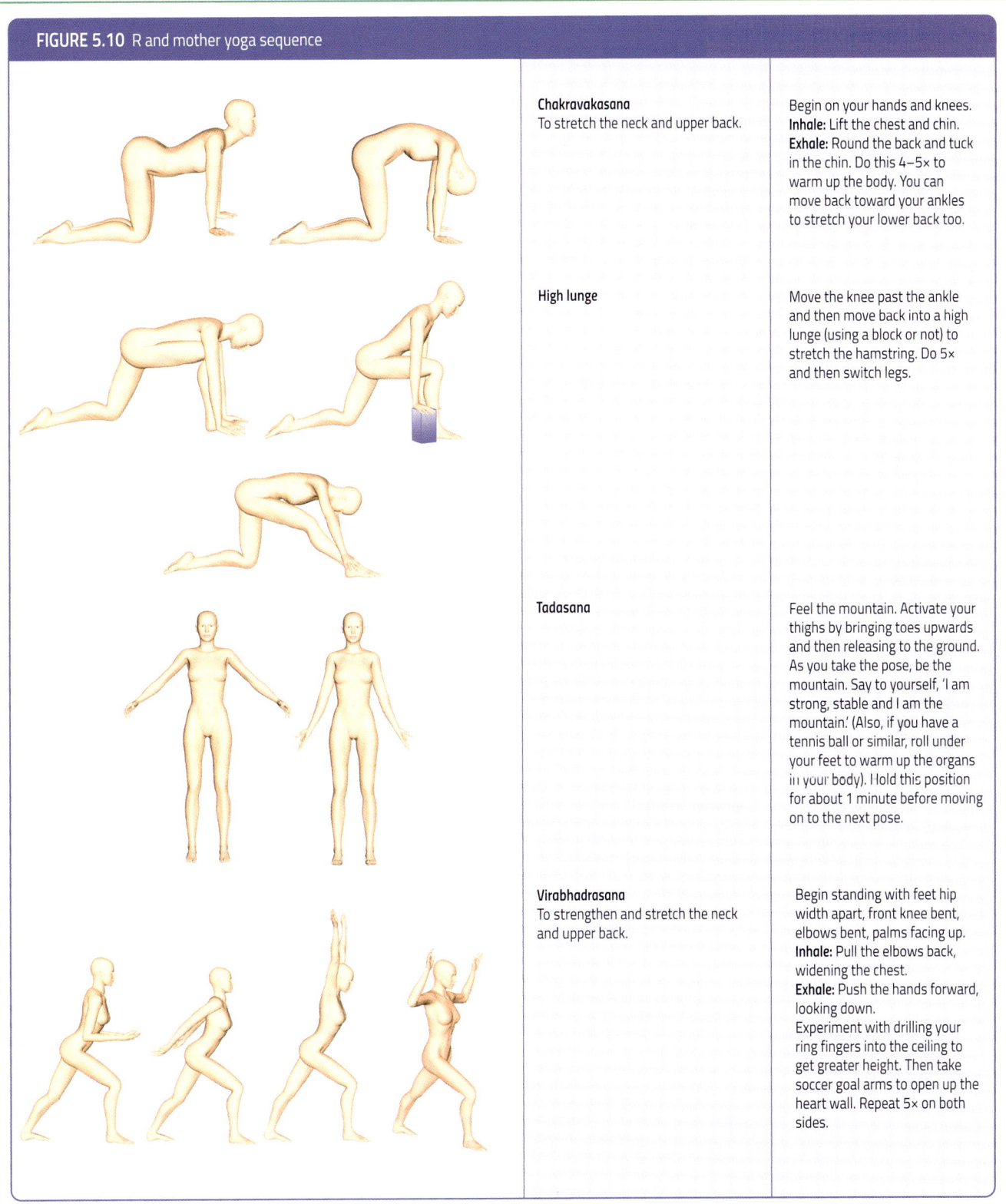

FIGURE 5.10 R and mother yoga sequence

Chakravakasana To stretch the neck and upper back.	Begin on your hands and knees. **Inhale:** Lift the chest and chin. **Exhale:** Round the back and tuck in the chin. Do this 4–5× to warm up the body. You can move back toward your ankles to stretch your lower back too.
High lunge	Move the knee past the ankle and then move back into a high lunge (using a block or not) to stretch the hamstring. Do 5× and then switch legs.
Tadasana	Feel the mountain. Activate your thighs by bringing toes upwards and then releasing to the ground. As you take the pose, be the mountain. Say to yourself, 'I am strong, stable and I am the mountain.' (Also, if you have a tennis ball or similar, roll under your feet to warm up the organs in your body). Hold this position for about 1 minute before moving on to the next pose.
Virabhadrasana To strengthen and stretch the neck and upper back.	Begin standing with feet hip width apart, front knee bent, elbows bent, palms facing up. **Inhale:** Pull the elbows back, widening the chest. **Exhale:** Push the hands forward, looking down. Experiment with drilling your ring fingers into the ceiling to get greater height. Then take soccer goal arms to open up the heart wall. Repeat 5× on both sides.

Chapter five

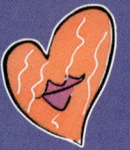 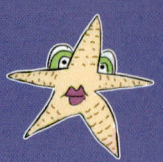

FIGURE 5.10 continued

	Parsvokanasana (pyramid pose)	Come forward with as straight a back as possible. Use block if needed and bend forward over front leg. Do 5× each side.
	Ardha Matsyendrasana To stretch the neck and strengthen the upper back	Begin in a seated position with the right knee bent and crossed over the extended left leg. Place the left elbow on the outside of your right knee. **Inhale:** Lengthen up through the top of the head. **Exhale:** Turn to your right, look back. Stay in position. **Inhale:** Lengthen up. **Exhale:** Use abdominal contraction to deepen the twist. Look back for 3–4 breaths, then turn your head and look forward for 3–4 breaths while maintaining the twist. Do on both sides.
	Heron pose and compass pose	Using the belt, extend one leg forward, bend elbows to sides using the belt to raise the leg upwards and straight. Hold for 5 counts, and do 5× total. Switch sides. In order to come into compass pose, take belt in one hand, bending elbow and raising the leg. Other hand goes in front of upward extended leg.
	Savasana	Take rest pose for a few minutes. Then sit up in sukhasana (easy cross-legged pose), say namaste, and if time, sit for a few minutes in meditation.

Clinical cases: adolescents

Alpha waves become engaged when you learn how to deploy these four basic types of attention (Fig. 5.11): (1) narrow focus: unsynchronized brain activity – flight or fight mode, (2) diffuse focus: slows the brain activity in activities such as yoga/dancing, (3) immersion focus: the flow state (immersed in activity like art which increases the five senses), and (4) objective focus: you separate from the focus area by disengaging from the activity or object. The final aspect of open-focus is learning how to immerse the brain in all four aspects simultaneously. Combining these attention states simultaneously is an awareness of awareness: the primal, primo open-focus state (Fehmi and Robbins 2008).

Several months elapsed and R had lost 20 lb (9 kg) since engaging in softball practice. Father's baby was born and while she had a few visits at her father's home, that quickly came to an end. During therapy, she admitted that over a weekend visit he had become very verbally abusive towards her and forced her to go for a car ride, when he drove over 100 mph (160 km/h). Scared, she asked him to slow down, but he did not. When they eventually arrived back at his home, he further threatened her by demanding that she not tell her mother about the weekend. She was palpably scared. But she told me this in therapy. I recommended that we have a family session with mother so that I could help her discuss this. She didn't want to continue to visit her father, even though that meant not seeing her baby half-brother.

Simultaneously, mother had just submitted a subpoena to the court in order to extract monetary support for R. I communicated my findings to the judges, and based on father's past physical and

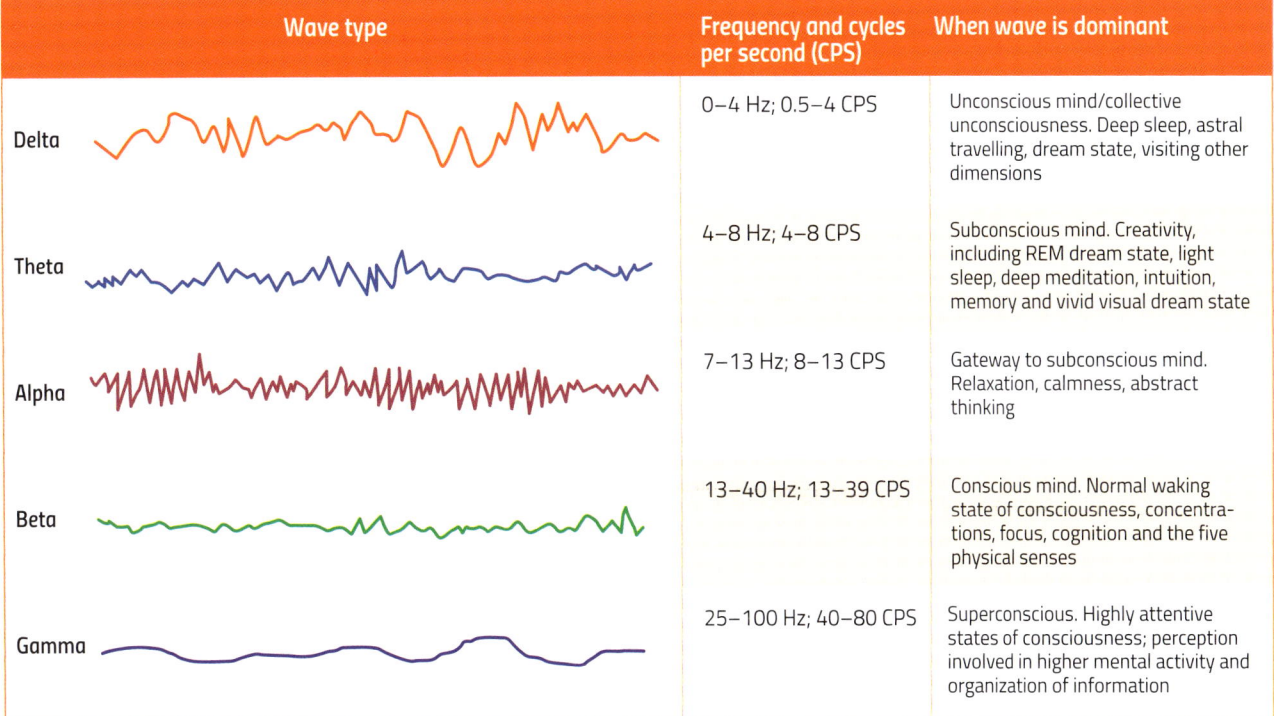

Wave type		Frequency and cycles per second (CPS)	When wave is dominant
Delta		0–4 Hz; 0.5–4 CPS	Unconscious mind/collective unconsciousness. Deep sleep, astral travelling, dream state, visiting other dimensions
Theta		4–8 Hz; 4–8 CPS	Subconscious mind. Creativity, including REM dream state, light sleep, deep meditation, intuition, memory and vivid visual dream state
Alpha		7–13 Hz; 8–13 CPS	Gateway to subconscious mind. Relaxation, calmness, abstract thinking
Beta		13–40 Hz; 13–39 CPS	Conscious mind. Normal waking state of consciousness, concentrations, focus, cognition and the five physical senses
Gamma		25–100 Hz; 40–80 CPS	Superconscious. Highly attentive states of consciousness; perception involved in higher mental activity and organization of information

FIGURE 5.11 Brain wave chart by author

Chapter five

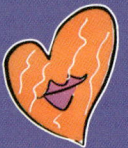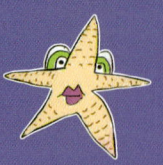

emotional abuse of R's mother, and his recent psychological abuse of R, I suggested that supervised visitation with the father was warranted. The judges agreed and awarded monetary support for R's care. While R was saddened by not seeing her father or the new baby, she was relieved that she no longer had to visit him.

Speed ahead to the diabetes summer camp. R made friends with other T1DM children from all over the state and soared by being away from her home for one independent week. She did wonderfully, loved the experience and was asked to return for a second week to be a counselor to other T1DM and T2DM children. This was a turning point for R. Once she returned from this experience and was able to distance herself from some of the last year's events, she did well in making up her failed coursework during summer school, and began to make friends with a girl in her neighborhood.

Once the school year started, I suggested that R needed more individual sessions where the focus could be on her issues and struggles. One day I received a text from R that she was, 'taking a break from all phone/ social media', and if necessary, to contact her via her mother. I applauded her decision. R continued to stay more physically active, forming healthier face-to-face friendships and limiting her online activities. In short, R had discovered JOMO (the joy of missing out), was staying healthy and physically active, keeping up with her homework and forging towards her goals.

While there might be some bumps ahead, R seems better equipped to handle her T1DM, adolescent angst and stress, and move forward towards her goals to graduate high school and attend college.

Present situation

While therapy has not directly involved R's biological father to date, much work has been done from letter writing to art therapy and psychotherapy, that has aided in putting some of her feelings to rest. As of this writing, after both R and I wrote to the father, he agreed to come to 'one session'. The session he attended was illuminating and helpful for R.

Surprisingly enough, R's mother decided to marry the stepfather even though there seemed no sign that she was less conflicted. When I asked about the mother's reasoning for this decision, she simply stated, 'It was the next step'. Some of this might have been bundled into what she and stepfather surmounted together with all of the past obstacles (particularly the house fire). Nevertheless, she also took the stepfather's name so everyone in the family (save R) now shares the stepfather's surname. R also wants to change her last name to her stepfather's so that the entire family will have the same last name. Her desire to adopt the stepfather's name seems to reflect her urgency to have a family, and to belong to something greater than herself. Unfortunately, due to state laws, R has to be 18 years old to do this and/or get the written permission from both parents. It is unlikely that R's biological father will consent to R changing her name: he has been quite adamantly opposed to the idea and was also opposed to her mother marrying the stepfather.

R continues to make strides, diligently working hard to complete her homework assignments (although certainly not working to her full potential and capacity). But for now, the T1DM seems to be well under control. R has a new Dexcom monitor which allows for continuous glucose monitoring, she is continuing to exercise, practicing yoga and artmaking on a regular basis, spends more time inhabiting her (chosen) 'aloneness' and less time in relationships that are not serving her. R is also investing more time in healthy F2F relationships while curtailing her online activity. While the therapy is by no means finished, R has come a long way in her trajectory towards health and well-being.

Clinical cases: adolescents

Reflection exercise 5.1

Exercise in open-focus thinking

Based on the work of Fehmi and Robbins (2008:65–69), let's try an exercise in open-focus thinking but add a twist at the end.

Imagine the distance or space between your eyes. Now close your eyes; next imagine the space inside your nose as you naturally inhale and exhale. Try and imagine your breath flowing behind your eyes as you inhale and exhale. Try and drop in a little deeper: can you imagine the space inside your throat and the space inside your nose? Can you imagine the space inside your ears... and between your ears? Can you imagine that as you inhale naturally your breath fills the entire volume of your face and scalp and head, including your eyes and ears? Stay with that for 30 seconds to a few minutes and relax into that space. Censor nothing, welcome it all. When you open your eyes, draw what you witnessed or write about how you felt in that space. Sit with that for a few moments. Let that fill your senses. Come back to that awareness as often as you like. This may help center you whenever you are feeling anxious or agitated. Remember, your breath breathes you.

Case study 2

17-year-old male with bipolar disorder (and co-morbidity of addiction disorder)

Addiction and yoga

Yoga has been recommended as an adjunct treatment for alcoholism and addiction (Hallgren et al 2014, Khanna and Greeson 2013, Khalsa et al 2008, Previc 2009, Zschucke et al 2012). In addition, several controlled studies demonstrated positive association between yoga and specific health outcomes including epilepsy, high blood pressure, pain and mood disturbances, and stress (Kohn et al 2013, Mackenzie et al 2013). Current theoretical models suggest that self-awareness, learned through yoga and mindfulness practice, targets multiple psychological, neural, physiological and behavioral processes implicated in addiction and relapse.

There have been some small (albeit well-designed) clinical trials and experimental laboratory studies on smoking, alcohol dependence and illicit substances. While more research is needed to understand what types of yoga and mindfulness-based interventions work best for what types of addiction, which patients, and under what conditions, the clinical effectiveness and hypothesized mechanisms of action of mindfulness-based interventions for treating addictions has been viewed positively. Current findings support yoga and mindfulness as promising complementary therapies for treating and preventing addictive behaviors (Khanna and Greeson 2013).

The American Psychiatric Association (APA) (2013) identifies drug addiction as a 'substance use disorder'. The result is a 'cluster of cognitive, behavioral, and physiological symptoms indicating that the individual continues using the substance despite significant substance-related problems' (APA 2013:483). Interaction between drugs and the brain is apt to cause problems associated with substance abuse. These include craving,

Chapter five

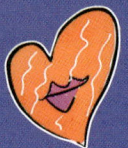

compulsive drug-seeking behaviors, impaired control over use, and chronic relapse (APA 2013, Blum et al 2012).

Blum et al (1996) discussed addiction in terms of reward deficiency syndrome (RDS). The RDS definition described actions associated with genetic antecedents, that resulted in a hypodopaminergic state and pre-disposition to obsessive, compulsive and impulsive behaviors. Further, Blum et al (2012) stated that, 'vulnerability to addiction differ(ed) from person to person and… [was] influenced by both environmental (home, family, nutrition, availability of drugs, stress, and peer pressure in school, early use and method of administration) and genetic risk factors' (Blum et al 2012:139).

According to Blum et al (2012), known holistic modalities that could induce dopamine release and promote well-being were yoga, exercise, diet, music therapy, relaxation using audio therapy, acupuncture, meditation (Kjaer et al 2002), and potentially hyperbaric oxygen therapy (HBOT). Furthermore, Blum et al (2012) purported that, 'agents that reduce stress such as known natural dopamine agonists should have benefits for craving reduction, relapse prevention and quite possibly prevention of other RDS behaviors, especially in adolescents'. This study further suggested that cognitive behavioral therapy (CBT), motivational incentives, motivational interviewing and group therapy coupled with, 'treatment medications and whole-body testing (adrenal and thyroid function, etc.) might provide clinicians with a blueprint for success' (Blum et al 2012:141).

High rates of psychiatric comorbidities are typically found in patients with bipolar disorders. For example, in a study of 288 outpatients with bipolar disorders, McElroy et al (2000) found that 42% met criteria for a comorbid anxiety disorder, 42% for comorbid substance use disorder, and 5% for an eating disorder (Juruena 2012).

A promising and noninvasive treatment for addiction is transcranial magnetic stimulation (TMS): it delivers electric field (E-field) pulses into the brain (Diana et al 2017). Magnetic fields efficiently pass through the electrically insulated skull and allow magnetic stimuli to induce strong and moderate spatially focal intracranial currents in the underlying brain tissue. Delivering many TMS pulses in sequences can cause long-term changes that facilitate or impede neuronal excitability and specific behaviors, depending on the stimulation site, sequence parameters and other factors, but of course one would need access to a facility where these whole-body treatments could be tested. Unfortunately, my private practice is not set up for such testing, which was a direct disadvantage (more will be stated about that in the significant sessions section below). However, Diana's studies suggest that neuroimaging tools could be useful in predicting which patients will benefit from TMS and which are likely to relapse, as well as guiding target selection to pinpoint treatment.

Regarding addiction: (1) males are more likely than females to become addicted to alcohol, drugs or two substances combined (US Department of Health and Human Services 2008), (2) adolescents and individuals with comorbid mental disorders are at greater risk of drug abuse and addiction than the general population (Pickens et al 1991), (3) the 12-step program has been proven to have merit; Comings (2008) and associates identified the role of a specific gene in spirituality (the dopamine D4 receptor gene (DRD4) was found to play a role in novelty seeking), and (4) Hamer (2005) found evidence of a 'God gene', the dopamine vesicular transporter gene (VMAT2), which was reported to be associated with spirituality. The latter research was of great comfort since it confirmed what I postulated in 2002 and subsequently (Horovitz 2002, 2017).

It is difficult to work with addicts when they are in denial, unwilling to view their addictions as problematic and averse to change. Homeostasis often rules the day, as it is easier to remain ill than move towards wellness. In this case, this patient's addiction was his equilibrium. So, given that, let's now turn towards his treatment and how the work unfolded.

Background and history

This was a very complicated and high-profile case. There seemed to be so much pathology in the family system that even though 'M' was the designated patient, it became clear that despite his comorbid diagnosis/issues (substance abuse disorder, bipolar 2 disorder, oppositional defiant disorder, traumatic brain injury at age 14 and suicidal history x 3), there was much to be unraveled in M's upbringing and his mother and father's psychosocial history. Therefore, the focus included family sessions with the father, telehealth sessions with the mother (who lived on the opposite side of the country), individual sessions with M and one home visit with M (while his father was out of town). While M's genogram (Fig. 5.12) attempts to summarize these issues, including the multiple suicide attempts, hospitalizations and medications, I will briefly relay M's background and those of his immediate family members.

At intake age 18, M was living with his father and paternal grandfather (having been kicked out of his mother's home). At his grandfather's house M basically had his own pad – a walkout basement living room, bathroom and bedroom area. His grandfather and father lived on the above floors and all shared the communal living and cooking space. However, father often travelled to New York for business and left M for multiple days at a time. These separations led to numerous drug and alcohol binges where M got into various untoward situations, such as forging checks from the grandfather's account (a felony charge), stealing from his father's account and getting into physical fights with other adolescents. In short, he was mostly out of control in terms of decision-making and his social circle of friends.

Developmentally, M had a rather checkered past, for example, refusing to remain tethered to his seat belt, he tried to exit his mother's moving vehicle (aged 4 years), fell from a roof at a playground (aged 8 years) and at 14 years suffered a traumatic brain injury (TBI) while surfing, which resulted in seizures for 2 months post-accident.

At age 15 he attempted suicide via alprazolam (Xanax) and psilocybin. At age 16, a second attempt was relayed by his father, who stated that he was telepathically drawn to the exact location in a nearby forest where M was attempting self-injurious behavior. At age 17, M attempted suicide by gun, but the gun malfunctioned. All of these actions led M into temporary inpatient hospitalizations with multiple diagnoses, and psychotropic interventions. During this time, there had been a few residential rehabilitation treatment settings, all without impact on M's drug and alcohol abuse.

Understanding this in context helps. Father had been traveling all over the world after he lost his job on the stock market in New York. While the family resided in California, father lived in New York City, London, Singapore, Tokyo, Dubai, Kuwait and Bahrain. Previously, the family travelled in high social circles and when the father lost his job in New York, the family went from riches to rags (the family home was sold, etc.). Due to M's behavior and suicidal ideations, his mother flew him across the country to live with his father and paternal grandfather (PGF).

M's father also relayed that he had a history of depression. In session, the father masked his depression with narcissistic self-adulation and was prone to bouts of mania. Meanwhile, mother was living across the country and had moved into a new, opulent home that was her fiancé's. Having

Chapter five

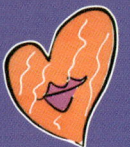
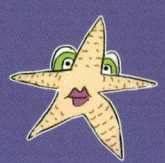

hailed from major ivy league colleges, both undergraduate and graduate, mother procured employment as an Assistant Dean at a university. Father stated that mother had a history of alcoholism and borderline personality disorder, but this was all based on his report, not hers.

In sum, M struggles with comorbidity of bipolar disorder, previous suicidal ideation, TBI (from multiple injuries as a child), PTSD, sexual abuse (which was revealed during Session 27) and substance abuse. Both M and his father have presented with suicidal ideation and depression (see Fig. 5.12). At M's age 16, during a family session, M accused his mother of having an affair. She admitted that this was in fact true and thus, shortly thereafter, the parents uncoupled. Around this time the father's brother (also diagnosed with bipolar disorder) died from brain cancer and the father's financial situation deteriorated. M also witnessed several of his mother's trysts with various sexual partners.

Significant sessions

There were 29 sessions with M. Five sessions included his father and two included his mother and father using a telehealth video platform. Initially, as in most cases, there was a 'honeymoon period', where M responded extremely well to therapy and was also complying with attendance at an outpatient substance abuse treatment program while concurrently seeing me. His verbal associations to the artwork produced during art therapy sessions also yielded a trove of clinical information.

The reason for requesting attendance at the outpatient substance abuse treatment program

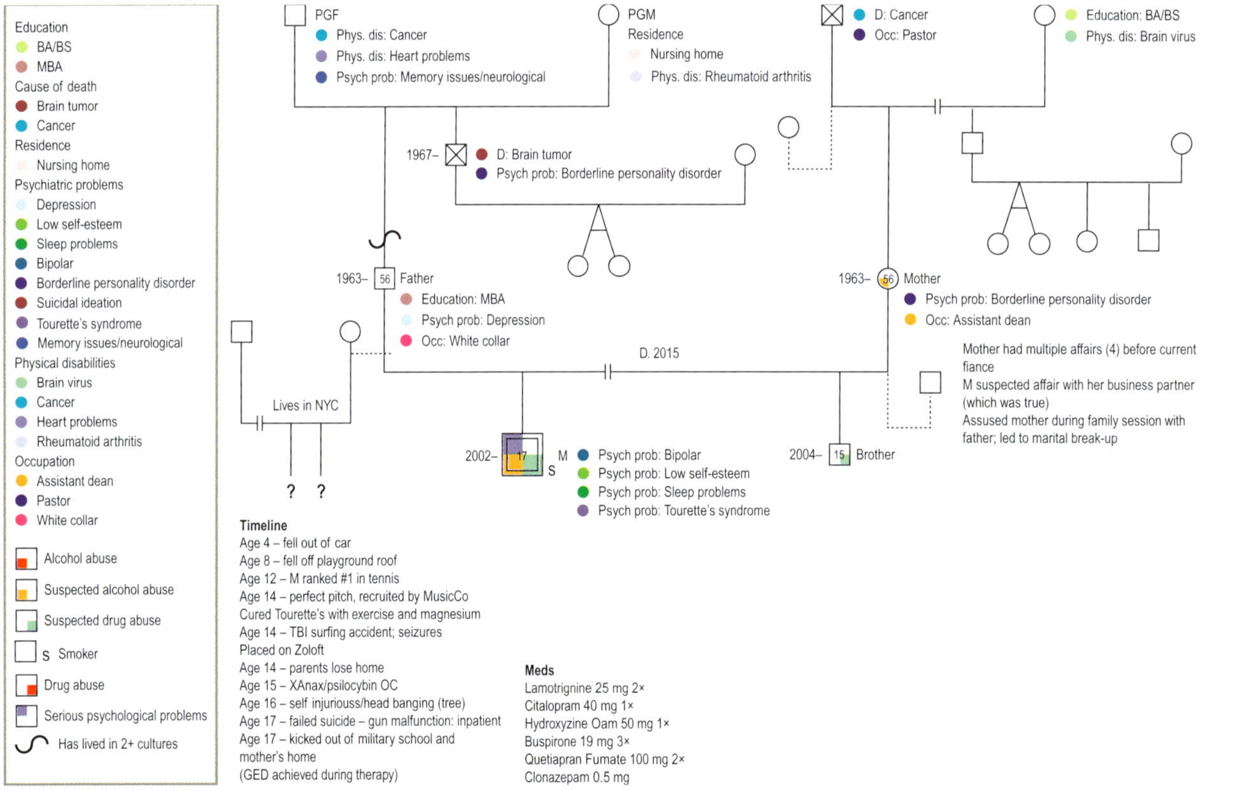

FIGURE 5.12 M's genogram

Clinical cases: adolescents

is that I lacked the ability to monitor his sobriety (e.g. weekly drug tests). He was also able to attend group therapy sessions specifically addressing substance abuse issues. I had releases to communicate directly with the staff at the outpatient substance abuse treatment program so that 'splitting' would not occur.

Prior to Session 2, I had conducted the DASS-21. His results post-session yielded normal range for depression and anxiety and moderate range for stress. During the session, M stated that he felt worthless, and defined himself as 'a bad person'. Based on his affect, I decided to start with yoga. I taught him *pratilomā ujjayi* (alternate nostril breath and ocean/victorious breath), mountain pose (*tadāsana*) and breath of joy. This was assigned as daily homework. Figure 5.13 details *pratilomā ujjayi* and breath of joy.

M struggled with family issues during his individual therapy sessions and many of his art pieces reflected his struggle around these issues. The kinetic family drawing (KFD) (Fig. 5.14) conducted post-yoga therapy during Session 2 depicted his struggles. Beyond the obvious agitation (line quality), the faceless entities and stick figures reflected his view of this impoverished family system. He drew his family sledding (he is on the upper left and father is pushing his brother down a hill). When I asked about his mother (drawn in the lower left-hand corner) he remarked that she was dead to him. Nevertheless, it became clear throughout our work together how much he missed his mother and longed for her attention, although his verbal association denied this.

The second session also provided a window of what it was like to work with a drug addicted, bipolar 2 individual who swung from affective, cognitively based work to impulsivity and lying, within a single session. Challenging doesn't even begin to describe that shift.

At the end of session, M went outside to get money from his father (who was waiting in his car). I only took part of the cash, based on their insurance. M seemed anxious, asked to use the bathroom and then pocketed the remaining money. Next, he texted me (within a few minutes) and asked me not to tell his father that he had the money, fabricating a story about owing money to a friend. I basically told him that I couldn't lie to his father and that I was just about to contact his father and tell him that I only took part of the money. I agreed to give him 20 minutes to own up. He did and our texts crossed.

He wrote, 'Thank you. I don't understand why I do things like that. I want to be a person of such high integrity, but my impulsivity gets in the way. Frequently things like this happen and I really want to put a stop to it'.

His father later texted me and thanked me for my work. He wrote, 'I am sorry to say his behaviors continue to be dishonest at times. He had the money stuffed in his sock and when he realized he was going to be caught, scrambled to alert you and come clean with me. I write to provide a lens into behaviors he neither likes about himself nor understands... On the positive side, he seems to greatly benefit from your sessions.... Step by step he is making progress. But it's fair to say it's not easy'.

By session fourteen M's DASS-21 scores were in the normal range for depression, anxiety and stress. Yoga and art therapy seemed to be having an effect on M. However, the vigilant eye that topped the clay container that he made (Fig. 5.15) seemed to reflect hypervigilance and paranoia, a precursor of things to come (Case and Dalley 2014, Horovitz 2017, Kramer and lager 1984, Oster and Crone 2004).

There were several sessions with the father that incorporated partner yoga and art therapy. During session 17 I had them make 'Self-boxes' (via origami). Because M's father had been 'cloaking' his relationship with his girlfriend in New York, I sug-

Chapter five

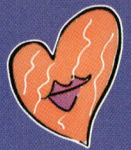
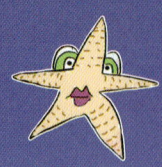

FIGURE 5.13 Yoga practice Session 2

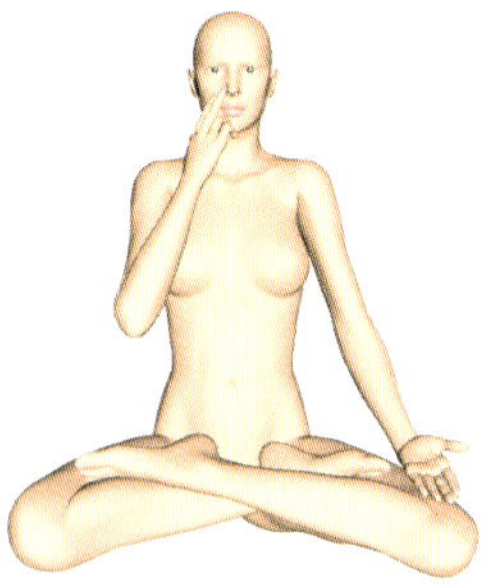	**Pratiloma ujjayi** Balancing effect, useful for mind centring	Inhale using ujjayi, exhale through the left nostril; inhale through the left nostril; exhale using ujjayi. Inhale using ujjayi, exhale through the right nostril; inhale through the right nostril; exhale using ujjayi. 1 cycle.
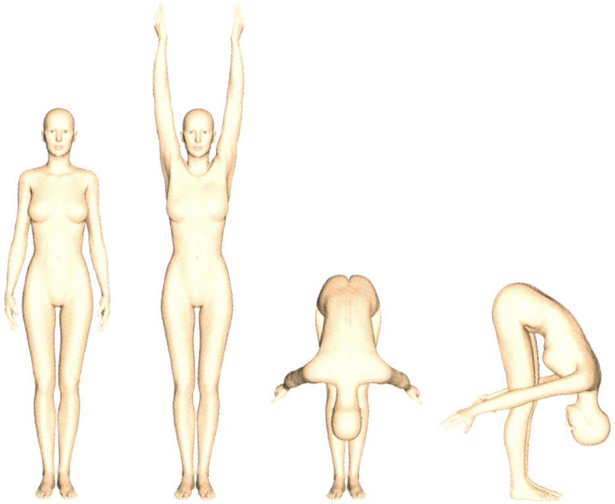	**Breath of joy**	Start in tadasana. Raise hands to side (like conducting an orchestra); next, take hands overhead as close to ears as possible with straight arms. Then come forward with a straight spine (bending at the waist), take head towards thighs and say 'Ha!'. Repeat 10×.

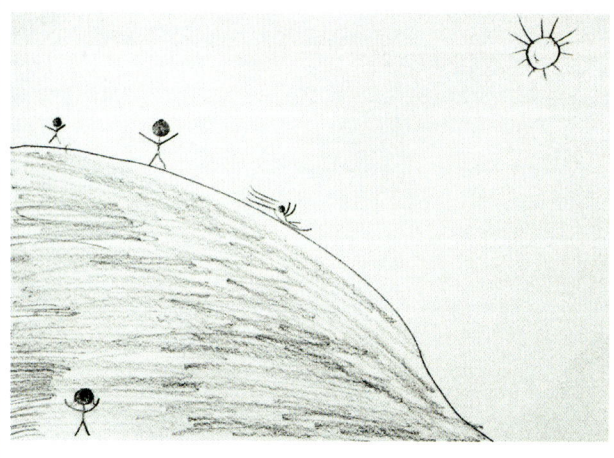

FIGURE 5.14 M's kinetic family drawing

gested that inside the box they place items, pictures or secrets that they had not shared with each other. His father's only response was 'V', which stood for the first name of his girlfriend (Fig. 5.16, left).

M's responses in his box (Fig. 5.16, right) were 'WPM' (weed pot marijuana) and his clean date of May 20th) M shared that he was high the day he took the general education development (GED) test, even though he 'nailed the test'. With tears in his eyes, M added 'never good enough', 'burden' and 'failure', to a scrap piece of paper. He stated that he felt like he was holding his father back from what he could pursue (the black dot that he added next) and that he knew about his father's girlfriend, but didn't

Clinical cases: adolescents

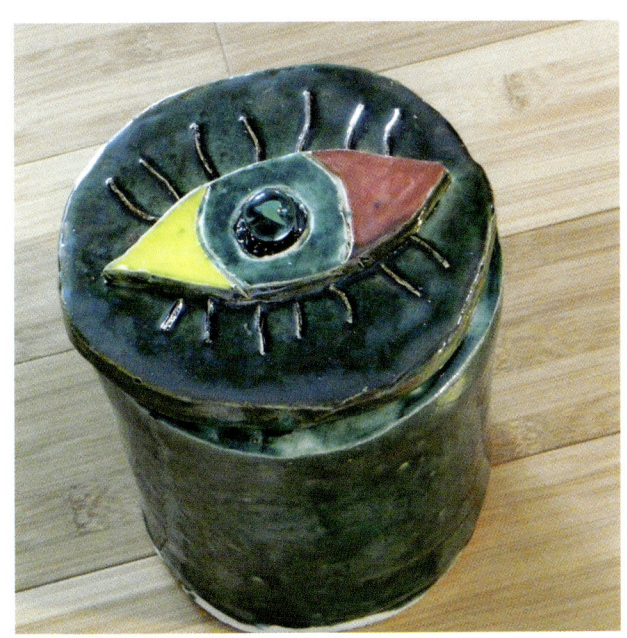

FIGURE 5.15 M's clay container

want to 'jinx' it. He explained that he had not asked for details since he wanted his father to be happy. M also opened up about his mother's previous lovers, how he had sabotaged those relationships and didn't want to disappoint his father. I suggested that perhaps he was holding his father hostage by not truly committing to sobriety and focusing on getting healthy. Of interest is that post this session his father privately relayed that M's mother became pregnant with M when they were engaged. The father had been contemplating breaking off their engagement but due to the pregnancy did not. It was wholly possible that M's feeling of not being wanted were deeper and more visceral than words could express. His father's parting statement that he 'can't see a way out', allowed me to weave this into their recap and homework.

Shortly thereafter M began to unravel and was 'dismissed' from his outpatient substance abuse group for 'harassing' his therapist. He also stopped taking his medication and deteriorated into a heightened manic episode: this resulted in property damage, theft in his grandfather's home and escalation of substance abuse. He refused to take responsibility for his actions and showed little to no remorse for his actions. At this time, his behavior escalated, and he no longer complied with our behavioral contract. It was during that time that I made it clear to both M and his father that he needed a higher level of care (e.g. rehabilitation placement). In essence, I fired the case until M was compliant with embracing sobriety.

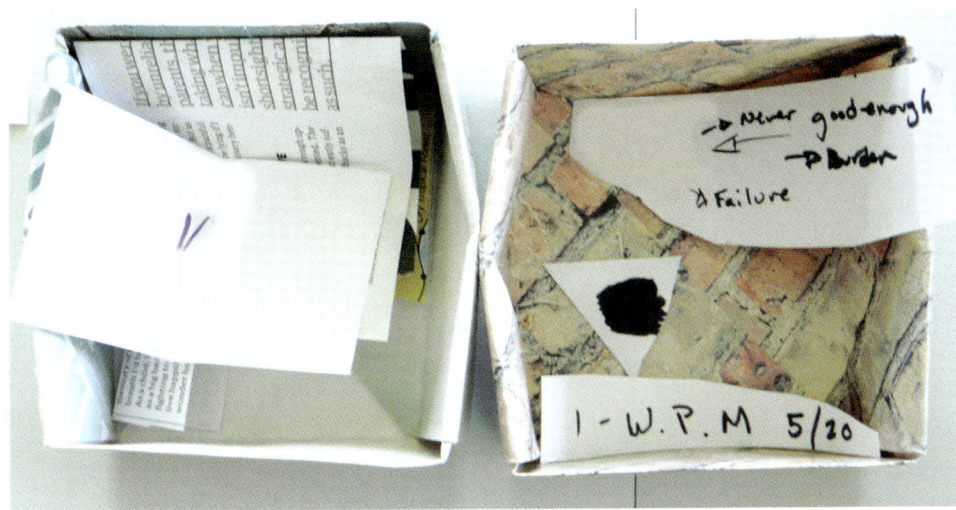

FIGURE 5.16 Self-boxes by father (left) and M (right)

Chapter five

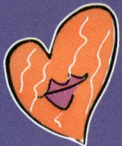
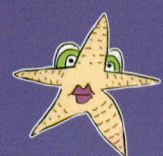

M's last session yielded assessment scores in the normal ranges for depression, anxiety and stress, which may have reflected his acceptance of his need to 'detox' and resolve his issues. I also conducted the opioid risk tool (ORT) during our final meeting before he entered his rehab treatment. Based on the results, M was at high risk for aberrant behavior (91%).

However, despite his dual diagnosis and familial struggles, he had extraordinary musical talent, and with proper medication and cessation of substance abuse, he could be an enormously successful and productive citizen. I had high hopes that perhaps this time the rehabilitation treatment would work. Nevertheless, his past history of TBI, substance abuse and familial dysfunction was a clear liability.

Final meeting while in treatment for drug and alcohol rehabilitation

Due to a hurricane in Florida (where his treatment facility was), M had to make a rare return to the area. His father asked if I would see him during this time. He was currently sober and not using drugs, sleeping about 5 to 6 hours per night. He mentioned fighting with another peer, but overall he was doing much better since being in the drug and alcohol treatment setting. Since he was on day 38 of sobriety, I suggested he create a bridge using his hands as a template. He delineated his 'before' (left hand), 'now' (thumbs touching) and 'future' (right hand) self (Fig. 5.17).

Of interest was how he described the bridge drawing: the left hand was his 'dark past' and the

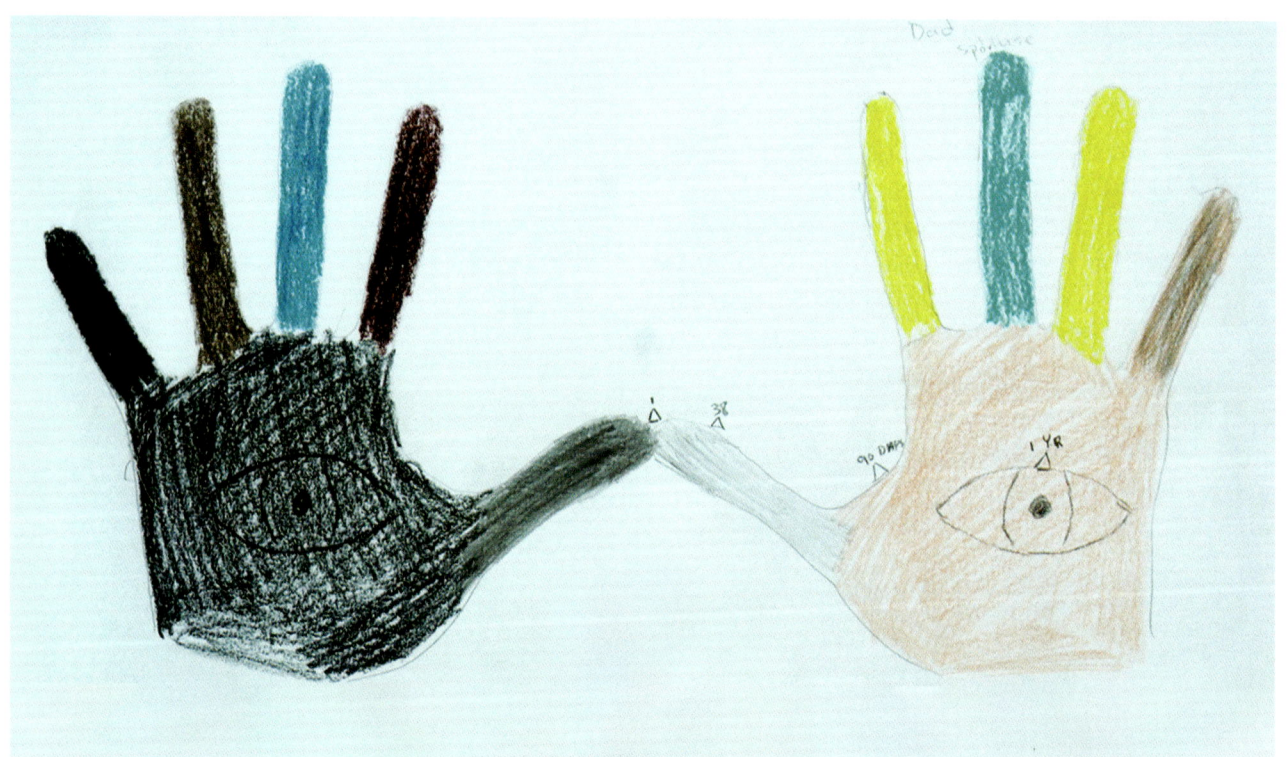

FIGURE 5.17 M's bridge drawing of sobriety, with his 'dark past' (left hand) and future self (right hand)

Clinical cases: adolescents

right his future self. He described this as being 'caught in a spiral', and the eye in the middle of the left palm was described as not being able to see since he was 'addicted to chaos' (which I found particularly poignant). He drew himself crossing over the right thumb at day 38. Next he detailed himself before the right thumb at 90 days. The right palm represented 1 year into sobriety and above the right middle finger he wrote his supports: 'Dad, halfway house, sober support, 38 days clean, weather, beach in FL, sponsor'. The right hand was how he envisioned the future (quite realistically), with the yellow fingers representing 'consistency', the blue 'better' than the left hand blue, but still clouded a bit and the peach/gray as those 'blech' days. His father, whom he later explained this to, pointed out that this was just like real life.

Next I had him write a letter from his current self to his 90-day-sober self. I then had him place it in an envelope and I told him I would mail it to him right before he reached that mark (Fig. 5.18).

Update and conclusion

I learned that M finally made it through to sobriety and after becoming clean, returned to the west coast in the hopes of attending a college which specialized in music.

Given my experience with this case, in the future I would only accept patients with severe addictions post-rehab treatment. The reasons are multifold, but the main reasoning is that an addict cannot truly be responsive to any kind of treatment until sober. It became clear (despite M's enthusiasm for both yoga therapy and art therapy) that he would be unable to make sufficient gains until he reached sobriety. Ultimately, I was able to get M into inpatient substance abuse treatment, and this in itself was a small measure of success, but you cannot be 'present' when self-medicating

> Dear Future Self,
>
> I am 38 days clean today and I'm already seeing clearly. You are now 90 days clean and that must feel incredible. You powered through the toughest 90 days in your recovery and I totally knew you could do it. I know it wasn't easy for you... It's not supposed to be. Everyone doubted your ability to stay clean for this long but you had the strength & willpower to do it. Keep on moving forward! You're in the right place @ the right time and by now I'm sure you already know that. You have an extraordinary life ahead of you. Keep pushing and lets make the next goal your 6 months! You can do it one day at a time.
>
> —Love—
> Present Self

FIGURE 5.18 M's letter to his future self

and thus I had to let go of any illusions that I could truly help M before he met that mark.

During the writing of this book, M's father contacted me and asked me if I could see M for an emergent session over this past Christmas holiday. M's younger brother had just committed suicide. I met M twice during the 5 days that he was back in town and communicated a report to his therapist on the west coast. While M was clearly raw and at great risk since he felt responsible for not watching his brother more closely (and preventing his death), to his credit he was not abusing drugs and was committed to living, no matter how painful.

Chapter five

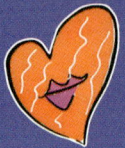 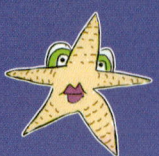

Reflection exercise 5.2

On being broken

There is a Japanese art form called *Kintsugi* or golden joinery, which uses gold-infused glue to reconnect broken pottery pieces. When the glue dries, the gold shines through the seams. The metamessage is that with the brokenness illuminated, the repaired object is considered to be more beautiful. Imagine if we were human *Kintsugi* pieces. We are all shattered and broken in some ways, but facing and accepting our brokenness takes courage in order to heal. And accepting that brokenness is the first step in recovery.

First, meditate on something that is broken in yourself and your life. Accept this *Kintsugi* concept within, then create yourself anew, cracks and all, in some form of artwork. Display this *Kintsugi* representation in a place of honor, so you can view the beauty within this aspect of yourself and embody that in your yoga and meditation practice.

Case study 3

17-year-old, from transgender to transsexual

Mental health, transgender issues and gender dysmorphia

According to Khalsa (2013) yoga treatment for a variety of psychiatric conditions can be both adjunctive and primary. Yoga therapy, art therapy and cognitive behavioral therapy (CBT) were the primary formats used in this case. However, before diving into this case, it is important to understand some basic concepts around working with transgender patients, as well as the cultural attitudes toward transgender people 'of color'. The term 'trans' is an umbrella term that refers to all of the identities within the transgender identity spectrum.

Gender identity refers to a person's deeply held sense of their own gender, which is not necessarily established by the assigned birth sex (Lev 2004). Clinicians, rarely trained in this area, are often ignorant and insensitive to such issues (Shipherd et al 2010, Carroll et al 2002, Lev 2004). According to Benson (2013) there are significant gaps in the mental health literature regarding transgender experiences and this subject is largely absent in couple and family therapy literature (Coolhart and Torres Bernal 2007). If you operate in the area of yoga therapy and art therapy (as I do) the chasm seems endless. According to Benson (2013), 'clinical literature tends to explore sexual orientation and fails to fully include emphasis on gender identity' (Benson 2013:18).

People experiencing gender dysphoria often feel a mismatch between their physical/assigned gender and the gender with which they identify. Self-described gender dysphoric people often experience discomfort with their body (particularly during puberty) and/or the expected roles of their assigned gender. People with gender dysphoria are often conflicted about how they feel and think about themselves (expressed gender) and their physical or assigned gender. Diagnostic criteria for gender dysphoria also centers on incongruence between gender and secondary sex characteristics, rather than gender identity *per se*.

Clinical cases: adolescents

Yet another problem exists in the DSM-5 diagnosis of gender dysphoria. Such limited diagnostic criteria were generally defined for medical treatment, which included prescriptions for hormones or surgery (Hanssmann et al 2008). Using a psychiatric diagnosis, which manifests into treatment, to legitimize access to medical treatment for transgender people, has required a diagnosis of 'psychological disease' and is in fact ethically questionable (Lev 2005). For the transgender or gender-dysphoric patient, therapeutic intervention has not been viewed as a place to address life challenges, but rather has served as an access point to medical intervention (Lev 2004). As the standards of care (SOC) have become more flexible, clinical practice has shifted from a primary focus on diagnosis and transition, to more inclusive quality-of-life issues (Coleman et al 2012). Indeed, health professionals can use the SOC to help patients consider the full range of health services open to them, in accordance with their clinical needs and goals for gender expression.

A review of mental health and gender dysphoria (Dhejne et al 2016) indicated that trans people attending transgender healthcare services appeared to have a higher risk of psychiatric morbidity (that improves following treatment), and suggested increased vulnerability of this population. As trans issues enter societal conscience (via social media, movies, TV and similar sources: think, Caitlyn Jenner, trans parent) more people will reflect on their assigned and experienced gender. The result may be an uptick of incongruence and questioning of cisgender status (previously taken for granted) (Bouman et al 2016). According to Bouman et al, 'the percentages of people reporting ambivalence and incongruence with their gender identity in the aforementioned population studies are simply staggering' (Bouman et al, p.1). Furthermore, Beek et al (2015) concluded that gender dysphoria and gender incongruence, currently considered as mental disorders in the DSM-5, may soon be viewed as a normal variation of human nature. Beek at al (2015) further suggest that in future revisions of the DSM-5 gender dysphoria and gender incongruence may be considered as mental conditions rather than 'diagnoses' *per se*.

Of import in this case is that this adolescent was of African American descent. Male to female or transgender women of color (African Americans, Latinas and Asian/Pacific Islanders) are considered at higher risk for suicidal ideation, depression and violent sexual and physical assault (Stotzer 2009, Nemoto et al 2006). In another study, more than two thirds of the transgender women of color (African American, number 235) reported being ridiculed or embarrassed by their family members because of their transgender identity or expression (Nemoto et al 2011). These facts are important to consider in review of this case. Transfeminine residents aged 15–34 years who were African American (black) or Latina were more likely to be murdered than were their cis-feminine comparators (Dinno 2017). So, given that dire statistic, let's review the case.

Background and history

'L' had an unusual upbringing. While very bright, she (her preferred gender identification) stated that she had suffered verbal and physical abuse at the hands of her biological father and mother. While both parents had been employed by the police, at intake they were divorced and both were on disability benefits. Mother's disability was due to her service post the September 11, 2001 attack and destruction of the World Trade Center in New York. The father had post-traumatic stress disorder (PTSD) and had been physically disabled prior to the 9/11 incident. While the mother had not been diagnosed post 9/11, she clearly had the hallmarks of PTSD. In addition, she had served in the police homicide division, and so may have also suffered PTSD during her employ.

Chapter five

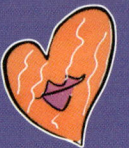 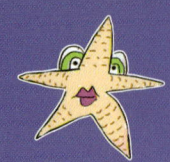

As can be seen by L's genogram (Fig. 5.19), mother had been involved in four different relationships (and subsequent divorces) and even though she was currently involved with a new boyfriend, she was still caretaking both her second husband and L's father (who were friends and living together). Complicated doesn't even begin to describe these relationships.

L had moved multiple times during her adolescence and was often the only black student in a predominantly white school. L was reportedly quite intelligent and so entered college early. Nevertheless, L left her first college placement due to extreme prejudice on the campus. L started seeing a psychiatrist at age 12 years when she identified as female. Due to her struggles with gender dysphoria and depression, she had undergone a short inpatient hospitalization while under the care of her psychiatrist. At intake, she was on Abilify and Wellbutrin for depression. Due to contracting Lyme

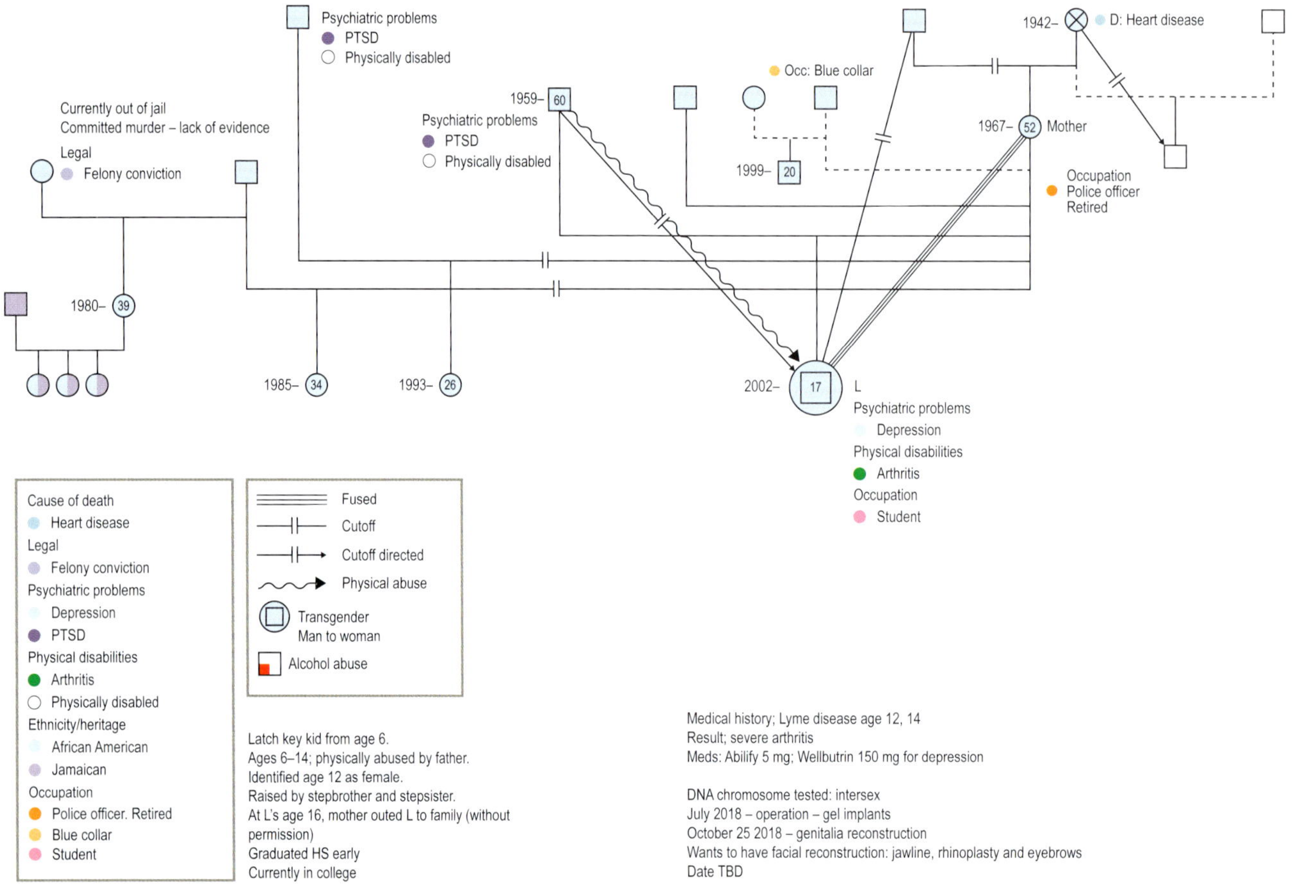

FIGURE 5.19 L's genogram

Clinical cases: adolescents

disease at her age 12 and 14, she allegedly suffered from arthritis, limiting her ability to exercise. At intake, her purpose in seeing me was to ascertain recommendations for multiple surgeries for her gender reassignment. However, as the treatment progressed, multiple comorbid issues came up including suicidal ideation, depression, hypersexual disorder, and agoraphobia.

These issues came up repeatedly throughout our 40 sessions. Initially some sessions were held twice weekly, with mother attending a total of four sessions, and there were also several telehealth sessions during her recuperation post-surgeries. Of interest is that a DNA test determined that she had been born intersex (a reproductive or sexual anatomy that doesn't seem to fit the typical definitions of female or male).

Significant sessions

According to Simons et al (2013) parental support of transgender adolescents translates into a higher quality of life and reduced depression. Therefore, interventions that promote parental support could positively affect the mental health of transgender youth. There was so much animosity between L and her mother that these sessions were strained, often reduced to screaming matches. Mother supported L financially, but their relationship was tempestuous, often turning into verbal and physical altercations. L was so eager to point out their screaming matches while traveling by car that she often recorded their conversations and then sent them to me via email. In all of these recordings, L remained calm, to the point of maddening her mother.

On a few occasions, I asked her mother to join in for family sessions. These sessions quickly escalated into heated arguments where mother constantly chewed out L for her behavior. Therefore, most of the sessions were individual. Session 6 was a family session. The overarching theme was that L refused to take responsibility for her actions, and as her mother put it, 'own her actions'. L continually relied on her mother for finances, and even though L had a vehicle, she was somewhat agoraphobic and relied on her mother to take her to all of her medical appointments. This resulted in her mother driving for 2 hours to pick L up and take her to an appointment in New York, 6 hours' drive away. L seemed unappreciative of mother's sacrifices.

Some of the artwork that rolled out of these initial sessions underscored L's gender dysphoria. In Figure 5.20, L described this feminine-looking tree as a 'self-portrait', but the tree lacked roots (read: lack of stability) and had 'dead limbs' suggesting a lack of blossom and growth. L and I were able to talk about this tree, how it truly reflected herself and how exercise (specifically yoga and breathwork) might help with a greater sense of Self.

Post this artwork, L's DASS-21 scores dropped into the normal range for depression, anxiety and stress. Prior to the session, her scores were in the moderate range for both anxiety and stress.

On her pain self-efficacy questionnaire (PSEQ), L's responses compared to other individuals with chronic pain suggested that L was less able to cope with discomfort. The pain was likely to cause significant impact on daily activities. Such

Chapter five

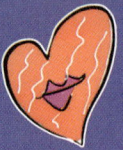
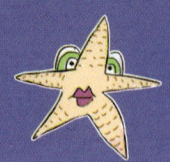

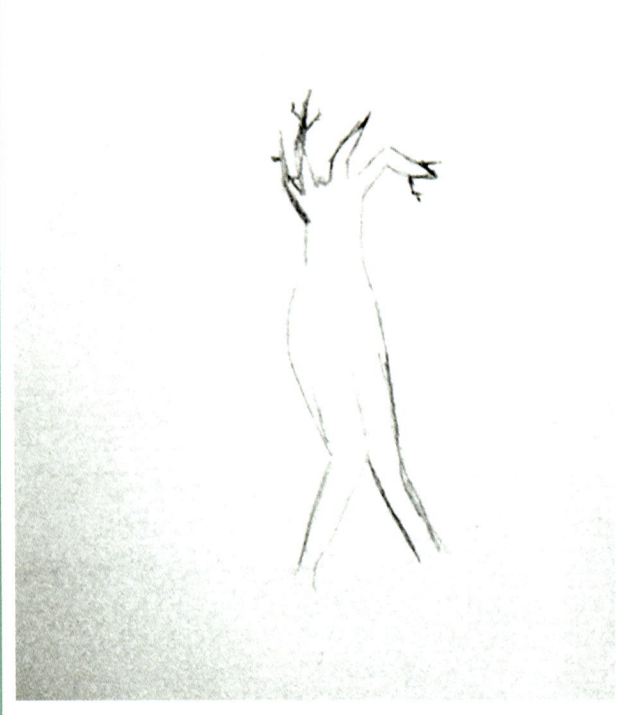

FIGURE 5.20 L's self-portrait

scores are often associated with chronic withdrawal from activities, and poor outcomes.

The recap reflected what we discussed in the session and L's need to exercise more to eradicate depression and prepare for her upcoming breast augmentation surgery. Her constant excuse for not exercising was the past arthritis caused by having Lyme disease twice. However, whenever L practiced yoga in sessions, the arthritis seemed non-existent. L responded positively to yoga and the art therapy; psychotherapy often brought up difficult and painful feelings. Yet, all were important parts of the treatment.

Recap homework:

1. You need to start an exercise regimen that you are comfortable with. You can find numerous workout videos on YouTube and we can work on a regimen that will leave you feeling refreshed and burn calories. Stretching is important and I am glad that you are doing that daily, but perhaps you could keep a careful journal of everything you eat for three days and show it to me the next time we meet. Then we can look at how nutritious (or not) your meals are. This would be good preparation for working with a nutritionist since you want to lose weight.

2. The main thing we need to work on is allowing for a deeper connection with others—that is, allowing others to actually see the real you and get close to you. A good place to start might be with your family. While you pride yourself on 'keeping your mom at bay', it would be in your interest to try and 'make friends' with her. In other words, allow yourself to let her in. While you struggle with that, she is your family, loves you, and would love to be a part of your life if you would allow for that. We need to explore why that is so difficult for you since it also affects your future ability to be in a healthy, caring and loving relationship.

3. Being able to bridge the above also affects your ability to trust me; it is all connected.

L's self-esteem (or lack thereof) was a running theme in our sessions and her artwork. A Self-box (made from fabric on an empty tin box) was reflective of her inner and outer issues. It was also meant to house her medication since L continually 'forgot' to take her psychotropic medication. Figure 5.21 is the Self-box. The top image shows the mirror on top of the box (which L shisha-embroidered around), which reflected her constant need to re-image herself. Inside, L stated that the skeletons represented her fear of death (middle image) and the stripes on the bottom (bottom image), her connection to the LGBTQ world.

L had a habit of uploading provocative images of herself on Facebook, Instagram and various

Clinical cases: adolescents

social sites several times a day. While unwilling to forge face-to-face (F2F) relationships, all of her interactions were born from online communications (Facebook, Instagram and Sugar Daddy meet-up sites). As a result, L initiated copious sexual interactions with relative strangers and exchanged these sexual favors for food, alcohol and sometimes money. It should be noted that none of these exchanges with men were actual dates. She preferred to receive these visits in her apartment and did not 'go out' with the 'Sugar Daddies'. While prostituting herself in exchange for these favors was suggested, she denied that she was in that category although her actions were similar. Getting her to stop this behavior was a large part of our treatment. Naturally, the yoga sessions were aimed at her honoring her body and treating it like a temple as opposed to a commodity to exchange for gifts.

Surgery and telehealth yoga

L turned 18 during our work together and since she was considered an 'adult', she scheduled her surgeries. First was her breast augmentation (top surgery), followed a few months later with her sex reassignment (bottom surgery). As surgery loomed near, L became more anxious, depressed, and agoraphobic. We continued to work on breathwork and mild stretching, since that was all she was willing to do. When L had her breast augmentation and sex reassignment surgeries a few months apart, those sessions which included yoga were conducted online while healing. Figure 5.22 is an example of some of the online yoga conducted to rebuild her strength and aid recovery.

L's bottom surgery was more difficult than her top surgery for a number of reasons. She was in excruciating pain post her bottom surgery and she had great difficulty with her new urethra and had to go to the emergency room twice. During her

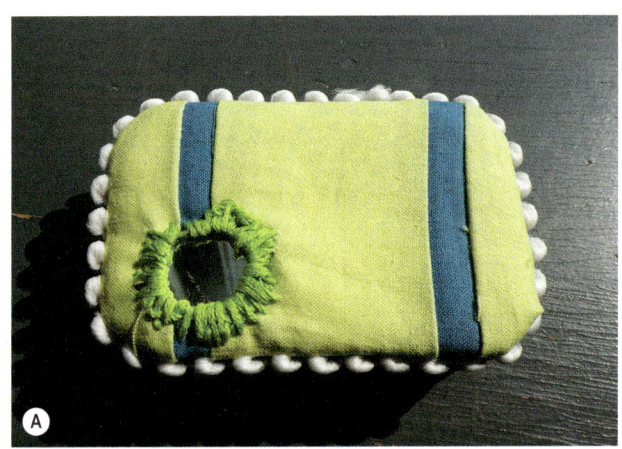
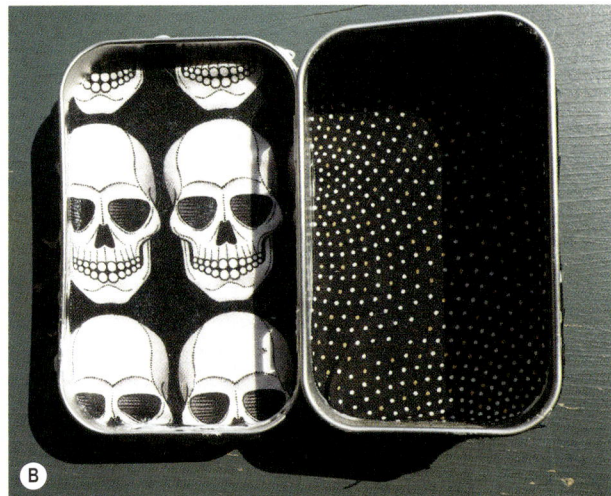
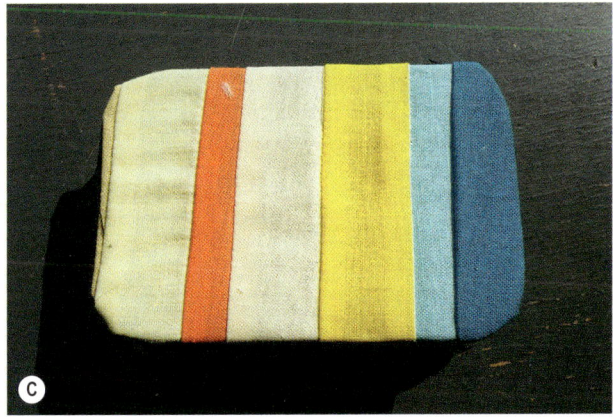

FIGURE 5.21 L's Self-box (top, inside, bottom)

Chapter five

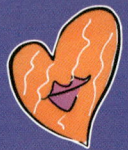 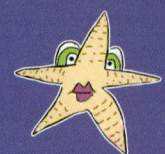

FIGURE 5.22 Yoga conducted during telehealth sessions

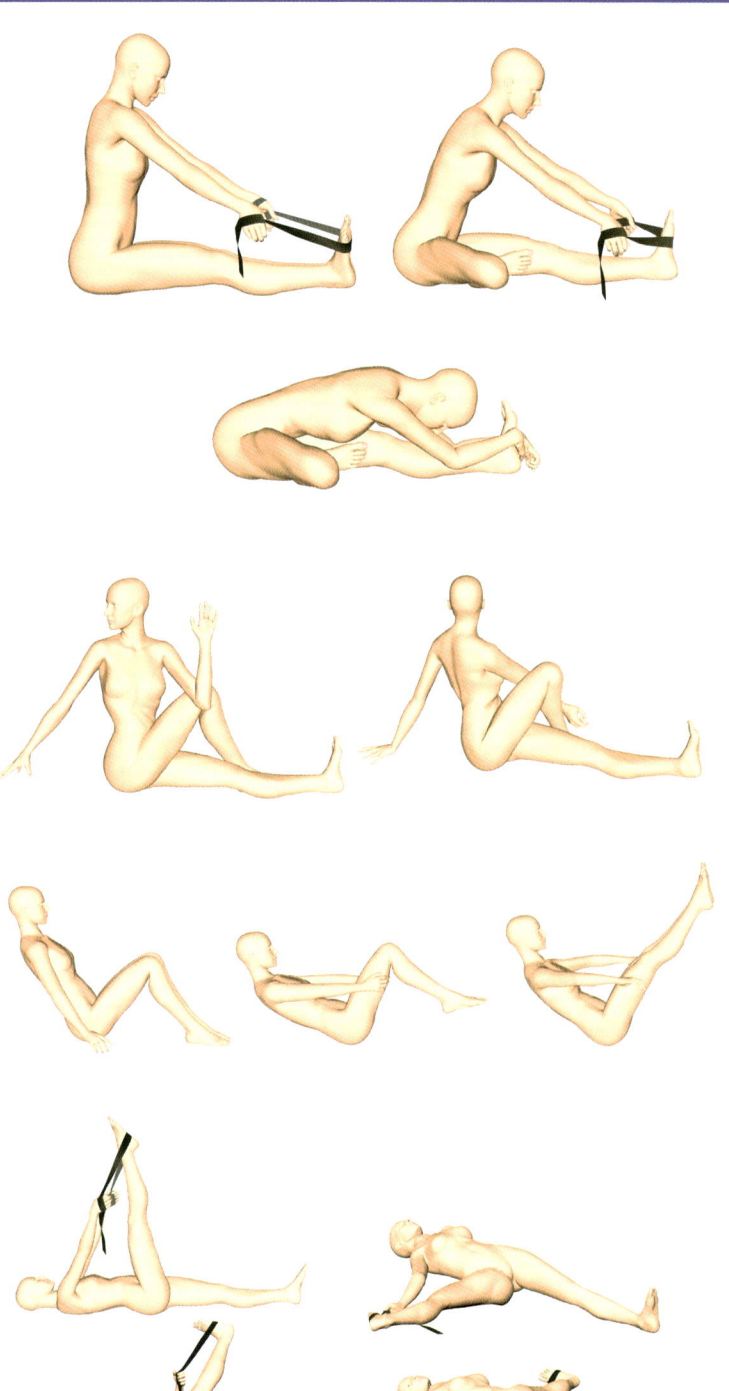

Using the belt around the bottoms of your feet, stretch forward to your level of flexibility. Then, take one foot to inside of thigh. Stretch over the extended leg as best you can with a straight back. Reverse legs – hold for up to 10 seconds.

Take one leg over the other. Flex foot of extended leg. Take opposite elbow to the outside of the bent leg and take the other hand behind you. Sit up tall and extend your back. Hold for 10 seconds.
Then, reverse arms (right arm goes over the right knee and left arm goes behind).

Boat pose for core work. Note position 1: You are using your hands at your sides as props until you can raise your legs and hold under your knees with a straight back. Final pose is number 3; work up to that; this will strengthen your core and lower back.

Supta Pādangusthāsana
Using a belt, extend one leg on the floor and take the other to your level of flexibility. Ensure extended leg has toes flexed towards the ceiling. Hold for 10 seconds. Then allow that leg to cross over the extended one. Hold for 10 seconds. Reverse legs. By the end of the session you are able to do this without a belt and have extraordinary flexibility. Aim for the last pose. Do on both sides.

recovery, L questioned her decision, but her comments of 'I'm not sure this was the right decision', quickly waned as she moved towards healing.

Once back in town she readjusted, but her agoraphobia increased. Some of this was pain-induced. While I encouraged her to get some moderate exercise (such as walking to rebuild her strength), she refused to get out of bed. As a result, I did several home visits which were illuminating. Despite how well put together L had been when she drove to my office, her small apartment reflected her inner chaos. Her home was a pigsty. The only time she attempted to clean her apartment was when she had a 'male visitor'. The healing from her bottom surgery limited her ability to have sexual relations for several months, which was actually a good thing, but she still entertained male suitors. She also had complications from the surgery (the vaginal opening was not wide enough, so she had to have a second operation to widen the area). All of this was a nightmare.

However, the good news was that I had convinced L to register for her next semester classes and none of the five classes were online. This forced her out of the house and into the world. Her agoraphobia disappeared as she began to go to classes and made friends. Still, while she was deathly afraid of any of her classmates finding out about her, her online postings were fairly transparent. It was an interesting pickle that she presented.

All the while, she was afraid to go into town alone for fear that she might be attacked. Just to note, L was almost 6 feet (1.8 m) tall, and quite large in stature. Diminutive she was not. While perfectly capable of handling herself, she still was at great risk. I suggested that when she went out that her friends accompany her. She was also attending a trans group (specifically for LGBTQ people of color) in the downtown area. Unfortunately, there was lots of drama attached to the group and so her socialization there was cut short. Yet things improved. Our sessions reduced from twice weekly to weekly and then every other week.

With continued yoga, psychotherapy and art therapy, L's DASS-21 results dropped to normal ranges for depression, anxiety and stress. Yet her mood and feelings questionnaire self-report (MFQ-Self) belied her DASS-21 results and suggested that she had clinically significant mood disturbance. I wanted to make certain that her medication was being monitored so I suggested that she see a nurse practitioner in town. The nurse practitioner and I were in close contact to make sure that no 'splitting' occurred.

Support for facial feminization surgery and discussion

Next, L decided to push ahead with facial feminization surgery (FFS). I understood her reasoning but thought given her recent surgeries that this was too soon. Nevertheless, I wrote a letter of support for a number of reasons, full knowing that it might take several months before her surgery would be approved by insurance.

At the time of my writing a letter of support, L was receiving cross-sex hormone therapy, was taking her medication as directed and living her life fully and openly in this role since at least 2014. She had received both breast augmentation and gender reassignment surgery, and the referral for FFS for the purpose of physiologic alignment with her female gender was to allow her to more effectively live in society in her asserted gender, with less instances of discrimination due to her typical masculine facial structure. By undergoing FFS, it was my hope that this would reduce significant gender dysphoria related to her masculine facial structure and facilitate her public recognition as a woman in all aspects of her life. This would enable

Chapter five

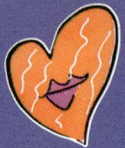

L to navigate education, career and social experiences with increased safety.

The World Professional Association of Transgender Health (WPATH), an internationally recognized body of medical and mental health professionals, has published extensively on the experiences of transgender individuals and published guidelines for treatment and support. There are significant data that conclude that individuals with gender dysphoria experience significant social oppression, discrimination and violence due to being visibly gender non-conforming. Transgender individuals are disproportionally denied housing and jobs when they are visibly seen as gender-variant through physical structures that do not change as a result of gender-confirming hormone treatments and other procedures. This population has been shown to experience staggering rates of harassment, discrimination and even violence in schools, jobs, public accommodations and homes due to their gender identity not aligning with their physical appearance. To be able to safely exist in a gendered society such as the USA, which is rigidly gender-binary, FFS is of utmost importance for many transgender individuals in order to maintain their safety, careers, and housing, and to be able to effectively and productively navigate interactions in everyday public and private life.

Since cross-sex hormone therapy alone could not reliably feminize L due to this treatment's lack of effect on the mature adult bone structure, the only choice for gender dysphoric adults with masculine facial structures (such as L) is to undergo FFS, to contour the facial bones to approach a more typically perceived feminine appearance.

For some transgender individuals, FFS is one of the most important medically necessary procedures in their gender affirmation process, since the face is one of the primary physically visible ways that gender is perceived and assigned in our society. Incongruence of the masculinized facial structure with the feminine identity and presentation of an individual leads to significantly increased risks of violence and discrimination in everyday life and functioning and severely inhibits the individual from participating in normal daily life, including the ability to secure and maintain employment and housing.

For L, a combination of extreme gender dysphoria (ICD-10 F64.9) and a need to ensure her safety in the world created a medical necessity for her to undergo this procedure. From a clinical standpoint, I saw no valid reason to deny her request for coverage of facial feminization surgery. She clearly met and exceeded the criteria for gender dysphoria under the DSM-5 guidelines (ICD-10 F64.9).

L's gender identity had been persistent since childhood and her having been born intersex established an additional veracity for this request. She met the criteria for gender dysphoria and had exceeded the requirements for the World Professional Association for Transgender Health Standards of Care (WPATH 2012). In order for this to be covered by insurance, I also diagnosed her as follows:

- F43.10, post-traumatic stress disorder, unspecified
- F64.9, gender dysphoria disorder
- F40.01, agoraphobia with panic disorder
- Z70.1, counseling related to patient's sexual behavior and orientation. Patient concerned regarding sexual orientation.

Around this time, due to a lecture commitment followed by a 2-week vacation, I prepared L for a break in our treatment. I felt confident that any issues that arose would be addressed by the nurse practitioner who L was also seeing twice monthly. Nevertheless, even though there would be a significant time-zone difference, I gave her the option of telehealth sessions, phone therapy or texting me. She chose none of those options. When I returned, she cancelled our next appointment and did not follow-up for another session. Some of this may have been due to her mother's decision not to continue to financially support our work together. Or it could be that she had gotten what she wanted from the therapy (the letters of support from me that she needed for all of her operations). Whatever the reasoning, given the constraints of HIPAA, my hands were tied. So, there I was unable to contact my patient again. I felt frustrated but needed to resign myself to the situation.

Reflection exercise 5.3

On being enough

Whether you are a healthcare professional or a yoga teacher reading this case, the way it ended was a hard pill to swallow. I turned to Perma Chodron's work. Chodron (2013) writes about accepting our shared humanity of suffering and compassion. She talks about Tonglen, a Tibetan meditation practice of giving and receiving, taking and sending. Practicing Tonglen, we take in the pain of the world with our inhalation, and expire our own comfort, healing and goodness. The practice is about opening your heart to suffering and offering compassion to yourself and others who suffer likewise. When you inhale sadness and exhale compassion, you discover a cache of kindness larger than yourself and your own suffering. When we hold others as healers, this is what we do – empathizing, mirroring and moving towards a trajectory of acceptance. This is interpersonal neurobiology, interoception at its best. In Buddhist language, one would say that this practice dissolves the fixation and clinging of ego. As Chodron describes it, you can breathe in feelings of inadequacy and exhale confidence and relief. At the end of the day, this is really all we can do.

Imagine practicing this perhaps for yourself, a patient or even an enemy. And then create some art around this perhaps to attend to how practicing Tonglen can inform your own well-being and those around you. As abruptly as this case ended, in practicing compassion for myself and L, I could live with the outcome, and let it go. And that is a gift.

Chapter five

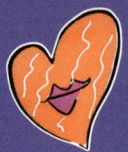
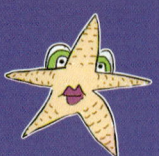

References

Admon G, Weinstein Y, Falk B, et al (2005) Exercise with and without an insulin pump among children and adolescents with Type 1 Diabetes Mellitus. Pediatrics 116(3): e348–e355.

American Psychiatric Association (2013) Diagnostic and Statistical Manual of Mental Disorders (5th edn). Washington, DC: American Psychiatric Association.

Anderson LH (1999) Speak. Harrisonburg, VA: RR Donnelly & Sons Company.

Beek TF, Kreukels BPC, Cohen-Kettenis PT and Steensma TD (2015) Partial treatment requests and underlying motives of applicants for gender affirming interventions. Journal of Sexual Medicine 12: 2201–2205.

Benson KE (2013) Seeking support: transgender client experiences with mental health. Journal of Feminist Family Therapy 25: 17–40.

Blum K, Sheridan PJ, Wood RC, et al (1996) The D2 dopamine receptor gene as a determinant of reward deficiency syndrome. Journal of the Royal Society of Medicine 89(7): 396–400.

Blum K, Chen A, Giordano J, Borsten J, et al (2012) The addictive brain: all roads lead to dopamine. Journal of Psychoactive Drugs 44(20): 134–143.

Bouman WP, deVries ALC and T'Sjoen G (2016) Gender dysphoria and gender incongruence: an evolving interdisciplinary field. International Review of Psychiatry 28(1): 1–4.

Carroll L, Gilroy PJ and Ryan J (2002) Transgender issues in counselor education. Counselor Education and Supervision 41(3): 233–242.

Case C and Dalley T (2014) The Handbook of Art Therapy, 3rd Edn. East Sussex, UK: Routledge.

Chodron P (2013) Living Beautifully with Uncertainty and Change. Boulder, Co: Shambhala.

Coleman E, Bockting W, Botzer M, et al (2012) Standards of care for the health of transsexual, transgender, and gender-nonconforming people, Version 7. International Journal of Transgenderism 13(4): 165–232.

Comings DE 2008 Did Man Create God? Duarte, CA: Hope Press.

Coolhart D and Torres Bernal A (2007) Clinical update: transgender in family therapy. Family Therapy Magazine 6(3): 36–42.

Dhjene C, Vlerken RV, Heylens G and Arcelus J (2016) Mental health and gender dysphoria: A review of the literature. International Review of Psychiatry 28(1): 44–47.

Diana M, Raij T, Melis M, Nummenmaa A, Leggio M and Bonci A (2017) Rehabilitating the addicted brain with transcranial magnetic stimulation. Nature Reviews of Neuroscience 18(11): 685–693.

Dinno A (2017) Homicide rates of transgender individuals in the United States: 2010–2014. American Journal of Public Health 107(9): 1441–1447.

Durlofsky P (2018) Pause before posting: the benefits of not over sharing on social media. Psych Central blog. Available at: https://psychcentralcom/blog/pause-before-posting-the-benefits-of-not-over-sharing-on-social-media/

Elliot S (2005) The New Science of Breath: Coherent Breathing for Autonomic Nervous System Balance, Health and Well-Being. Allen, TX: Coherence Press, LLC.

Fehmi L 2014 How do you pay attention – a look into what is 'open focus'. Available at: https://www.youtube.com/watch?v=tmgHDEyp-PAQ

Fehmi L and Robbins J (2008) The Open-Focus Brain: Harnessing the Power of Attention to Heal Mind and Body. Boston, MA: Trumpeteer Books, Shambhala Publications.

Hallgren M, Romberg L, Bakshi A-S and Andréassan S (2014) Yoga as an adjunct treatment for alcohol dependence: A pilot study. Complementary Therapies in Medicine 22: 441–445.

Hamer D (2005) The God Gene. New York, NY: Doubleday.

Hanssmann C, Morrison D and Russian E (2008) Talking, gawking, or getting it done: provider trainings to increase cultural and clinical competence for transgender and gender-nonconforming patients and clients. Sexuality Research and Social Policy 5: 5–23.

Higgs MM (2019) Why you should find time to be alone with yourself. New York Times (28 October). Available at: https://www.nytimes.com/2019/10/28/smarter-living/the-benefits-of-being-alone.html

Hong RY and Park SJ (2012) Impact of attachment, temperament and parenting on human development. Korean Journal of Pediatrics 55(12): 449–454.

Horovitz EG (2002) Spiritual Art Therapy: An Alternate Path. Springfield, IL: Charles C Thomas Ltd.

Horovitz EG (2005) Art Therapy as Witness: A Sacred Guide. Springfield, IL: Charles C Thomas Ltd.

Horovitz EG (2017) Spiritual Art Therapy: An Alternate Path, 3rd Edn. Springfield, IL: Charles C Thomas Ltd.

Innes KE, Selfe TK and Hecht FM (2016) Yoga therapy for diabetes. In: Khalsa SBS, Cohen L, McCall T and Telles S (eds) The Principles and Practice of Yoga in Health Care. Edinburgh, UK: Handspring Publishing, pp. 209–239.

Iyengar BKS (1979) Light on Yoga. New York, NY: Schocken Books.

Jeter P and McCall T (2017) Research Summary for Yoga Therapists: Yoga Therapy for Type 2 Diabetes Mellitus. International Association of Yoga Therapists. Available at: https://cdn.ymaws.com/iayt.site-ym.com/resource/resmgr/docs_Research_Summaries/4.Summaries_Diabetes_v2.pdf

Juruena MFP (2012) Cognitive behavioral therapy for bipolar disorder patients. In: Reis de Oliveira I (ed) Standard and Innovative Strategies in Cognitive Behavioral Therapy. Rijeka, Croatia: InTech, pp. 76–98.

Kahley-Isley LC, Peterson J, Fischer C and Peterson E (2010) Yoga as a complementary therapy for children and adolescents: A guide for clinicians. Psychiatry 7(8): 20–32.

Kay AB and Nelson LB (2015) Yoga and Diabetes: Your Guide to Safe and Effective Practice. Alexandria, VA: American Diabetes Association.

Khalsa SS (2013) Yoga for psychiatry and mental health: an ancient practice with modern relevance. Indian Journal of Psychiatry 55: 334–336.

Khalsa SB, Khalsa GS, Khalsa HK and Khalsa MK (2008) Evaluation of a residential Kundalini yoga lifestyle pilot program for addiction in India. Journal of Ethnicity in Substance Abuse 7(1): 67–79.

Khanna S and Greeson JM (2013) A narrative review of yoga and mindfulness as complementary therapies for addiction. Complementary Therapies in Medicine 21(3): 244–252.

Kjaer TW, Bertelsen C, Piccini P, Brooks D, Alving J and Lou HC (2002) Increased dopamine tone during meditation-induced change of consciousness. Brain Research Cognitive Brain Research 13(2): 255–259.

Kohn M, Persson Lundholm U, Bryngelsson IL, Anderzen-Carlsson A and Westerdahl E (2013) Medical yoga for patients with stress-related symptoms and diagnoses in primary health care: a randomized controlled trial. Evidence Based Complementary and Alternative Medicine 2013: 215348.

Kramer ES and Iager AC (1984) The use of art in assessment of psychotic disorders: changing perspectives. The Arts in Psychotherapy 11(3): 197–120.

Lerner RM and Steinberg L (2009) Handbook of Adolescent Psychology, Vol. 2: Contextual Influences on Adolescent Development, 3rd Edn. Hoboken, NJ: Wiley & Sons.

Lev AI (2004) Transgender emergence: Therapeutic guidelines for working with gender variant people and their families. New York, NY: Haworth Press.

Lev AI (2005) Disordering gender identity: gender identity disorder and the DSM-IV-TR. Journal of Psychology and Human Sexuality 17(3/4): 35–69.

Lotstein DS, Seid M, Klingensmith G, et al (2013) Transition from pediatric to adult care for youth diagnosed with type 1 diabetes in adolescence. Pediatrics 131(4): e1062–e1070.

Mackenzie MJ, Carlson LE, Ekkekakis P, Paskevich DM and Culos-Reed SN (2013) Affect and mindfulness as predictors of change in mood disturbance, stress symptoms and quality of life in a community-based yoga program for cancer survivors. Evidence-Based Complementary and Alternative Medicine 2013: 419496.

Mahler M (1968) On Human Symbiosis and the Vicissitudes of Individuation: Volume I, Infantile Psychosis. Madison, CT: International Universities Press.

Mayo Clinic 2020 Dissociative disorders. Available at: https://www.mayoclinic.org/diseases-conditions/dissociative-disorders/symptoms-causes/syc-20355215

McCoy K 2009 Emotional Support for Type 1 Diabetes. Available at: https://www.everydayhealth.com/type-1-diabetes/type-1-diabetes-emotional-support.aspx

McElroy SL, Atshuler LL, Suppes T, Keck PE, Frye MA and Denicoff KD (2000) Axis I psychiatric comorbidity and its relationship to historical illness variables in 288 patients with bipolar disorder. American Journal of Psychiatry 159: 420–426.

Nemoto T, Sausa LA, Operario D and Keatley J (2006) Need for HIV/AIDS education and intervention for MTF transgenders: responding to the challenge. Journal of Homosexuality 51(1): 183–202.

Nemoto T, Böedecker B and Iwamato M (2011) Social support, exposure to violence and transphobia, and correlates of depression among male-to-female transgender women with a history of sex work. American Journal of Public Health 101(10): 1980–1988.

Oster GD and Crone P (2004) Using Drawings Assessment and Therapy: A Guide for Mental Health Professionals, 2nd Edn. New York, NY: Routledge.

Pickens RW, Svikis DS, McGue M, Lykken DT, Heston LL and Clayton PJ (1991) Heterogeneity in the inheritance of alcoholism. A study of male and female twins. Archives of General Psychiatry 48(1): 19–28.

Previc F (2009) The Dopaminergic Mind in Human Evolution and History. Cambridge, UK: Cambridge University Press.

Ratner RK and Hamilton RW (2015) Inhibited from bowling alone. Journal of Consumer Research 42(2): 266–283.

Chapter five

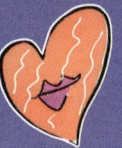
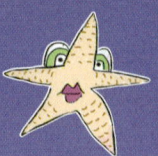

Sahay BK (1986) Yoga and diabetes. Journal of the Associations of Physicians of India 34:645–648.

Shipherd JC, Green KE and Abramovitz S (2010) Transgender clients: Identifying and minimizing barriers to mental health treatment. Journal of Gay and Lesbian Health 14(2): 94–108.

Simons L, Schrager SM, Clark LF, Belzer M and Olson J (2013) Parental support and mental health among transgender adolescents. Journal of Adolescent Health 53(6): 791–793.

Statista (2019) Most popular social networks of teenagers in the United States from fall 2012 to fall 2019. Available at: https://www.statista.com/statistics/250172/social-network-usage-of-us-teens-and-young-adults/

Stearns MN (2018) Healing anxiety depression and unworthiness: 78 brain-changing mindfulness and yoga practices. Eau Claire, WI: PESI Publishing & Media.

Stotzer RL (2009) Violence against transgender people: a review of United States data. Aggression and Violent Behavior 14(3): 170–179.

US Department of Health and Human Services (2008) Alcohol Alert Number 76: Alcohol and other drugs. US Department of Health and Human Services.

van der Kolk B (2014) The Body Keeps the Score: Brain, Mind and Body in the Healing of Trauma. New York, NY: Penguin.

Weintraub A (2012) Yoga Skills for Therapists: Effective Practices for Mood Management. New York, NY: WW Norton & Co.

Wellcome Trust Sanger Institute (2017) New type of stem cell line produced offers expanded potential for research and treatments. Science Daily. Wellcome Trust Sanger Institute, 11 October. Available at: https://www.sciencedaily.com/releases/2017/10/171011131722.htm

WPATH (2012) Standards of Care for the Health of Transsexual, Transgender, and Gender-Nonconforming People. Available at: https://www.wpath.org/media/cms/Documents/SOC%20v7/SOC%20V7_English2012.pdf?_t=1613669341

Yar S and Bromwich JE (2019) Tales From the Teenage Cancel Culture. New York Times, 31 October. Available at: https://www.nytimes.com/2019/10/31/style/cancel-culture.html.

Zinman R (2017) Yoga for Diabetes: How to Manage your Health with Yoga and Ayurveda. Rhinebeck, NY: Monkish Book Publishing Co.

Zschucke E, Heinz A and Strohle A (2012) Exercise and physical activity in the therapy of substance use disorders. The Scientific World Journal 2012(5): 901741.

Clinical cases: adults 6

The mind has great influence over the body, and maladies often have their origin there.

Molière (1622–1673)

The manner in which you, the provider, show up matters as much or more as how the patient arrives.

Matthew Taylor PT PhD E-RYT500 C-IAYT

Yoga therapy with older adults

In a recent quest, I researched the subjects of yoga therapy with aging adults. Oddly, the earlier scientific studies reminded me of how pearls are formed. An irritant – such as a parasite or grain of sand – somehow wedges its way into an oyster. The defense mechanism of that oyster is to produce a fluid which coats the irritant. This coating, called nacre, is deposited repeatedly until a lustrous pearl is formed. When researchers investigate unanswered questions, the process is akin to the irritant which wedges its way into our psyches until that nacre is formed and fueled into the workings of science. This is truly interoceptive research.

Back in the dimensions of yoga therapy and the Western medical model, Taylor was confronted with that same 'irritant'. Like many researchers that followed, he pointed out that the ancient healing modalities of yoga (the Indian doctrines of *Vedanta* – i.e. the sheaths or *kosha* models) provided the original prototype of biopsychosocial–spiritual rehabilitation. This *Vedanta* system offered an 'orderly and comprehensive system of addressing rehabilitation', which optimized not only health but also 'the social, emotional, psychological and spiritual aspects of the human experience' (Taylor 2012:93). That's a pretty tall order when you think about it. But that thinking also concretized everything that I had been reading for years. Finally, one of the pearls that Taylor tossed out in his article was that yoga therapy has the potential to rework and 'release cognitive patterns and limiting thoughts'. Given the neuroplasticity of the brain and what we have learned about the brain's ability to change (e.g. epigenetics) as we grow older, yoga makes even more sense regarding medical rehabilitation and aging adults.

As early as 1975, Blau and Berezin discussed the mild feelings of depression, anxiety, grief, and reduction of aspirations as symptomatic of working with an older adult population. Sable et al (2002) posited that cognitive impairment, memory and concentration difficulties, might also be more prevalent in older adult populations. So, what is an older adult? According to Wang (2009) an older adult can be anywhere from 55 to 100 years old (or older); it is important to note this is a 45-year range. This presents an enormously diverse group of persons that varies in experience and cultural and religious preferences. These factors affect appropriate and beneficial yoga practices for each individual (Wang 2009:95) (as well as motor integration skills for art therapy if one uses that modality).

As of 2020 there were an estimated 573,000 centenarians worldwide (Statista 2020), and this adds to the complication and diversity of working with older adults. In one of my yoga classes for 'seniors' I have a 99-year-old woman who uses the mat for her practice, so my guess is given the variability of people's abilities, this may become more prevalent than not. In fact, after one of my classes a member thanked me for not 'babying' them and offering them a class appropriate to their 'abilities'. And while I naturally adapt the *asanas* for whoever attends my yoga classes and private therapy sessions, her comment made me aware of how people feel. Of course, there are people that may be on the opposite spectrum, so as I always say, 'it depends'.

Tornstam's (2005) view on the concept of gerotranscendence breaks new ground by taking 'a phenomenological approach to reach a "from-within" understanding of what developments come with aging. The subjective meaning given to aging has been given preference before the meaning researchers ascribe to aging' (Tornstam 2005:187). It helps to look at Tornstam's views, as he casts aging into a different light. Tornstam divides gerotranscendence into three domains: (1) the cosmic dimension, which looks at past, present and the mysteries of finitude and beyond, (2) a self-dimension that surpasses puerile obsession with the body, and (3) social/personal relationships and asceticism and the attainment of everyday wisdom. When reading his theory, a lot of this smacked

Chapter six

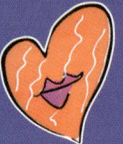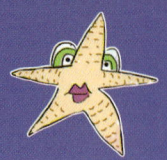

of the theoretical underpinnings of yoga. Applying gerotranscendence theory utilizes reminiscence therapy, dream analysis, meditation, respect for older adults' need for positive solitude (see Higgs' (2019) concept of 'aloneliness covered in Chapter 5), and acknowledges differences in older people's sense of spatial boundaries, time, cosmic communion, death and dying.

Still other studies touched on spirituality and religiosity when practicing yoga with older adults. Haber (1983) observed that minority elders reviewed their future in 'God's hands' (read: external control), which in turn influenced participation. Moreover, some elders perceived yoga as threatening to their spiritual and/or religious practices. In a recent study, Middleton et al (2015) underscored that yoga might be less acceptable for those with certain socioeconomic backgrounds or racial/ethnic identities. The authors warned that the yoga research conversation 'should be informed by the perspectives of those with differing opinions, without dismissing them as (an) isolated concern' (Middleton et al 2015:34).

Patel et al (2012) conducted a meta-analysis review of over 18 studies ($N = 649$ patients). Quantitative and qualitative synthesis unearthed that the benefits of yoga exceeded those of conventional exercise interventions for self-rated health status, aerobic fitness and strength. However, evidence was mixed for depression, sleep and bone-mineral density, a huge concern when participants have osteopenia or osteoporosis. Current recommendations are for 30 minutes of physical activity several times per week to prevent loss of abilities (Chodzko-Zajko and Proctor 2009, Physical Activity Guidelines Advisory Committee 2009).

My view on exercise for older adults has been colored by my own experience. I do *pranayama*, meditation and yoga *asanas* daily (I trained in the Iyengar method). I have also been a swimmer my entire adult life. I presently take total resistance exercise classes, barre classes and pump iron, kayak (in good weather) and I walk a lot, in addition to my yoga practice. In short, I love to exercise. For the last 5 years I have been conducting a 'Silver Sneaker Yoga' class, but I have not been adhering to the regulated script. For starters, I always start with an intention and brief meditation. Often, we '*Aum*' and include breath control, especially during the *asana* practices. I have also created my own methodology using the chair as a prop. I incorporate the principles from my Lakshmi Voelker Chair Yoga (Voelker 2020) training and for part of the class I have participants use weights (providing these seniors with much-needed bone mineral uptake). Chapter 7 gives a sampling of how I conduct these classes using the chair as a prop and sitting on the chair. Sometimes we use exercise balls, both small and large, and we always use yoga belts for some of the *asanas*, both seated and standing. If someone needs to sit on the chair, then I also teach to that, despite the fact that some of these members also use the mat for downward facing dog (*adho mukha śvānāsana*), etc. The last 10–15 minutes of class are either conducted in a chair (or on the mat for some) as they prepare for *savāsana* (relaxation/corpse pose). This is a twice-weekly yoga class, with approximately 26 participants, give or take the snowbirds who leave for a few months during the winter. The class continues to grow by word-of-mouth. The ages range from people in their sixties to their nineties. No surprise, this group has formed a *saṅga* (community). They check in on each other and socialize before and after the class. I really love this group and it's hard to believe I get paid to work with such wonderful, accomplished people.

According to the studies reviewed by Patel et al (2012) yoga improves health-related quality of life (HRQoL), enhances walking and balance, muscular strength, cardiovascular health, blood pressure, sleep and functioning of other systems (Patel et al 2012:902–903). It was also suggested that yoga may contribute to psychosocial benefits and emotional problems linked with aging. Loneliness has been touted as a factor in depression, especially among the elderly. Findings underline the importance of the social context of psychological well-being. Social isolation, whether subjective (loneliness) or objective (non-integrated social network) accounted for 70% of the prevalence of depressed mood in a study conducted by Golden et al (2009). Overall, Patel et al (2012) recom-

Clinical cases: adults

mended yoga for older adults with careful observation and monitoring for side-effects. According to Sims et al (2012), 'physical activity may assist both in the prevention and management of depression in older people' (p.115). While this is common knowledge for those that exercise, recent studies have demonstrated that people who exercise are less likely to be, or become, depressed (Brosse et al 2002).

In a study on chair yoga (Bonura and Pargman 2009), the chair yoga group demonstrated greater benefits than did the chair-exercise or walking groups. Bonura and Pargman proposed that, 'in a population of already active older adults, yoga provided additional mental health benefits above and beyond aerobics and walking' (p.84). In this study the chair was also used as a prop, where participants used it for seated, standing and balance poses. Beyond the scientific research, particularly useful was a sample chair-yoga class provided at the end of the article. The authors admitted that the participants consisted of predominantly elderly widowed women, but the results indicated that mindfulness-based exercise practices such as yoga might provide additional benefits beyond exercise alone (Bonura and Pargman 2009:86).

Art therapy and yoga for adults

Encouraging and supporting art-making can be effective in working with all ages, including older adults (Horovitz 2005, 2014, 2017a, 2017b, Kramer 1975, 2016, Rubin 2016). Some studies have focused on individuals with dementia who are coping with memory loss and/or a restricted ability to communicate (Abraham 2005, Alders and Levine-Madori 2010, Hattori et al 2011, Horovitz 2005, 2014, 2017b, Mimica and Dubravka 2011, Rubin 2016, Stallings 2010, Stewart 2004), or suffering from a life-long mental illness (Orr 1997). Stephenson (2013) reviewed a community-based art therapy program for older adults from a gerotranscendence perspective. This reinforced the notion of healthy adaptation when working in a communal atmosphere by using art materials for self-expression and communication. It appears that art therapy is most effective with older adults when approached with an understanding of 'what is healthy and adaptive during this remarkable developmental stage' (Kerr 1999:37). Again, healthy regulation was thematic in Kerr's work.

Morris (2014) reported that art therapy might be a viable addition to cognitive behavioral therapy (CBT) for patients with panic disorder with agoraphobia (PDA) and generalized anxiety disorder (GAD). A study on whether or not coloring mandalas could reduce anxiety demonstrated that, 'participants who colored on a blank piece of paper showed no reductions in anxiety, whereas those participants who colored a mandala actually decreased their anxiety levels to levels below that which they reported before the anxiety induction' (Curry and Kasser 2005:83).

Beyond my own previous work (Horovitz 2014, Horovitz and Elgelid 2015), Gibbons (2015) integrates yoga, meditation, *mūdras* and art therapy exercises in her book. My favorite take-away from Gibbons' book is her practice chart for intention-centered yoga and art (p.55–66). Also, exercises on mindful doodling as outlined by my colleague Isis (2016) may be helpful as starting points with patients who are not necessarily geared towards more creative art materials. Franklin (1999) also discussed art therapy and yoga. One of my favorite quotes is from an early article he wrote about art and its informative process.

Over and over again, I have been humbled by the creative process. It is much wiser than I could ever hope to be... Even when I think I am in control, I am not. I am not the doer, only a participant who is listening to the rhythms of the Self. Meditation and art are ways to listen

(Franklin 1999)

In 2011, Franklin went a bit further, suggesting that he could not 'separate art from yoga' (Franklin 2011:97). Years passed and Franklin crystalized his ideas in his 2017 opus. He suggested that art combined with meditation and service was akin to *sādhanā* (spiritual practice) and aided him into unfolding into its 'numinous content' (Franklin 2017:153). While art has often been saddled

Chapter six

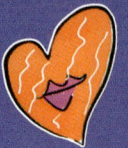 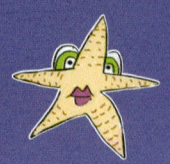

with the concept of rumination (and the seat of *citta*/mind), Franklin (2017) pointed out that, 'art and meditation reduced stress by creating visual representations of our thoughts'. He suggested that these two practices were plaited and 'uniquely untangle[d] enmeshment with shadowed unconscious material' (p.158).

Of course, this stance mirrors the earlier ideas of Csikszentmihalyi (1997), who discussed the flow state and the autotelic personality during this absorbed state of engagement. The autotelic state is fulfillment for the sake of oneself as opposed to an exotelic state which is goal-oriented, objective and outcome oriented. Satprem (1982) referred to this autotelic state as, 'cellular consciousness… no longer imprisoned within the net of a body', and coined this, 'the other state' (Satprem 1982:30–31). In conversation with 'Mother' (otherwise known as *Mirra Alfassa*) Satprem writes, 'it seems that one can truly understand only when one understands with the body' (Satprem 1982:10).

Colangelo (2003) likens this 'first container' (the brain) to 'our senses as perceived through our hands' (e.g. 'hold on to that thought') (p.13). Colangelo suggests that 'timing is everything'. She encourages that the reader practice activities that create a 'temporal millionaire', causing you to 'lose track of time and bring on a flow… performance trance'. She suggests to 'do those things often' (Colangelo 2003:198). She writes that 'Art is the form of the verb "to be"', and suggests that we, 'create and become'. So even yogis and yoginis are writing about art, flow states, meditation and yoga all being an embodied state of knowing.

Right brain theory, polyvagal theory and trauma

Of interest is Schore's recent work on relational therapy and how right brain activity (creativity) is enacted in psychotherapy. At the core of Schore's (2019) model is that relational, interactive regulation of affect informs and models the maturation of the right brain. Schore (2014) contends that the right brain interacts 'beneath the words', nonverbally communicating 'essential, non-conscious bodily-based affective relational information about the inner world of the patient (and therapist)' (Schore 2014:394).

Dana (2018) discussed this in terms of a 'mapping system' where therapists and patients create a shared understanding of the patient's autonomic profile. Dana talks about inviting the 'embodied sense of the autonomic state (right hemisphere bias) and then adding language to the experience (left hemisphere bias)'. She contends that this reshapes the 'patterns of engagement', and is 'supported by a ventral, vagal state and inhibited from states of sympathetic or dorsal vagal response' (Dana 2018:54). This brings us to the polyvagal theory as espoused by Porges (2011).

According to Porges (2011), 'the vagus is a family of neural pathways which enable bidirectional communication between the brain and internal organs' (p. 81). These fibers are efferent and communicate the brain's state to the body's internal organs (heart, stomach, etc.). This communication of the internal state of the body is what we describe as interoception (or 'feelings'). The vagal system digests this interoceptive information and decides how resources will be disseminated. The therapeutic goal is to engage the resources of the ventral vagus system and recruit the social engagement system (SES) (Porges 2009, 2011). The SES is the 'face-to-heart' connection: to engage, link the ventral vagus (heart) and striated muscles in face and head (facial expressions), which control how we listen (auditory) and how we speak (communication/vocalization) (Dana 2018:7).

According to Tracey (2002), 'hypnosis and meditation can significantly increase vagus nerve output and have been observed to inhibit immediate-type and delayed-type hypersensitivity responses' (p.861). However, if our more advanced vagal system is unavailable, we use our more primitive vagal system (think: reptilian brain). Dana (2018) states, 'polyvagal theory demonstrates that

Clinical cases: adults

even before the brain makes meaning of an incident, the autonomic nervous system (ANS) has assessed the environment and initiated an adaptive survival response. Neuroception precedes perception'. She talks about following the four Rs to avoid 'story-following state' of a perceived situation. They are:

- recognize the ANS
- respect the adaptive survival response
- regulate or co-regulate into a ventral vagal state
- re-story (Dana 2018:6–7)

Porges (2011) likens the vagal nerve to a car brake (stepping off the brake for challenges and pushing on the brake when able to regulate and return to a calmer state). Vagal tone (the interaction, let's say, between therapist and patient) can greatly influence this dialogue and move a patient toward regulation and/or dysregulation. Understanding the influence of vagal tone and immune system functioning is key in dealing with trauma and moving our patients toward wellness. This brings us full circle and back to Chapter 1, where we discussed the therapeutic bond and Wampold's (2001) theory. Now let's look at vagal tone, therapeutic bond and how this impacted this first case.

Important to note is that only mammals have a myelinated vagus, capable of regulating cardiac output to foster engagement and/or disengagement. Babies do not develop myelinated vagus and need to learn this self-soothing behavior from their caretakers. So, if their caretakers are not physically or psychologically present, then this myelinated vagus remains undeveloped. We witnessed this in Chapter 5, Case Study 1, where R's stepbrother (B) had been abandoned by his crack-addicted mother and lacked the ability to self-regulate.

Case study 1

78-year-old depressed male and his wife: couple's therapy

Background and history

At onset, the wife ('R') made it clear that she wanted to be engaged in all the yoga and art therapy sessions with her husband ('F'). This was not about control but rather concern for his welfare and F's increasing difficulties in cognitively navigating his world. R drove him to all his medical appointments and kept very detailed records of all his medications, supplements and therapies. Why she needed to be involved was understandable given F's past surgery. Post-surgery, F's right scapula had been damaged during a post-operative move. The pictures provided by R suggested that a muscle might have been torn as the right scapula was severely out of alignment. Blalock (1989, 1994) suggested that the immune system functions as a 'sixth sense' which detects microbial invasion, and in turn creates molecules that relay this information to the brain. At onset of treatment, F was seeing multiple health practitioners, including a physical therapist. The physical therapist and I worked very closely together on F's recuperation.

Both F and R were very accomplished, educated and interesting people who had been involved in the arts, specifically advertising. To boot, F was an incredibly talented photographer and had worked for numerous companies before he retired. He was amazingly gifted, as was R. Looking at F's genogram (Fig. 6.1), F had worked with R and they

Chapter six

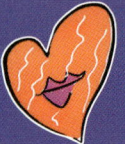 

eventually had an affair. Their liaison severed his marriage and F and R married shortly after that. Previous to their marriage, F had one son with his first wife, who he described as having an 'independent spirit' and distanced from F. In short, R was his world and F was hers (Figure 6.1).

Pearson et al (2020) warned that when a patient has pain warn that, 'negative cognitions increase suicidal ideation and disconnection from loved ones, which can create a downward spiral of fear, anger, depression and isolation'. Furthermore, they purport that, 'chronic pain disrupts emotional well-being by interfering with both physical and social function', and may increase loneliness and social isolation (Pearson et al 2020:31). So, having F's wife at the sessions not only lessened the possibility of social isolation but also insured that these practices would be replicated in between sessions (she monitored all of F's medication, appointments and the like). While having R in sessions created a family dynamic, it was also clear to me that R needed to be in these sessions as much as F did, but her pressure emanated from a greater fear – losing her husband.

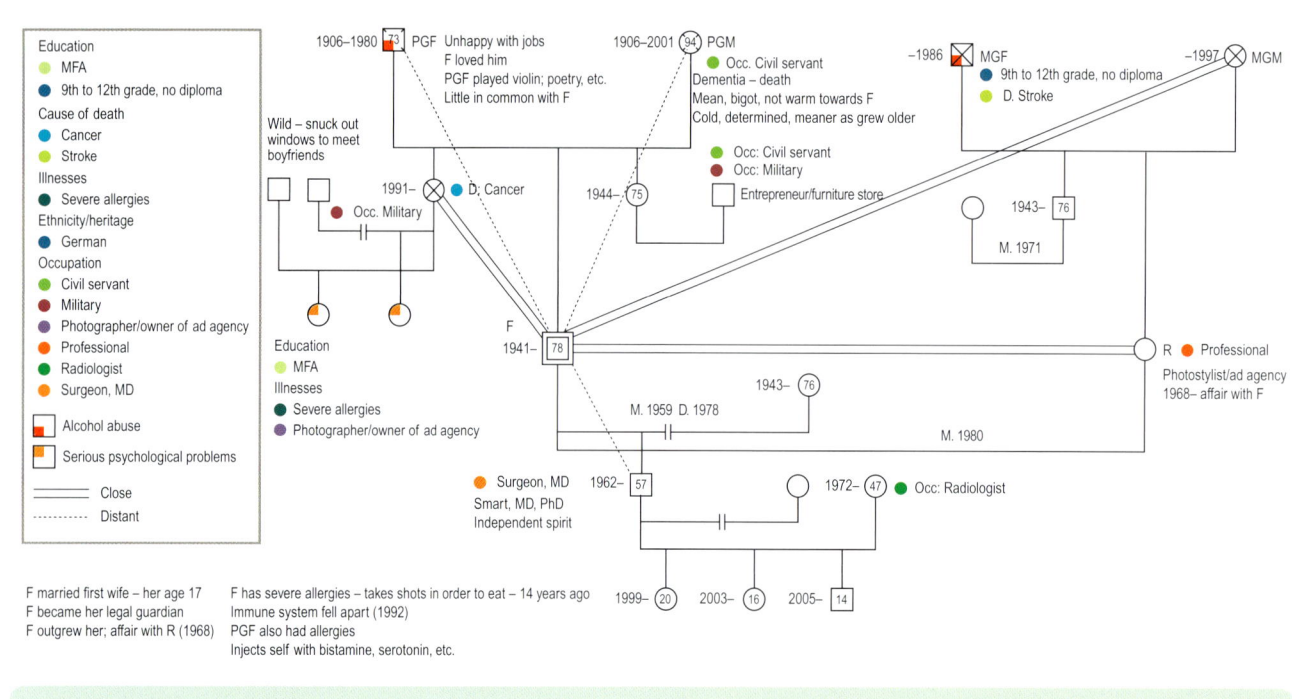

FIGURE 6.1 F's genogram

Clinical cases: adults

Significant sessions

I saw both F and R for 40 sessions over one and a half years. Figure 6.2 was created from a photocopied image that R gave to me as an indication of F's shoulder injury. Note the imbalance between his shoulders. The objectives in therapy were to repair F's right shoulder injury via yoga, while working on his cognitive decline and depression with art therapy. Both the yoga and artwork aided F in returning to normal physical functioning and alleviating cognitive decline and depression.

In some respects, it was helpful to have R present for the sessions. Meditation, in this instance kirtan kriya (Alzheimer's Research and Prevention Foundation 2013) was employed since research indicates great gains in older people and especially their caretakers (Lavretsky 2017). My favorite quote of Lavretsky's is, 'it really doesn't matter what you do in the study, it matters what

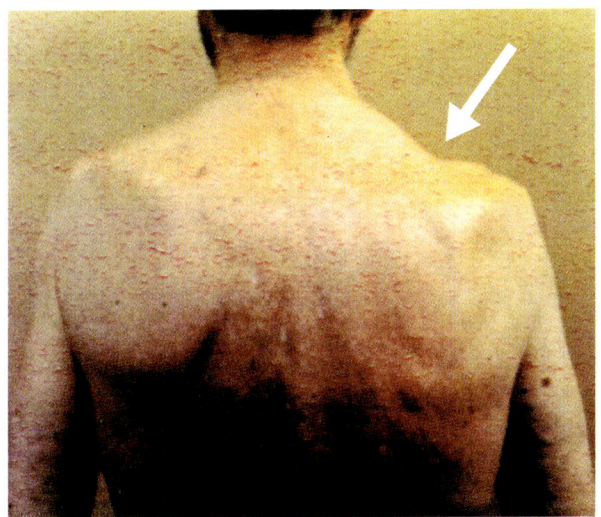
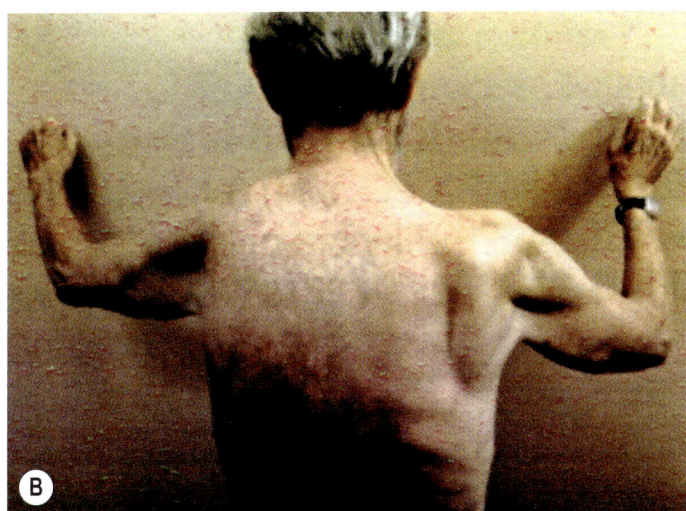
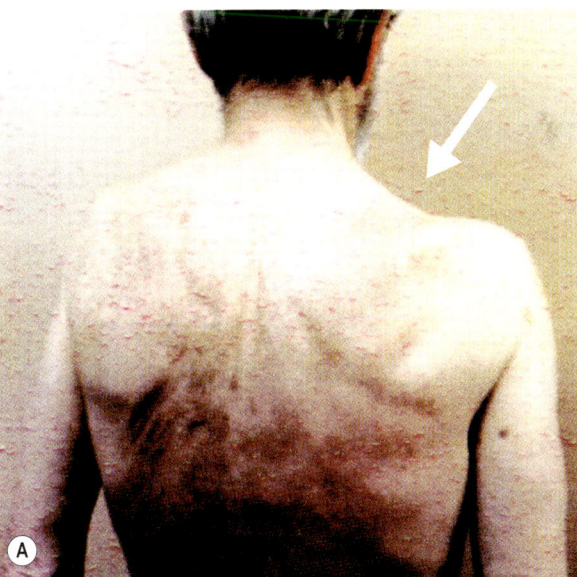

FIGURE 6.2 F's shoulder injury post-surgery

Chapter six

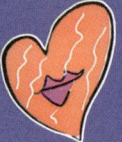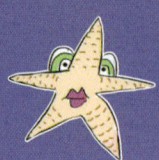

TABLE 6.1 Personal profile for F at 78 years-of-age, about 1 year into therapy

Test	Score	Below ave.	Normal	Above ave.	Standard fitness	Comments
Chair test (#)	12		X		Y	
Arm curl (#)	19 R 22 L			X (R + L)	Y	
2-min walk test (steps)	115			X	Y	'Superior' range for 60–64-year-old male
Chair sit/reach	R = 4" L = 7"			X	R, Y L, N	Work on L for more reaching, etc.
Back-scratch	R = 11" L = 8"	X (R)	X (L)		R, N L, Y	Work on this more
Get-up-and-go 8' (seconds)	6.75		X		Y	

Height = 136 cm. Weight = 5'7". BMI = 21.3, normal range.

they do after the study'. So, in essence, homework matters, and follow-through. I also used the senior fitness test (Rikli and Jones 2012) to determine abilities at various points during treatment (Table 6.1).

Some of the *asanas* included physical therapy-related exercises in order to free up F's shoulder, such as 'washing the wall' and in Figure 6.3, making a W at the wall and then raising the arms in an upward fashion. Given F's injury, I would often have R aid F into this position so she could assist him in practicing these moves in between our sessions. Therefore, in addition to the Sequence Wiz application, I often sent them actual images of F's progression. This aided in his recovery (however, it was a lot of extra work for me, see Fig. 6.5 and Fig. 6.6, below). Nonetheless, it paid off as by the end of our treatment, F's shoulder had returned to near-normal.

Of particular import was meeting Loren Fishman and attending his workshop at a conference, Symposium on Yoga Therapy and Research, in 2015. I learned multiple ways to aid F's shoulder injury

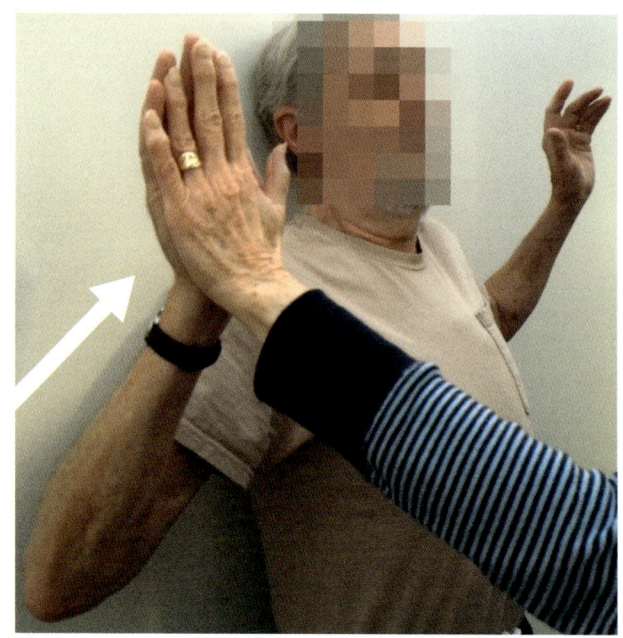

FIGURE 6.3 R is aiding F by holding his hand and helping him push his shoulder against the wall (the W-move in an upward movement). While I have full permission to use F and R's facial images, I have edited these so that their identities are still protected

Clinical cases: adults

including headstand at the wall (building up the time; see Figure 6.5) followed by pumping arms in conductor fashion. This was exceptionally helpful in returning F's shoulder to normalcy. Reading Fishman's (2015) text was particularly informative, especially the section on rotator cuff and shoulder injuries. Figures 6.4 and 6.5 are indicative of some of the *asanas* and exercises that were performed over the period F was in yoga therapy, and Figure 6.6 shows the homework sheets. Additionally, I loaned an individual co-operative blanket to F in order to aid his shoulder repair while exercising in between our sessions.

Simultaneously, F was keeping a journal (sketching from his dreams) and often combining art therapy in the same session. Mostly we combined the art therapy to enhance F's cognitive functioning and I was tracking psychosocial regulation using the DASS-21 and other psychological instruments to assess F's pain. After all yoga therapy sessions, F's and R's depression, anxiety and stress lowered to normal states. This was very affirming and informed me what worked and what didn't. Psychotherapy was left on the backend and instead yoga therapy and art therapy were intermingled to inform right brain functioning (Schore 2014, 2019). According to Sims et al (2012), depressed older adults benefit from physical activity since being active offers a therapy 'where negative events are minimal, and benefits

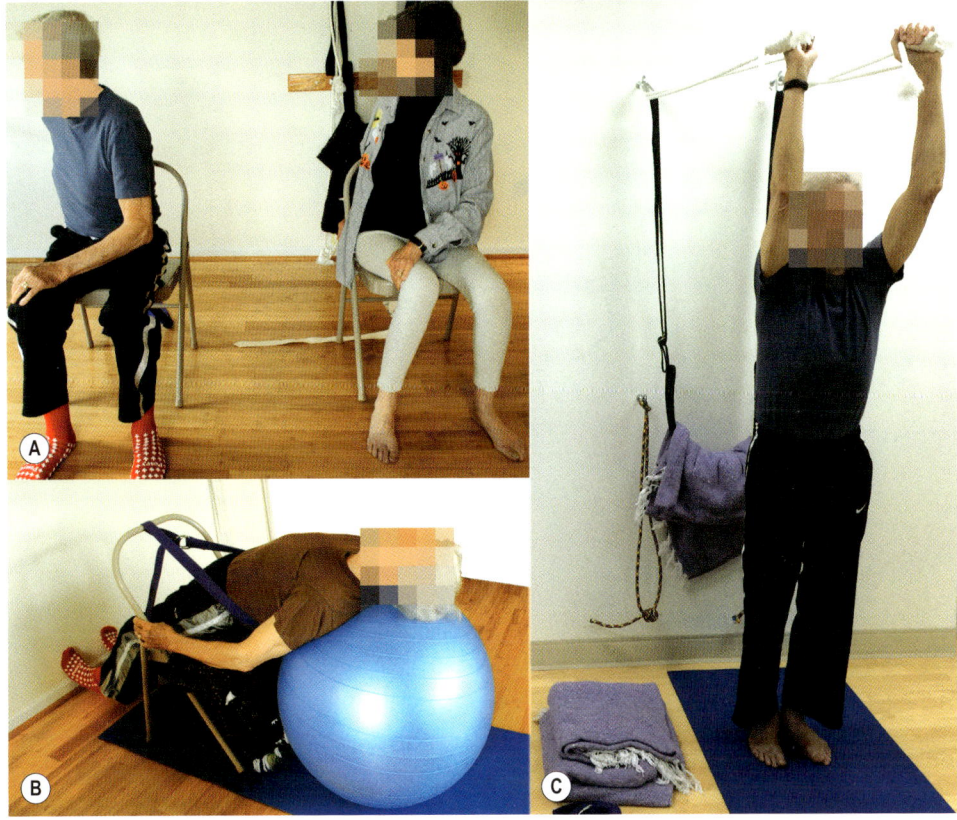

FIGURE 6.4 Opening sample of exercises with F and R

Chapter six

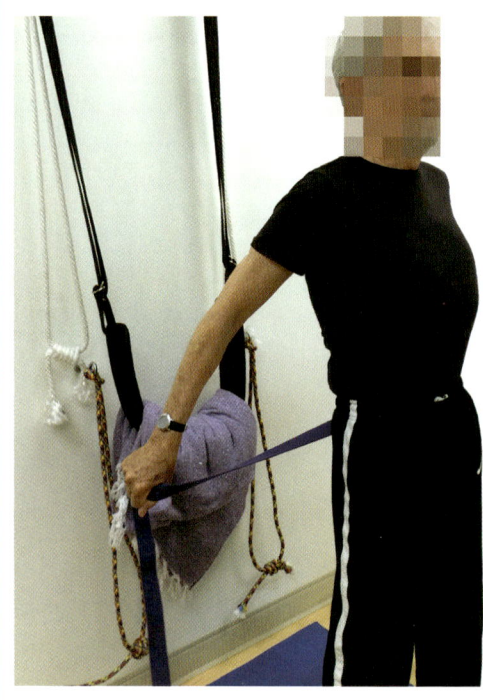
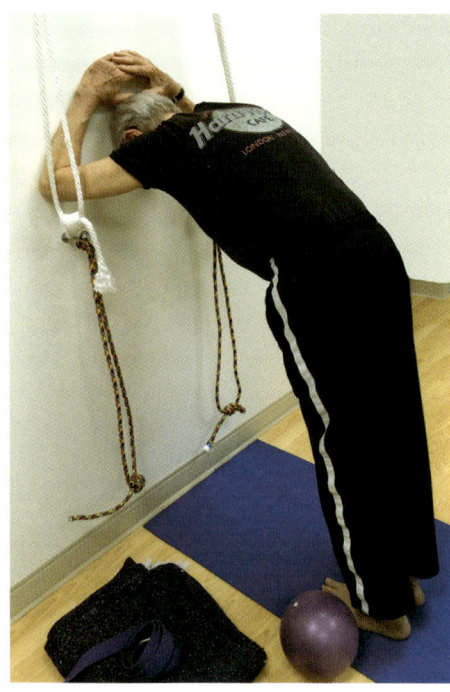

FIGURE 6.5 F opening up his chest wall and scapular area using the yoga belt (left). F in headstand at the wall (based on Fishman 2015)

can accrue for both physical and mental health status' (Sims et al 2012:115).

Figure 6.7 is an example of F's journal sketch (top) prior to yoga therapy. He described this dream fugue state as feeling trapped by his pain and age-related cognitive decline. The *savāsanā* image (end of session) below the sketch shows R and F (left to right) in a state of relaxation. When F did the DASS-21 post the therapy session, his previous scores of depression, anxiety and stress (which were moderate to severe) all returned to a normal range of functioning. Clearly, F's ventral vagus system had returned from his dorsal state post-session (Dana 2018, Porges 2009, 2011). Psychological markers like the DASS-21 and/or other instruments can truly measure efficacy from session to session. And as each day changes, no matter one's age, it is helpful to ascertain what works and what doesn't.

Clinical cases: adults

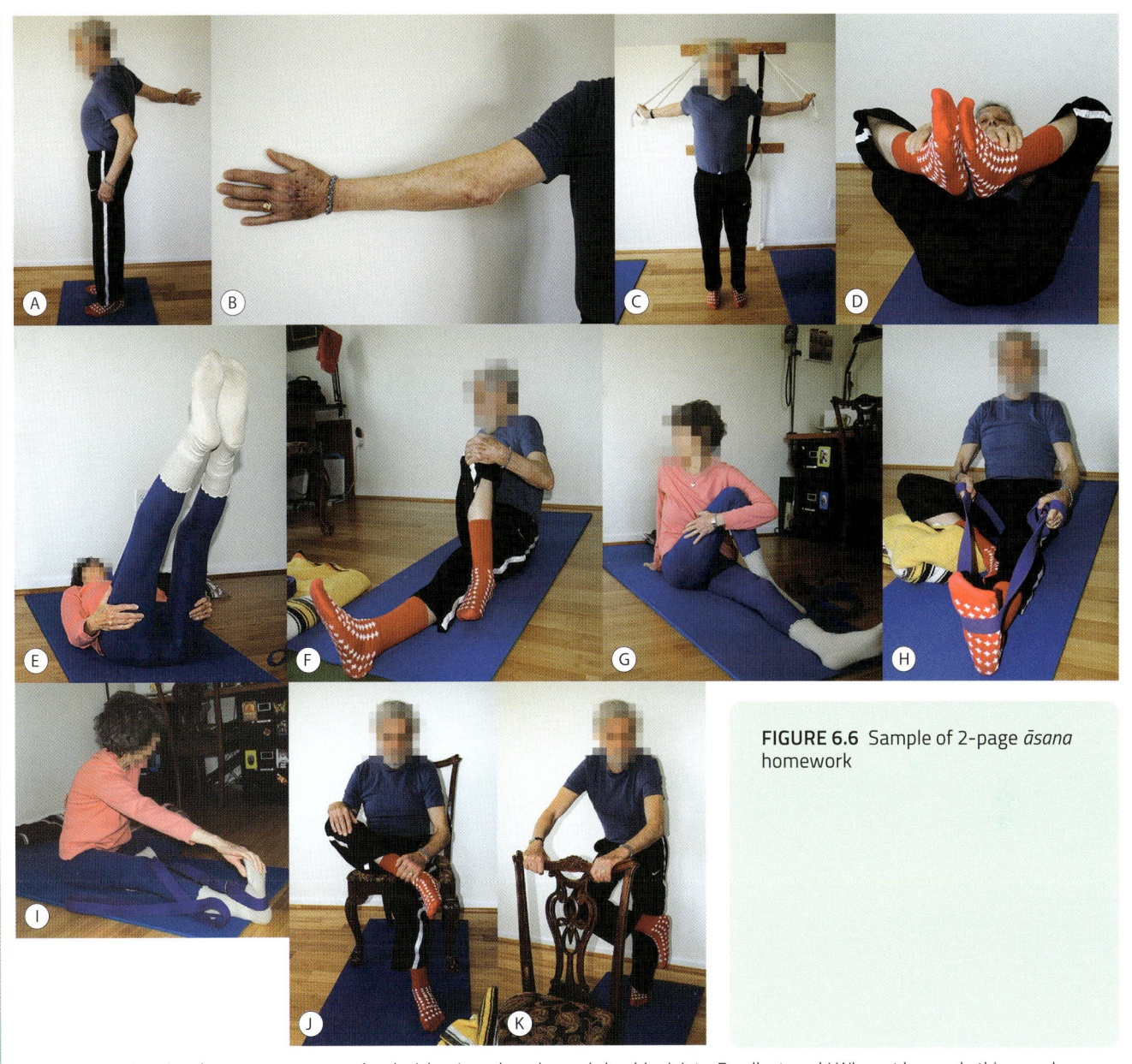

FIGURE 6.6 Sample of 2-page *āsana* homework

In image C, F is using the ropes to open up the clavicles. Lymph nodes and shoulder joints. Excellent work! When at home, do this on a door frame as F is doing in image A. In image B, post warm up that we did with the belt, doing the finger exercise to floss the wrist and alleviate pain by isolating fingers (which is not shown); begin the wall work to begin to straighten the right (and left) elbows. Remember to keep the feet parallel, move hand away from shoulder joint and rotate the opposite shoulder back. Here you are doing an excellent job to strengthen your muscles. Look how straight the elbow is on your left arm. In Image D, F is placing his feet together and then doing a sit up bringing hands towards his feet; do 10–20×. In image E, R demonstrates another core exercise. Feet move from 90 to 45 degrees, hovering above the floor and back up again. Do 10–20×.

Images F and G, excellent job with twists. Remember to flex the straight leg.

On images H and I, make sure you use a blanket or bolster at home to support your bent leg, F. (Note that R has such flexibility that she need not use the belt.) In images J and K: excellent work doing the number 4 exercise using a chair (image J) and standing (image K). Remember, you can do this anytime when you are sitting. Always maintain a seed of a backbend. Do this as often as you can to open up your hip flexors and develop strength in your IT band.

Chapter six

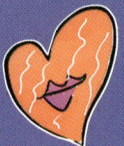 

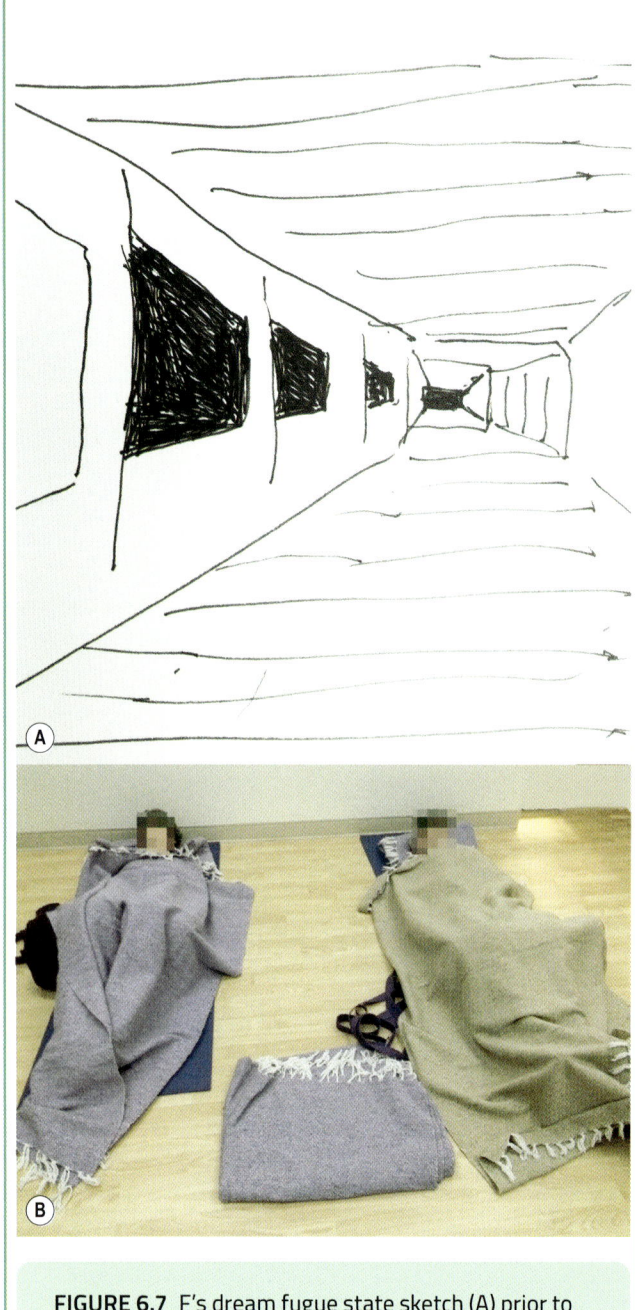

FIGURE 6.7 F's dream fugue state sketch (A) prior to yoga therapy

Reflection exercise 6.1

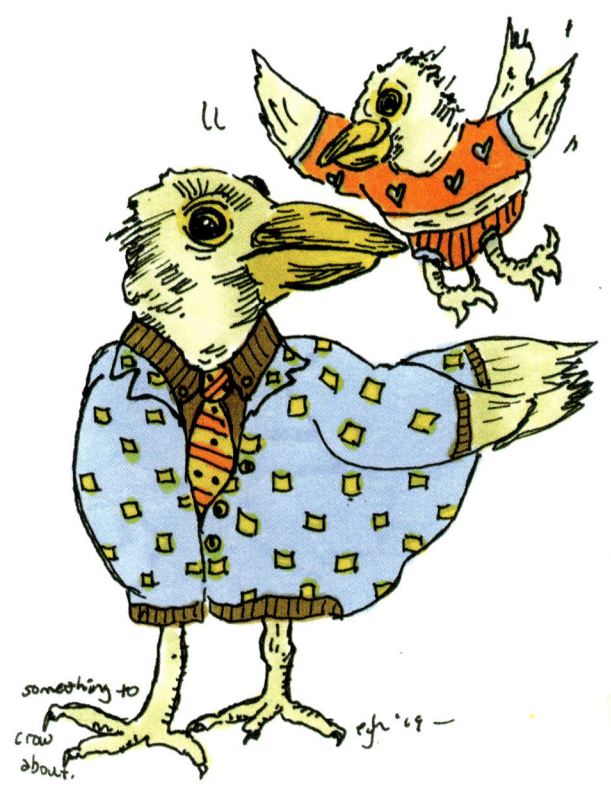

FIGURE 6.8 'Something to crow about'. Stoking the ventral vagal tone, drawing by author

Judith Lasater, the 'Queen of Rest and Relaxation', in discussing Patanjali wrote that Patanjali uses yoga to mean 'a state of wholeness'. She goes on to write that, 'when you are in a state of yoga, or wholeness, you rest in your own true nature' (Lasater 2000:5). Take out a piece of paper. Draw yourself in profile as a person, animal, sea creature, bird or whatever your fancy. Next invite your ventral vagal system in, as a similar person, animal, sea creature,

Clinical cases: adults

> **Reflection exercise 6.1** (Continued)
>
> bird or the like. Draw that image facing your constructed image on the paper. Imagine that this sentient being is activating your safe/social construct and influencing your ventral vagal system. Perhaps that sentient being represents a person with whom you are in relation in your life. Or maybe that last being is your Higher Self (Fig. 6.8). Whoever or whatever it is, know that you have the option to come to this image, just as you do your yoga mat, to calm yourself down in times of high anxiety. If you have time, practice a round of kirtan kriya meditation and arrive to your present Self refreshed.

Case study 2

23-year-old female with comorbidity (vesicoureteral reflux disorder, eating disorder and PTSD)

Background and history

A brief synopsis of this case was presented in Chapter 3 and the genogram is presented in Figure 3.18. The most difficult aspect of this case is the fallout from the Identified Patient's (IP's) struggle with her vesicoureteral reflux disorder (American Academy of Pediatrics 2019). Also, while this patient no longer was an addict, she had an addiction to ecstasy and cocaine during her adolescence but went 'cold turkey' with her father's help and kicked her addiction. Teicher et al (2010) purported that early trauma impairs the development of the hippocampus and corpus collosum. These areas relate to emotion, memory and reasoning. According to Quinn (2020), the effect of earlier abuse may not be seen until much later when it can lead to addiction (and can) undermine the efforts to get sober.

Because vesicoureteral reflux disorder was so traumatic for this patient, this resulted in a lifelong struggle with anything to do with sex, and later morphed into an eating disorder. In a nutshell her kidneys backed up from her obstruction: the ureterovesical junction obstruction impeded the flow of urine down to the bladder, causing the urine to back up into and dilate the ureters and kidney. If not dealt with, it could be life-threatening.

Particularly traumatizing for IP was that she would be taken to the hospital by her parents, who had to endure watching her scream as a catheter was inserted into her urethra to unblock the obstruction (this occurred from her age 6 months through 9 years, when she finally outgrew the condition). As she got older, these procedures became further apart, but she always knew that one was coming when her name was called over a loudspeaker to come to the school office. I can only guess that her parents felt that preparation for this procedure would only cause IP more stress and thus, never pre-warned her of the next appointment. Clearly, IP's dorsal vagal system engaged during these times and no matter how soothing her parents might have been, neither were allowed in the procedure room, thus amplifying her dorsal vagal system collapse (Dana 2018).

Of interest is that by age 12, IP had become an expert swimmer and was ranked number one in her state for her age in competitive swimming. However, this became so important to her father

Chapter six

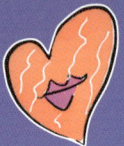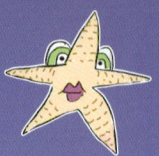

that IP would often binge-eat and purge to get out of her swim meets – thus began her eating disorder courtship. Nonetheless, she described herself as always being 'large-bodied' and was used to receiving taunts for being 'fat' from her cousins and schoolmates. This caused a cyclical response of controlling her eating habits through exercise, bingeing, purging and basically non-caloric intake. However, for all her efforts, her body mass index was in the obese range. I suggested testing her thyroid, which yielded normal results.

Regarding her body, IP referred to anything vaginal as 'down there', so labeling her body parts (e.g. vagina as opposed to 'down there', breasts as opposed to 'boobs') required re-education and discussion around everything from masturbation to sex, and how to insert a tampon. And yes, we discussed all of this in therapy.

When IP went away to out-of-state college she saw a different therapist. I sent reports to the other therapist, but the other therapist sent nothing back to me. When IP returned in between semesters to the area, our work resumed and thus, there was a 4-month lapse between our ninth and tenth session. As of this writing, I have seen IP for 10 individual sessions and one family art therapy session, which was presented in Chapter 3.

Assessments conducted were the appearance anxiety inventory (AAI), depression, anxiety, stress scale, short form (DASS-21), eating attitudes test (EAT-26), and the generalized anxiety disorder test (GAD-7).

After reviewing the AAI inventory results with IP, I learned that sometimes she was so preoccupied with her appearance that she would skip classes. After reviewing her AAI in the eighth session before she returned to college, her scores had lowered. Nonetheless, we had a lot to work on, including her self-esteem issues, eating disorder and PTSD regarding her past vesicoureteral reflux disorder and resulting fear around sexual relations.

Significant sessions

During our second session we reviewed her genogram (see Fig. 3.18). This was when IP revealed that her sister's best friend and 13-year-old daughter had moved into her parents' home while she had been away at college. To make matters worse, her sister's friend had overtaken her room, moved out all of IP's belongings, and her father had taken a 'shine' to the 13-year-old daughter. 'The boarders' were supposed to leave before IP came home but still had not exited when she arrived.

IP's father wanted her to work another job on top of the 40 hours she was already doing. She suggested that her father was always critical of her. In inquiring more about this, IP stated that they all had 'compartmentalized' areas for their respective food areas. She felt she had no place of her own. We talked about getting 'the boarders' out and how that might be accomplished. I suggested a physical calendar on the wall (or refrigerator) to remind all that the time for their departure was drawing near. Her parents were also resentful that 'the boarders' had 'overstayed their welcome,' but hadn't pushed them to leave.

We did some breathing exercises (belly breathing and coherent breath) and then we did some yoga (Fig. 6.9) to calm her anxiety. Her DASS-21 scores dropped significantly post-session to the normal range for depression, anxiety and stress (Fig. 6.10).

After the family session covered in Chapter 3, our fourth, yoga and poetry journaling continued for a few sessions. Discussion continued about sexuality, IP's desire to 'lose' her virginity (and concomitant fear), as well as her need to ask her parents for increased financial assistance with schooling and her living expenses. Session 7, conducted a few weeks before IP returned to college, touched on many of these issues, so I sent her the following recap:

1. When you thank your parents for what they are doing for you, try something like

Clinical cases: adults

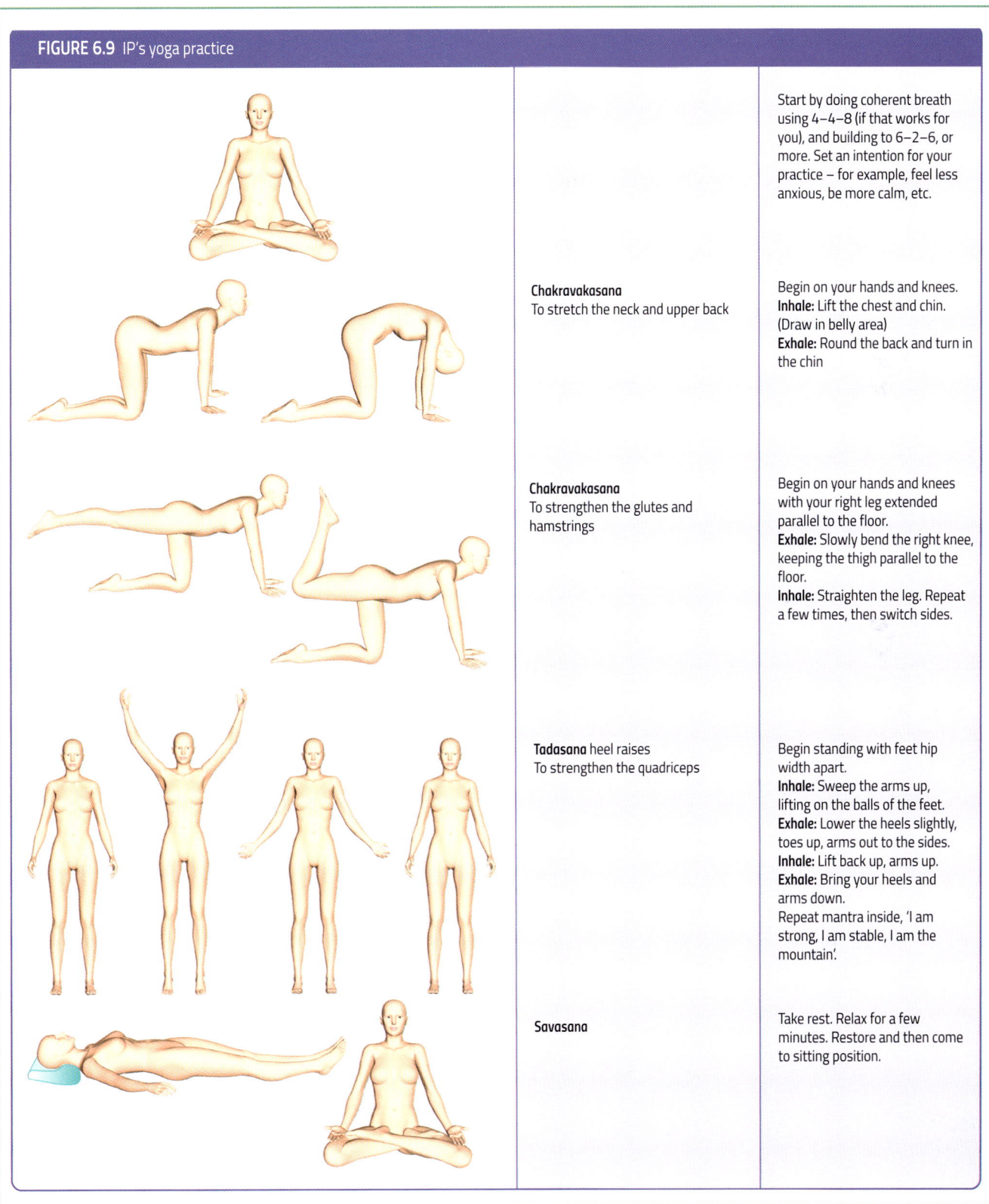

FIGURE 6.9 IP's yoga practice

Chapter six

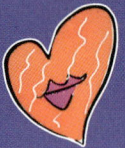
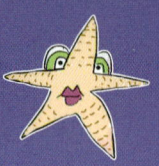

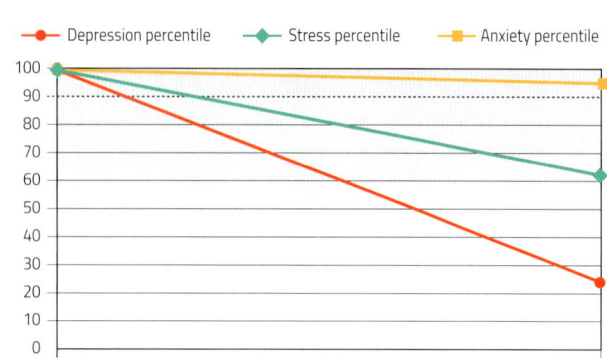

FIGURE 6.10 IP's DASS-21 scores post-session

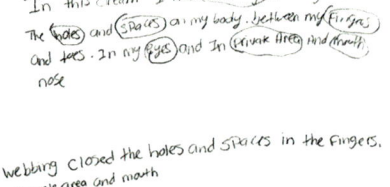

FIGURE 6.11 IP's dream

this: 'I want you to know that I really appreciate how much you are helping me with financial assistance towards my education and paying for my therapy with Ellen. It means a lot to me that you are investing in me and love me'. That is entirely different than just saying thank you.

2. Call your primary care physician ASAP and see if you can get an earlier appointment just in case she wants to run some diagnostic tests on you: given the fact that you are restricting your caloric intake, exercising so much, and not dropping weight, you want to rule out thyroid issues and the like. Also ask her whether or not you should see a nutritionist, since you really are trying to lose weight.

3. Try and do yoga for at least 10 minutes/day and do 2/4 of those breathing exercises that I sent. You will feel calmer and more relaxed.

Her next session was our last before returning to college. As expected, her DASS-21 results skyrocketed as she was anxious about returning to school. She also revealed that she had been communicating with a young man from school and they had been texting over the summer. They were both 'looking forward to losing [their] virginities' with each other. This was the first I had learned about him. Door-knob therapy again.

IP stated that she had been having dreams that plagued her, so I suggested that she draw her dream, then write a paragraph about it, whittle down the paragraph to a cluster of meaningful words, and then hone those words into a single sentence (inserting necessary words to make it read cogently). This is a shorthand version of the art therapy dream assessment that I designed (see Horovitz and Elgelid 2015). After that was done I mirrored her, reading the paragraph, cluster of words and final sentence back to her. Doing this with ventral vagal tone allows for the patient to hear the inner message of the dream (Fig. 6.11).

The paragraph read, 'In this dream, I had webbing, covering all the holes and spaces on my body, between my fingers and toes, in my eyes and in private areas and mouth and nose'. The cluster of words were circled next. They were, 'webbing, holes, spaces, fingers, eyes, private area, mouth'. Her final sentence was, 'the webbing closed the holes and spaces in the fingers, eyes, private area and mouth'. This sentence allowed us to have a frank discussion of her need to close-off orifices and entrances into her sexuality. I was able to link this to her trauma from the procedures sustained during her childhood, her current eating disorder

Clinical cases: adults

and fear of sexual intercourse. As can be imagined, this was a lot to process during our session before she left for her fall semester. I was worried about her return and reattachment with her therapist.

While she expressed attachment to her other therapist, they had never discussed sexual topics or many of the subjects that we had in our short time together. I also had the advantage of conducting a family art therapy session with her parents. IP's connection to me was clearly different. I wondered about her re-connection to her previous therapist, so naturally I wrote a detailed summation of our work and shared it with her therapist before their forthcoming appointment.

Four months later

A few weeks before IP returned home for the winter break, she texted me to make an appointment. This signaled to me that she might be unduly anxious. Her pre-session DASS-21 results were in the extremely severe range for depression; anxiety and stress. Her EAT-26 (eating attitudes test) had a raw score of 30 (20 or above is considered to have a high level of concern about dieting, body weight or problematic eating behaviors). This placed IP into the category of a diagnosable eating disorder. When I saw her, it was clear that she had ballooned even more since our last meeting. She admitted she had been in a routine of bingeing, vomiting and taking laxatives, especially when she returned home briefly over Thanksgiving break. She also admitted that she had been somewhat depressed and returning home from college on most weekends (a 3-hour drive/commute). IP relayed depression over the fact that her 'potential' boyfriend had slept with two girls and so broke things off with her explaining that he 'didn't want to hurt her'. She was devastated by this and decided to only see him as a 'friend', but when they met, returned to kissing and fondling, so she decided to break off all contact with him. In part of the session, we reviewed possible outpatient clinics for eating disorders. I printed out materials for her to review with her mother.

In the next session, I learned that her mother's response when IP presented the material on eating disorder treatment was, 'our whole family are stress eaters', thus ignoring IP's cry for help. IP pleaded further and pointed out the clinic also offered family therapy, but her mother was adamantly against joining her or discussing the matter. I was quite frank with IP that I was truly worried about her health and the damage she was doing to her body. I suggested that she have her mother join us for the final session before returning to school. In the next session, I discussed the polyvagal system. In short order, using Dana's ladder system (Dana 2018:68), I helped IP identify her triggers (and glimmers) associated with the systems that ruled her from her infancy (6 months to 9 years). Dana (2018) suggests assigning a color and/or symbol to each area of the ladder and then filling in the glimmers and triggers next to each stage. IP's chosen symbols were a hot pink smiley face, red stop sign, and a turquoise door.

While creating the ladder system (Fig. 6.12), she described the ordeal of having to 'pee the catheter out' as excruciating. I asked her what her parents would do after the procedure and she answered as I suspected: they would take her 'out for a treat' (food). I pointed out how food had been paired with this horrific experience and became her go-to since neither parent was available for ventral vagal tone/soothing each time the procedure was repeated. That enabled her to talk about her compulsion with 'everything in twos'. She recalled that her parents would offer her a cookie for each hand – she had no memory of ever having one cookie. This led to her admission of grocery shopping and buying everything in twos: two bags of chips, two bags of kale, etc. This was a true 'aha' moment for IP as she was able to piece together her eating disorder with her vesicoureteral reflux disorder procedures.

Chapter six

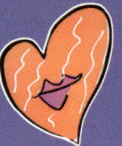 

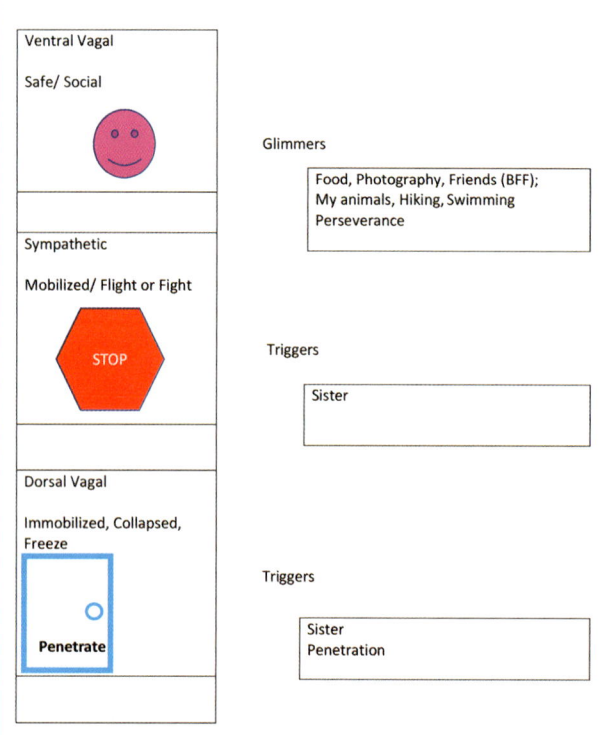

FIGURE 6.12 Graphic rendition of IP's ladder system

In sum, this case continues to be challenging and complex due to the co-morbidity of addiction, eating disorders, PTSD and vesicoureteral reflux disorder. While IP clearly needs continued treatment to aid her with these issues, the combination of yoga therapy, art therapy and cognitive behavioral therapy is being used to aid IP in re-wiring her systems-processing thinking and functioning. This case supports the research that yoga, cognitively based psychotherapy and art therapy interventions are effective in modulating stress and sensitively engaging traumatic memory processing utilizing a nonverbal and right-hemisphere dominant approach.

Update on the case: IP recently texted that her mother agreed to support her outpatient treatment at an eating disorder clinic when she returns from school as well as seeing a specialist in eating disorders while at college.

Reflection exercise 6.2

FIGURE 6.13 'Patience with the questions', created by Audrey Omenson during the author's 5-day yoga and art therapy retreat in Petaluma, CA, in September 2018

As previously mentioned, babies do not have fully developed myelinated vagus, and cannot regulate their emotions. Even if their caretaking is replete with ventral vagal tone and soothing, it requires years to learn how to self-regulate and generally occurs around early adulthood (NurrieStearns 2018). In this case, IP turned to drugs, food and other compulsions to mitigate an untenable situation that resulted from her medical trauma. It might be impossible for you to empathize with this situation. But in this case, IP needed to develop self-compassion

Clinical cases: adults

> **Reflection exercise 6.2   continued**
>
> and love herself. This may be akin to taking a vow. And, sometimes, a vow involves a ritual, like selecting a specific date, location, or time to take that vow. It could involve lighting a candle, reciting a poem or selecting a piece of jewelry for the occasion. Imagine yourself or a patient in a similar predicament. Perhaps you could help your patient or make that vow to be there for yourself, in sickness and in health. Imagine how you (or your patient) might feel in holding that promise sacred. Perhaps you (or your patient) could journal about that as an initial preparation. And then take the plunge into that higher space that is truly aligned with your Self and create an artwork or poem to represent that (see Fig. 6.13).

Case study 3

64-year old female stroke survivor

Stroke: some definitions

A stroke is the result of reduction or disruption of bloodflow to the brain. There are two main categories of stroke: (1) ischemic stroke, caused by blockages in an artery, and (2) hemorrhagic stroke, the result of bleeding in the brain caused when an artery's wall is torn. Within the category of ischemic strokes, there are three types: thrombotic (blood clot in the brain blood vessels), lacunar (a series of small strokes occurs) and embolic (blood clots that travel to the brain). About 60% of all strokes are thrombotic and are caused when clots form and interfere with blood supply to the brain as they slowly choke off an artery. This type of stroke is a result of atherosclerosis – a thickening and hardening of the arterial wall.

Approximately 30% of stroke patients are afflicted with aphasia. Wernicke's aphasia, identified in 1847 by Karl Wernicke, is a language impairment marked by fluent verbal output and impaired verbal comprehension.

In Broca's aphasia, often identified as non-fluent aphasia, anterior aphasia, motor aphasia and expressive aphasia, speech is greatly reduced with short, agrammatic phrases, difficulty 'finding' words, and impaired repetition. This was the kind of aphasia that this patient, 'L', experienced. While word comprehension is generally preserved, patients with Broca's aphasia are often frustrated by their inability to speak. Stroke can leave many survivors with ongoing cognitive deficits that contribute to the challenges and dilemmas that present after stroke. Participation in daily life and activities of daily living (ADL) skills are greatly impaired by the resulting hemiparesis and cognitive deficits. According to Garrett et al (2011) and Horovitz (2005, 2017a), stroke can leave many survivors with ongoing cognitive deficits that contribute to challenges in daily life. Ellis-Hill et al (2000) noted that in stroke, 'the body, separated from the self, takes on the nature of an object' (p.728). This was described as a sense of detachment from their body. Dysfunctional body parts and limbs were viewed as 'dislocated from other aspects of [their] life... jobs, friends, and general independence' (Garrett et al 2011:2408). Considering this, let's see how this played out in L's case.

Chapter six

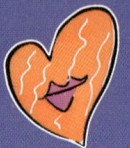 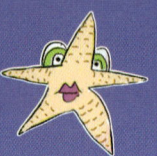

Once upon a time

Long ago, before I practiced yoga therapy, I was working solely as an art therapist. My yoga teacher journey with Sri François Raoult was unplanned and occurred during a sabbatical. When I returned completely altered from this experience, I approached my Dean and told her I wanted to incorporate yoga in the art therapy clinic where I worked. She agreed to this, since years before we had combined art therapy and speech therapy in the clinics.

As it turns out, the patient herein named L (Fig. 6.14) had been attending group art therapy with five other members (male and female, approximately the same age), all of whom had suffered varying types of strokes. Most had lost their speech, some could no longer read and comprehend the words in front of them, and some suffered from global aphasia, where their words were often garbled and sounded like gibberish. Just imagine how frustrating it would be to one day find yourself unable to communicate your thoughts, feelings, needs, and perhaps, suffer partial paralysis. L's inability to verbalize, compounded by hemiparesis on her dominant (right) side, affected her gait and to some degree her frontal lobe functioning. This resulted in severe speech problems, changes in her personality, poor coordination and difficulties with impulse control. In short, she was a very changed woman. Despite this, she was never irritable and always joyful to be around.

Working with L was so early in my 'yoga' career that I pretty much flew by the seat of my pants, since this work was conducted over 20 years ago. This is exactly why I am presenting it herein: sometimes, even without much scientific knowledge, our work as clinicians is intuitively based. So, this work preceded all the apps that I use today. I also did not communicate with L in between sessions, or send her recaps, or create photographic images to share with her. However, I did videotape many of our sessions and while I have complete permission to use L's images and those videotapes for publication on the Internet, as with Case Study 1 in this chapter, I have pixellated facial images to obscure her identity. I worked with L for over 4 years and watched her skillset change from the very first introduction to yoga therapy.

How it began

One day, I brought some tennis balls into the group art therapy setting and sat down with all six members of the group. I asked the members if any of them had done yoga or were interested in trying it. None had previous experience with yoga and so I gave each of them a tennis ball and had them roll the ball on a table from their elbow to their fingertips with their functioning (unimpaired) arm. Figure 6.15A shows an example of me doing this with L, and her affected (hemiparetic) arm (B,C).

After telling the group members that they had actually just done yoga, they were surprised. While not an *āsana*, per se, this had set the stage for what yoga could be as opposed to the glossy images featured in the *Yoga Journal* magazine ads. At this time, L's speech, when prompted, was

FIGURE 6.14 L's genogram

Clinical cases: adults

completely halted and occasionally was a one-word response.

The next week, as the members walked up the corridor to the art therapy clinic, L practically ran towards me. Her gait appeared more balanced and as she drew near me, she pulled her tennis ball from her purse, and said (in staccato fashion), 'I... want... yoga!' I am not sure who was more amazed, L or me.

Progress: flying by the seat of my pants

And so it began. My wheels started turning and I soon recognized that for L, yoga primed her speech. Getting her speech therapists to recognize this was more of a struggle. I invited my Dean (who wore two hats, including Director of the Communication and Science Disorders Department) to come observe us. While I later published my results (Horovitz 2005), when I began yoga with L in 1999 I had little to go on save my intuition. Years later when reading Garrett et al (2011), Harris and Eng (2010) and Schmid et al (2014), I was delighted to learn that I had been on the right track. Participants generally described their participation in the yoga program in positive terms (Garrett et al 2011). Particularly affirming was reading that scapular ROM movements had been part of the Schmid et al (2014) study, since (as seen in Fig. 6.16) I too incorporated these kinds of movements in order to open up the anterior deltoid and increase L's ROM. Schmid and Van Puymbroeck (2019) have since published an entire book dedicated to yoga therapy and stroke. A wealth of topics (including the use of *prāṇayāma*, *mudrās* and meditation) is peppered throughout and their sample yoga practices are useful to the emerging practitioner.

It became clear to me that as I worked with L, her speech was improving. I likened this to 'priming the pump' (her brain). Her speech improved as did her comprehension of words and ability to form sentences. Below are some samples of how

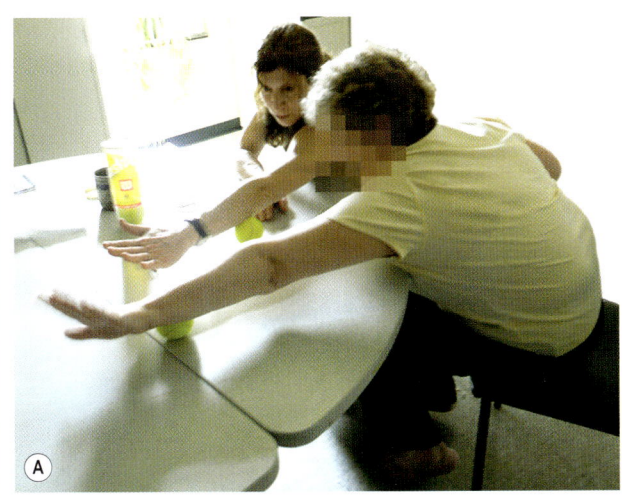
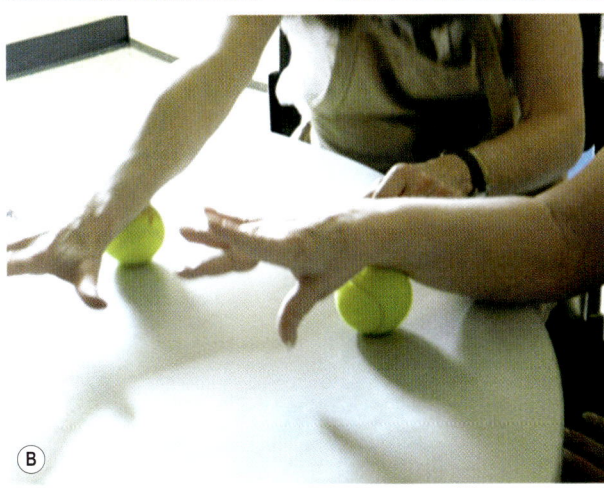
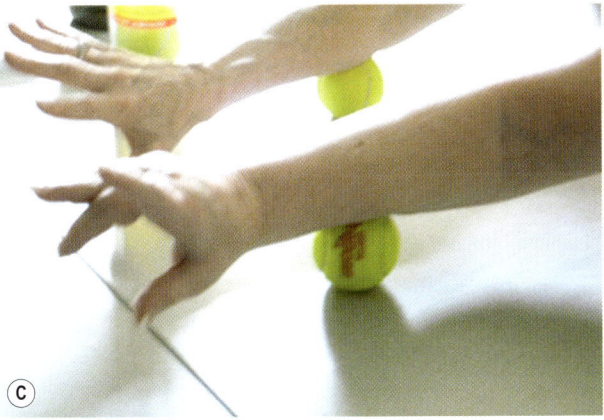

FIGURE 6.15 L and I practice with a tennis ball to stimulate the left hand muscles (**A**) and close-ups of practice using the affected hand (right dominant (**B,C**)). Note fingers increasingly relaxed in (**C**).

Chapter six

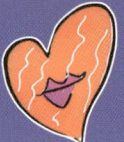
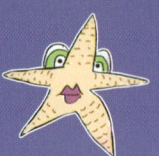

L progressed from one-word answers to whole sentences. These are extracted from conversations during some of our sessions.

- *'I want yoga!'*
- *'My daughter had an accident yesterday.'*
- *'She got run into by a car.'*
- *'My son gave them to me for Christmas.'*
- *'I had ice coffee.'*
- *'I used the microwave!'*
- *'These are men's shoes.'*
- *'I got a permanent last Thursday.'*

While this may not seem like much to someone who has never suffered a stroke and experienced Broca's aphasia, for L and her husband this was little short of a miracle. I am fully convinced that the combination of meditation, breathwork and regular practice of *āsanas* improved L's communication, balance, ADL skills and overall function. Her fine motor coordination also improved in the art therapy.

I helped L use the wall as a prop (see Fig. 6.16). This opened up the function in the hemiparetic right side, in addition to her anterior deltoid and scapular region. Figure 6.16C shows progress months later, when L could do these movements independently.

We also used a foam roller to extend L's arms; Figure 6.17 shows her progress.

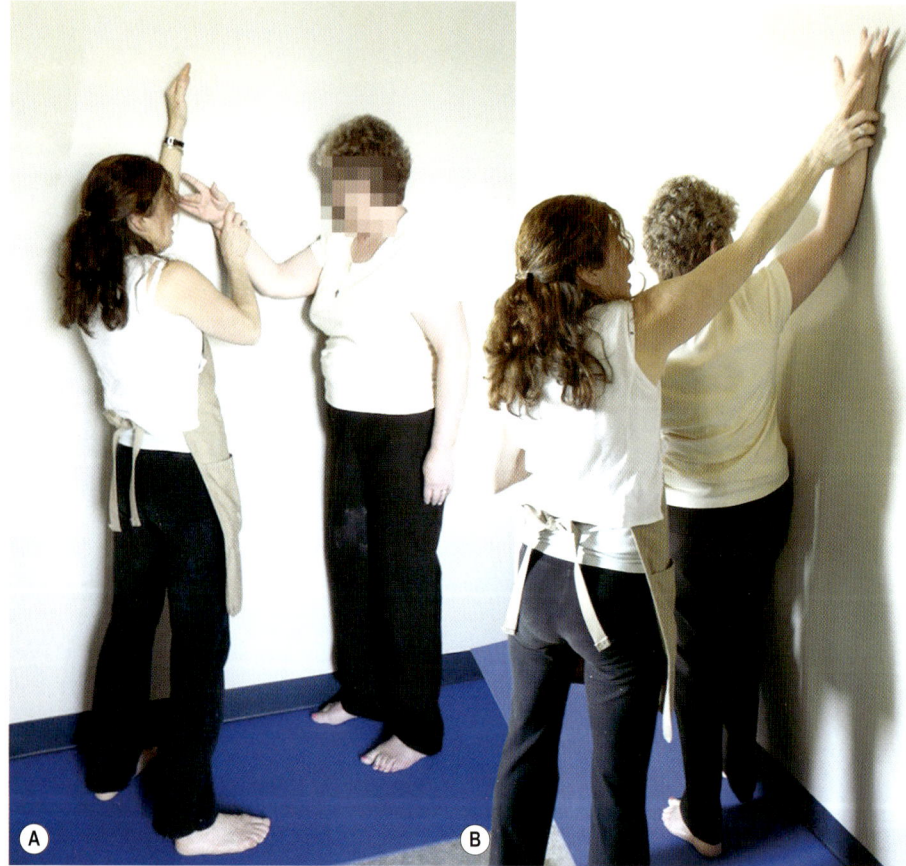
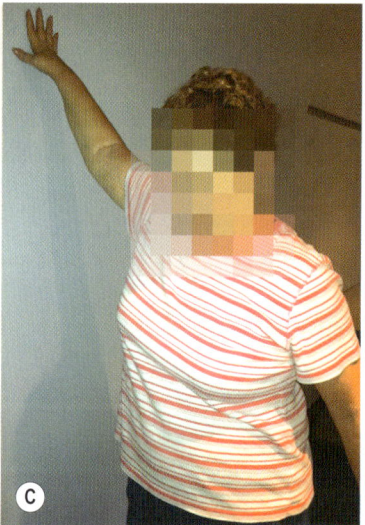

FIGURE 6.16 L and author using the wall to increase ROM. **(C)** progress months later

Clinical cases: adults

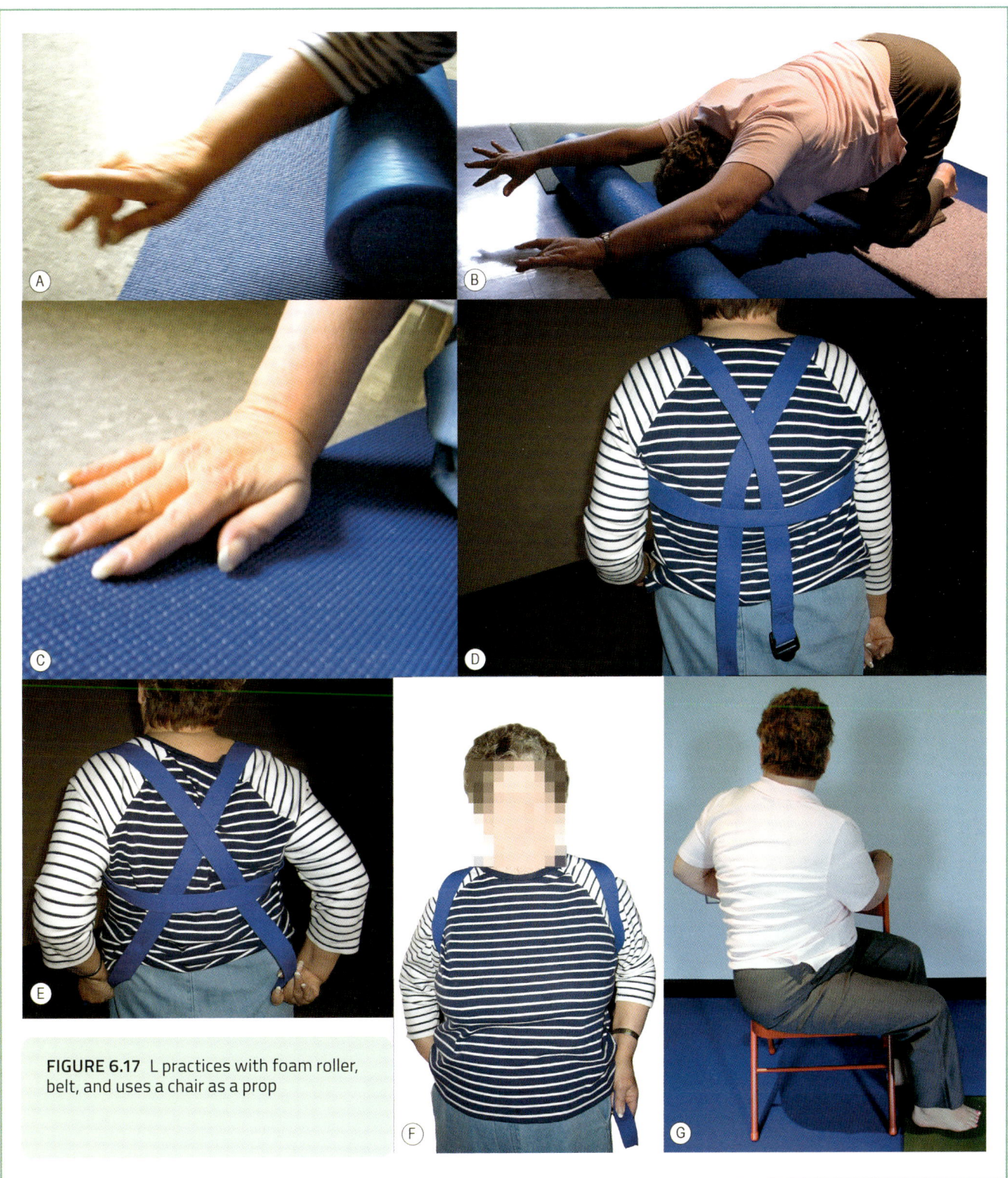

FIGURE 6.17 L practices with foam roller, belt, and uses a chair as a prop

Chapter six

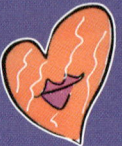

Figure 6.17C shows how much her right hand relaxed after using the roller; Figs 6.17A and B show the progression. Also, a 10-foot yoga belt was used to open up her chest wall, stretch her anterior deltoid muscles and improve her posture (Figs 6.17D–F). Here you can see how the belt is strapped, and L's command of her posture via holding onto the belt ends as she practiced walking with the belt. In Fig. 6.17G, L is using a chair to do twisting poses.

Initially I also used a tennis ball in order to aid L with her balance on her feet. She would roll the tennis ball under the ball of her foot, arch and sides. This required aid from me to hold her in place as she attempted this exercise. A chair was always available if she tired. In time this improved her gait and balance. We also used a larger ball (Fig. 6.18) and L would lean against the wall, squat, and return back up the wall. At first, she needed my aid to do this but as seen in her progressions in Figure 6.18A, not in the end. This improved her quadriceps strength and also aided in her balance. Fig. 6.18B shows L using the wall to perform tree pose (vṛkṣāsana).

In Figure 6.19, L beamed as she was able to hold the large medicine ball above her head with both hands. Figure 6.20 shows L in *supta pādāṅguṣṭhāsana* (A), using the belt overhead to aid right arm (B) and in the C and D I am adjusting her for meditation. Finally, L relaxes in *śavāsana* (Figure 6.21). Often, I would also perform Reiki on her hands, and I have videos of her hands completely unfurled and relaxed. These are just a sampling of L's work during of our time together.

It became clear that L's communication improved when she received yoga therapy before speech therapy, so L's yoga therapy sessions preceded her speech and art therapy sessions. This was based on the norms of developmental

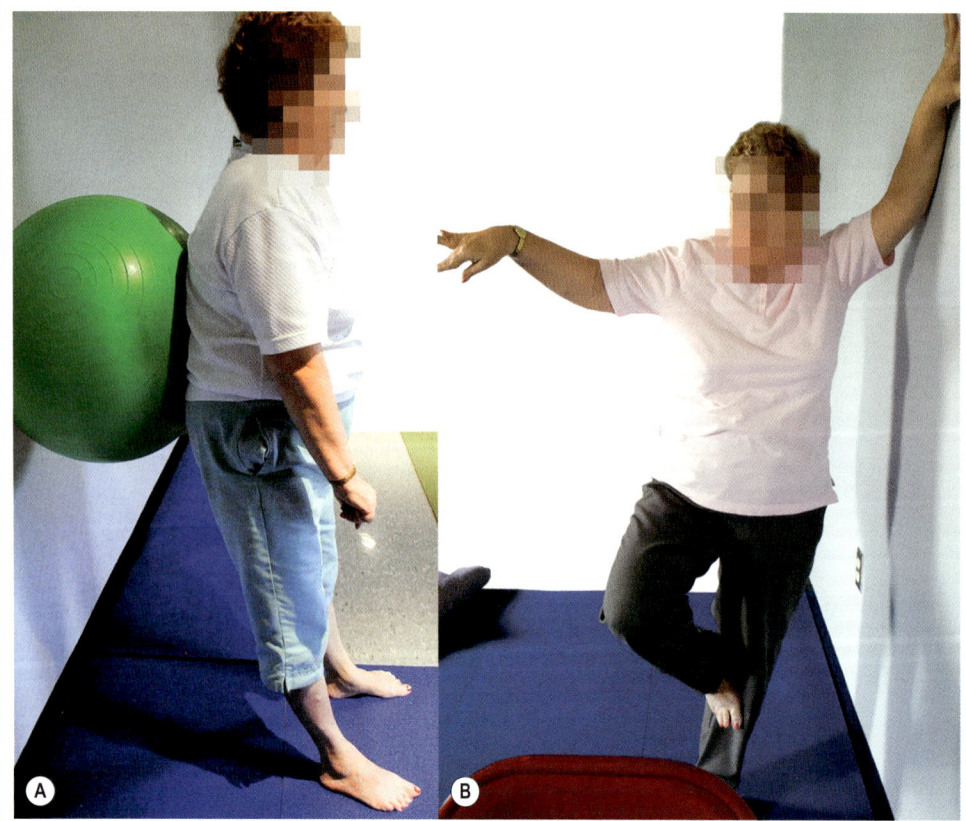

FIGURE 6.18 L using the large ball to improve quadriceps strength and practice tree pose (vṛkṣāsana)

Clinical cases: adults

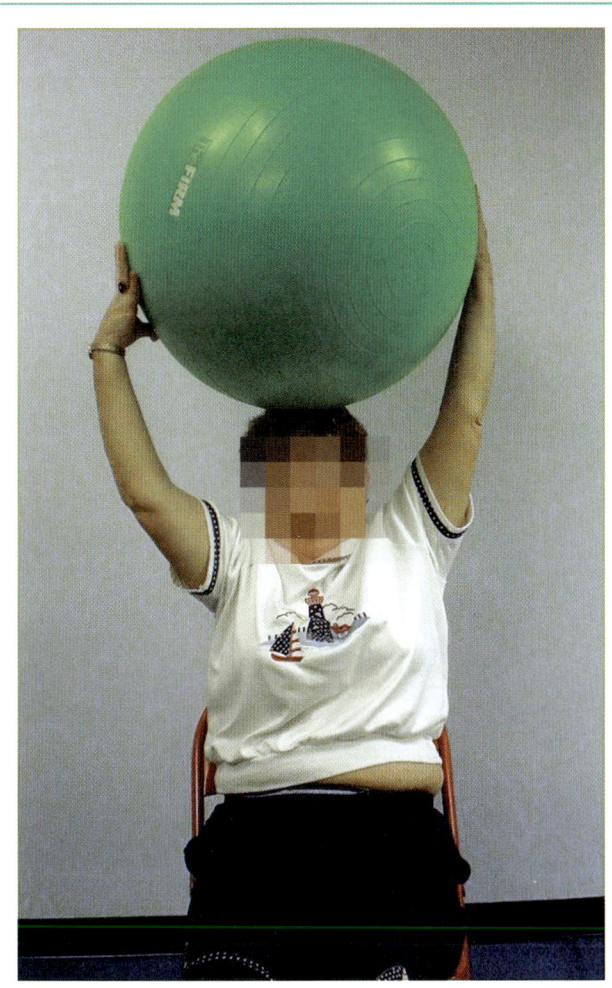

FIGURE 6.19 L holding medicine ball with arms stretched overhead

art (Lowenfeld and Brittain 1987), as well as my own hypothesis of connecting the visceral body to executive function. This resulted in improved fine and gross motor control and skill. One day, while painting seemingly without purpose, an angel appeared in L's artwork. As it formed in the paint swirls, she turned to me with a large smile on her face and said, 'I made an angel!' (Fig. 6.22). And so she had. Working with L was one of my greatest gifts. It gave me an opportunity to truly appreciate the miracle that she was and that could unfold from the power of combining yoga and art.

This was the beginning of my journey as a yoga therapist. I knew then that my work could never be the same, and to this day I am amazed at how seamlessly these two creative therapies work together in restoring both physical and emotional function. This reminded me of a passage that I recently read. Sterios (2019) talks about 'two of the most powerful approaches to the practice of yoga in the face of resistance... are patience and kindness toward yourself'. He stated that 'no matter what circumstances took you into your current situation... the experience of compassion for yourself... can help you develop a childlike curiosity, free from results... leading you to discover something unknown about yourself' (Sterios 2019:50). This is true for our patients but more importantly for ourselves as 'healers'. It is in that mix that we truly co-create with our patients and discover that font of well-being.

Chapter six

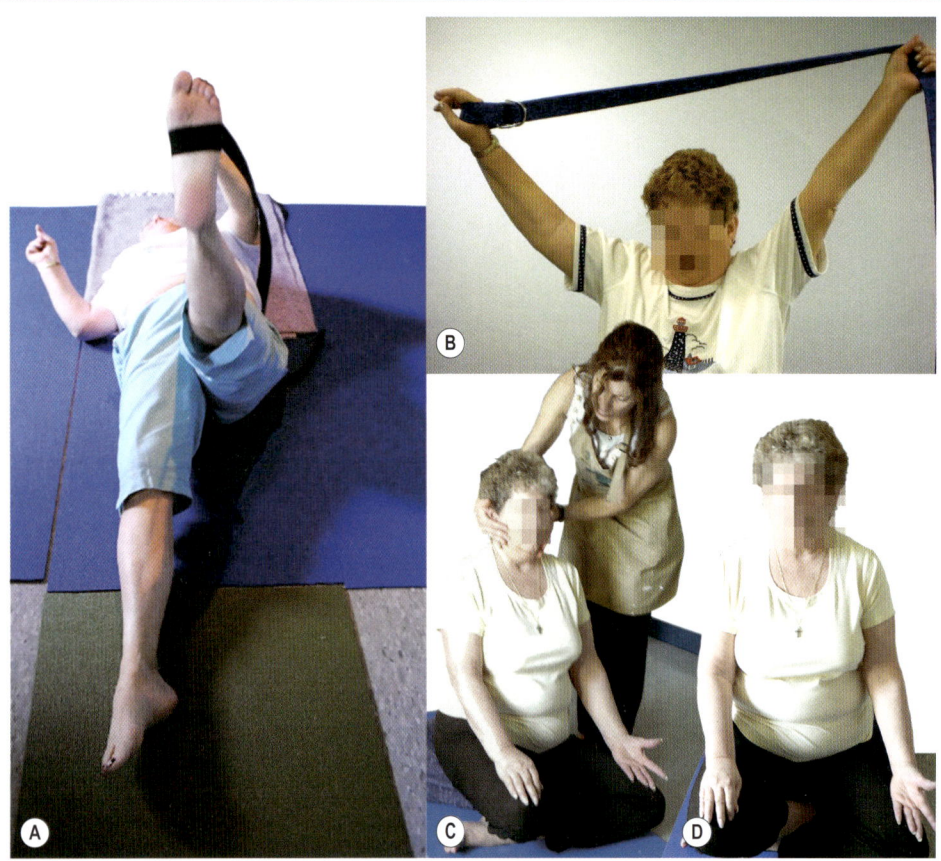

FIGURE 6.20 L in *supta pādāṅguṣṭhāsana* (left) using a belt and meditation (with author assist)

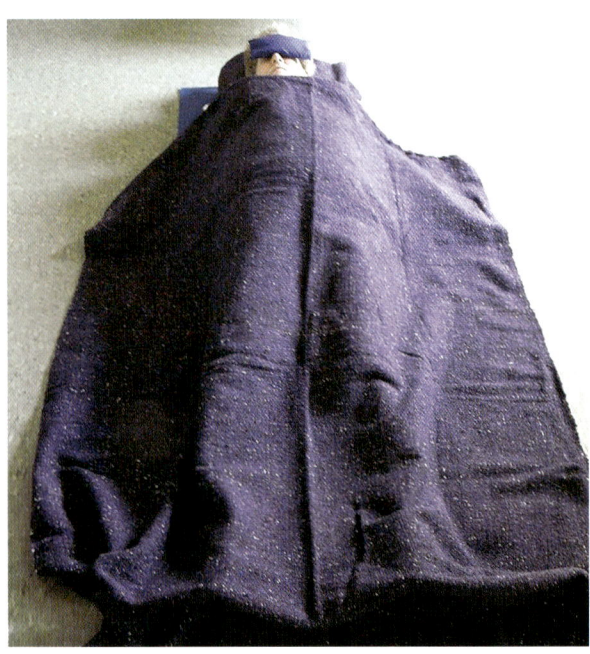

FIGURE 6.21 L in *śavāsana*

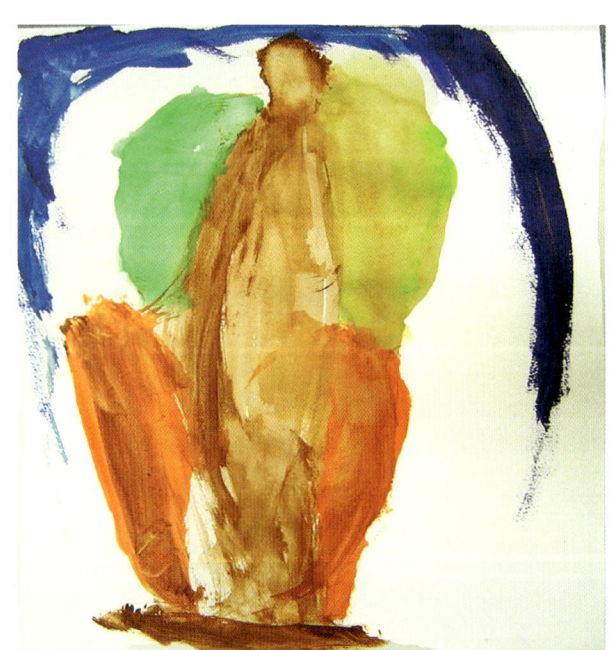

FIGURE 6.22 L's angel

Clinical cases: adults

> ### Reflection exercise 6.3
>
> In thinking about this case I wished Sanford's (2006) work had been published when I started working with L. Many of Sanford's words struck me, post the loss of his father and sister in a car accident that left him paralyzed. He wrote, 'it is easy to see how yoga clarifies the connection between mind and body... Take one part away... and the overall experience changes significantly' (Sanford 2006:26). It is hard to imagine one's body and mind as a stroke survivor or in Sanford's case, paralyzed from the waist down. And while one would never wish to be in this situation, when working with another stroke survivor (Horovitz 2005) I entered the art therapy room with my right hand in a sling and continued to function one-handed for months. The reasons were myriad for doing this, including demonstrating that artmaking could be fashioned using my sinistral (left) hand. This empathic decision aided that patient (and me) in understanding his predicament. It also encouraged him to persevere. He eventually made beautiful artwork.
>
> Having suffered significant losses in my life I don't take much for granted; but I truly wonder if I could have been as gracious as L was and persevere without wallowing into depression. So, for this exercise, perhaps make a list of your strengths and gifts. Imagine your life without one of these riches. Perhaps create some artwork to reflect how you might cope. Be gentle with yourself: as Sanford writes, 'the splendor and subtlety of living is most apparent in the conscious presence of the silence... Progress is what you make of it' (2006:168).

Final thoughts

These clinical case studies in Chapters 4, 5 and 6 are representative of some of my work where I have combined the disciplines of yoga therapy and art therapy. While only a smattering of my cases, I hope it gives you a taste of the possibilities of working in this manner.

In thinking about this last case, where I operated from my innermost visceral being, I am again reminded of Sanford's words, 'feeling without knowing, that is our fate' (Sanford 2006:46). Sterios (2019) discussed his interpersonal challenges and wondered whether he could consciously breathe into his stored stress and with each exhale, release the pain. In discovering the 'yes' to that question, he discovered that all he had to do was, 'show up in the moment... [listen] to a quiet voice inside... and stay present... how we meet resistance on the mat is a beautiful reflection of how we meet resistance in life' (Sterios 2019:46).

Sometimes this becomes wholly obvious in words spoken or released through a deep sigh. The clues are always there hiding in the body, the buried images and the undeclared words. All we need do is listen to that prescient sound, always bubbling up inside of us, just waiting to be received, understood, and unleashed into deliverance. To pay attention to that wellspring is the work, and in that is *sattva*.

References

Abraham R (2005) When Words Have Lost Their Meaning: Alzheimer's Patients Communicate Through Art. Westport, CT: Praeger.

Alders A and Levine-Madori L (2010) The effect of art therapy on cognitive performance of Hispanic/Latino older adults. Art Therapy: Journal of the American Art Therapy Association 27(3): 127–135.

Alzheimer's Research and Prevention Foundation (2013) Kirtan Kriya Yoga Meditation, information sheet. Available at: http://alzheimersprevention.org/wp-content/uploads/2013/11/Kirtan_Kriya_Instructions.pdf

American Academy of Pediatrics (2019) Vesicoureteral Reflux (VUR) in Infants & Young Children. Available at: https://www.healthychildren.org/English/health-issues/conditions/genitourinary-tract/Pages/Vesicoureteral-Reflux-in-Infants-Young-Children.aspx

Blalock JE (1989) A molecular basis for bidirectional communication between the immune and neuroendocrine systems. Physiology Reviews 69: 1–32.

Blalock JE (1994) Shared ligands and receptors as a molecular mechanism for communication between the immune and neuroendocrine systems. Annals of the New York Academy of Sciences 741: 292–298.

Chapter six

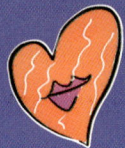
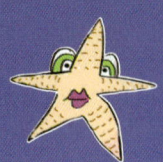

Blau D and Berezin M (1975) Neurosis and character disorders. In: Howells J (ed), Modern Perspectives in Psychiatry of Old Age. New York: Brunner/Mazel, pp. 201–233.

Bonura KB and Pargman D (2009) The effects of yoga versus exercise on stress, anxiety and depression in older adults. International Journal of Yoga Therapy 19: 79–89.

Brosse AL, Sheets ES, Lett HS and Blumenthal JA (2002) Exercise and the treatment of clinical depression in adults: recent findings and future directions. Sports Medicine 32: 741–760.

Chodzko-Zajko WJ and Proctor DN (2009) American College of Sports Medicine position stand: Exercise and physical activity for older adults. Medicine & Science in Sports & Exercise 41: 1510–1530.

Colangelo J (2003) Embodied Wisdom: What Our Anatomy can Teach us About the Art of Living. Linclon, NE: iUniverse.

Csikszentmihalyi M (1997). Finding Flow: The Psychology of Engagement with Everyday Life. New York, NY: Basic Books.

Curry NA and Kasser T (2005) Can coloring mandalas reduce anxiety? American Journal of Art Therapy 22(2): 81–85.

Dana DA (2018) The Polyvagal Theory in Therapy: Engaging the Rhythm of Regulation (Norton Series on Interpersonal Neurobiology), 1st Edn. New York, NY: WW Norton & Co.

Ellis-Hill C, Payne S and Ward C (2000) Self–body split: issues of identity in physical recovery after stroke. Disability and Rehabilitation 22: 725–733.

Fishman L (2015) Healing Yoga: Proven postures to treat twenty common ailments – from backache to bone loss, shoulder pain to bunions, and more. New York, NY: WW Norton & Co.

Franklin M (1999) Becoming a student of oneself: activating the witness in meditation, art and supervision. American Journal of Art Therapy 38(1): 2–13.

Franklin M (2011) The yoga of art and the creative process: listening to the divine. In Farrely-Hansen M (ed) Spirituality and Art Therapy: Living the Connection. New York, NY: Jessica Kingsley.

Franklin M (2017) Art as Contemplative Practice: Expressive Pathways to the SELF. Albany, NY: State University of New York Press.

Garrett R, Immink MA and Hillier S (2011) Becoming connected: the lived experience of yoga participation after stroke. Disability and Rehabilitation 33(25–26): 2404–2415.

Gibbons K (2015) Integrating Art Therapy and Yoga Therapy: Yoga, Art and the Use of Intention. Phildelphia, PA: Jessica Kingsley.

Golden J, Conroy RM, Bruce I, et al (2009) Loneliness, social support networks, mood and wellbeing in community-dwelling elderly. International Journal Geriatric Psychiatry 24: 694–700.

Haber D (1983) Yoga as a preventative health care program for white and black elders: An exploratory study. International Journal for Aging 17: 169–176.

Harris JE and Eng JJ (2010) Strength training improves upper-limb function in individuals with stroke: a meta-analysis. Stroke 41(1): 136–140.

Hattori H, Hattori C, Hokao C, Mizushima K and Mase T (2011) Controlled study on the cognitive and psychological effect of coloring and drawing in mild Alzheimer's disease patients. Geriatrics and Gerontology International 11(4): 431–437.

Higgs MM (2019) Why you should find time to be alone with yourself. New York Times, 28 October. Available at: https://www.nytimes.com/2019/10/28/smarter-living/the-benefits-of-being-alone.html

Horovitz EG (2005) Art Therapy as Witness: A Sacred Guide. Springfield, IL: Charles C Thomas Ltd.

Horovitz EG (2014) The Art Therapists' Primer: a Clinical Guide to Writing Assessment, Diagnosis and Treatment, 2nd Edn. Springfield, IL: Charles C Thomas Ltd.

Horovitz EG (2017a) The Guide to Art Therapy Materials and Methods: A Practical, Step-by-Step Approach. New York, NY: Routledge Press.

Horovitz EG (2017b) Spiritual Art Therapy: An Alternate Path, 3rd Edn. Springfield, IL: Charles C Thomas Ltd.

Horovitz EG and Elgelid S (2015) Yoga Therapy: Theory and Practice. New York, NY: Routledge Press.

Isis P (2016) The Mindful Doodle Book: 75 Creative Exercises to Help You Live in the Moment. Eau Claire, WI: PESI Publishing & Media.

Kerr C (1999) The psychosocial significance of creativity in the elderly. Art Therapy: Journal of the American Art Therapy Association 16(1): 37–41.

Kramer E (1975) Art Therapy With Children. New York, NY: Schocken books.

Kramer E (2016) Sublimation and art therapy. In: Rubin J (ed) Approaches to Art Therapy, 3rd Edn. New York, NY: Routledge.

Lasater J (2000) Living Your Yoga: Finding the Spiritual in Everyday Life. Berkely, CA: Rodmell Press.

Lavretsky (2017) Integrative Therapies For Mood And Cognitive Disorders Of Aging (Video). Available at: https://www.semel.ucla.edu/cimmh/video/helen-lavretsky-md-integrative-therapies-mood-and-cognitive-disorders-aging

Clinical cases: adults

Lowenfeld V and Brittain WL (1987) Creative and Mental Growth, 8th Edn. New York, NY: MacMillan.

Middleton KR, Andrade R, Moonaz SH, Muhammad C and Wallen GR (2015) Yoga research and spirituality: A case study discussion. International Journal of Yoga Therapy (25): 33–35.

Mimica N and Dubravka K (2011) Art therapy may be beneficial for reducing stress-related behaviours in people with dementia: Case report. Psychiatria Danubina 23(1): 125–128.

Morris FJ (2014) Should art be integrated into cognitive behavioral therapy for anxiety disorders? The Arts in Psychotherapy (41): 343–352.

NurrieStearns M (2018) Healing, Anxiety, Depression and Unworthiness: 78 brain-changing Mindfulness and Yoga Practices. Eau Claire, WI: PESI Publishing & Media.

Orr P (1997) Treating the whole person: a combination of medical and psychiatric treatment for older adults. Art Therapy: Journal of the American Art Therapy Association, 14(3), 200–205.

Patel NK, Newstead AH and Ferrer RL (2012) The effects of yoga on physical functioning and health related quality of life in older adults: a systematic review and meta-analysis. Journal of Alternative and Complimentary Medicine 18(10): 902–917.

Pearson N, Pearson L and Byron E (2020) Pain and yoga therapy Part 2: the lived experience of persisting pain. Yoga Therapy Today, Winter 2020: 30–33.

Physical Activity Guidelines Advisory Committee (2009) Physical Activity Guidelines Advisory Committee Report 2008. Part A: Executive summary. Nutrition Reviews 67: 114–120.

Porges SW (2009) The polyvagal theory: new insights into adaptive reactions of the autonomic nervous system. Cleveland Journal of Medicine 76(Suppl.2): S86–S90.

Porges SW (2011) The Polyvagal Theory: Neurophysiological Foundations of Emotions, Attachment, Communication, Self-regulation. New York, NY: WW Norton & Co.

Quinn P (2020) Art Therapy in the Treatment of Addiction and Trauma. Philadelphia, PA: Jessica Kingsley.

Rikli RE and Jones CJ (2012). Senior Fitness Test Manual, 2nd Edn. Champaign, IL: Human Kinetics.

Rubin J (2016) Approaches to Art Therapy, 3rd Edn. New York, NY: Routledge.

Sable J, Dunn L and Zisook S (2002) Late-life depression: how to identify its symptoms and provide effective treatment. Geriatrics 57: 18–32.

Sanford M (2006) Waking: A Memoir of Trauma and Transcendence. Emmaus, PA: Rodale Press.

Satprem (1982) The Mind of the Cells or Willed Mutation of Our Species (translated by Venet L and F). New York, NY: Institute for Evolutionary Research.

Schmid AA, Miller KK, Van Puymbroeck MV and DeBaun-Sprague E (2014) Yoga leads to multiple physical improvements after stroke, a pilot study. Complementary Therapies in Medicine 22(6): 994–1000.

Schmid AA and Van Puymbroeck MV (2019) Yoga Therapy for Stroke: a Handbook for Yoga Therapists and Health Professionals. Philadelphia, PA: Jessica Kingsley.

Schore JN (2014) The right brain is dominant in psychotherapy. American Psychological Association 51(3): 388–397.

Schore JN (2019) Right Brain Psychotherapy. New York, NY: WW Norton & Co.

Sims J, O'Connor D and Browning C (2012) Management of depression in older people: a role for physical activity. In: Abdel-Rahman E (ed) Depression in the Elderly. New York, NY: Nova Science Publishers Inc, pp. 115–139.

Stallings JW (2010) Collage as a therapeutic modality for reminiscence in patients with dementia. Art Therapy: Journal of the American Art Therapy Association 27(3): 136–140.

Statista (2020) Number of people aged 100 and older (centenarians) worldwide from 2010 to 2100. Available at: https://www.statista.com/statistics/996597/number-centenarians-worldwide/

Stephenson RC (2013) Promoting well-being and gerotranscendence in an art therapy program for older adults. Art Therapy: Journal of the American Art Therapy Association 30(4): 151–158.

Sterios P (2019) Grace and Gravity: How to Awaken your Subtle Body and the Healing Power of Yoga. Boulder, CO: Sounds True.

Stewart EG (2004) Art therapy and neuroscience blend: working with patients who have dementia. Art Therapy: Journal of the American Art Therapy Association 21(3): 148–155.

Taylor M (2012) Creating a biopsychosocial bridge of care: linking yoga therapy and medical rehabilitation. International Journal of Yoga Therapy 22: 93–94.

Teicher M, Samson J, Sheu Y, Polcari A and McGreenery C (2010) Hurtful words: association of exposure to peer verbal abuse with elevated psychiatric symptom scores and corpus callosum abnormalities. American Journal of Psychiatry 167(12): 1464–1471.

Chapter six

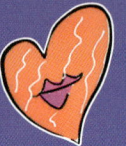
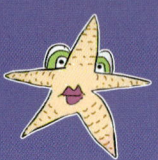

Tornstam L (2005) Gerotranscendence : A Developmental Theory of Positive Aging. New York, NY: Springer.

Tracey K J (2002) The inflammatory reflex. Nature 420(6917): 853-850.

Voelker L (2020) Lakshmi Voelker Chair Yoga. Available at: https://getfitwhereyousit.com/

Wampold BE (2001) The Great Psychotherapy Debate: Models, Methods and Findings. Hillsdale, NJ: Lawrence Erlbaum.

Wang D (2009) The use of yoga for physical and mental health among older adults: a review of the literature. International Journal of Yoga Therapy 19: 91–96.

A sampling of *āsanas* for seniors 7

Yoga does not just change the way we see things, it transforms the person who sees.

B.K.S. Iyengar (2005)

As stated in Chapter 6, an older adult can be aged anywhere from 55 to 100+ years old, and this 45-year range presents an enormously diverse group of persons that varies in physical ability and life experiences.

Beyond my training as a yoga teacher and yoga therapist, I am also trained as a Silver Sneaker Yoga Teacher (aimed at people over 55) and a chair yoga teacher (under the tutelage of Lakshmi Voelker (2020)). Naturally, I developed my own manner of working, as seen in the Chapter 6 Case study with L. This was long before my Silver Sneaker Yoga and Voelker chair yoga training. Herein, I present some *āsanas* that one can use with this population, and when I am using the skillset learned from Voelker, I will specify. It is important to note that Voelker's method teaches people to sit on the chair: sometimes, I have people sit on the chair and other times I use the chair as a prop. The reasons are myriad and are also not part of Silver Sneaker Training nor Voelker's training, and as I repeat throughout this book, it depends on the individual.

Each body is different no matter age or physical function. As a practitioner (even when working with large classes of 26 seniors or more), one has to assess the variations in the room, evaluate abilities and be prepared to offer modifications. All of this happens quite quickly (formal diagnostic evaluation is not possible). As Amy (2019) suggested (see Chapter 2), use your eyes.

In the description of Silver Sneaker Yoga, participants do not get down on the mat, but I have seniors that choose to do this in a class when everyone else is either using a chair (as a prop) or sitting on the chair. So, I may have several modifications within that class for each *āsana*. I could be rigid and suggest that the person not attend the class if they decided to use the mat, but I tend to be adaptable and fluid. If I feel someone is unsafe, I attend immediately to that person, so my internal compass is externally dialed to the needs of the participants.

I also note quite quickly when seniors need to sit, and so to avoid strain, the class might consist of sitting on the chair and using the chair as a prop (standing poses).

During a recent senior yoga class where I taught this method, a woman came up to me after we ended and said, 'Thank you for not treating us like babies; I so appreciate how you challenged us'. That sealed it for me and made me realize how empowering it is to offer choice and variability, especially with this population that in her words was 'sick of being handled with kid gloves'.

None of us look forward to becoming infirm, sick or less able. But sometimes due to disease, accident (Sanford 2008), or just age-related breakdown of our parts, our bodies change. I am not suggesting that one ignore this and 'push' through *āsanas*, military style. *Āsanas* do not define yoga, yoga defines us. As Sterios (2019) suggested, 'Is your practice of yoga supporting you to be kinder and more open toward the people close to you? At its core, yoga is bonding. Yoga is union. Yoga is one' (2019:51). Sterios (2019) suggested that if we 'let pain be our guide', and respond without emotion, in turn that opening will create more space for our bodies' healing to work. I agree.

In the past, after undergoing a surgical intervention, my doctor eschewed all exercise for 6 weeks (to allow my body to heal). Naturally, movement and walking were encouraged. But I know my own body. I practiced yoga post-surgery on day one. I am not talking about hatha yoga, handstands, headstands or the like. Lasater's work (1995) was key as I eased my body back into shape. But I also heeded the words of my doctor and never pushed myself. When I finished my practice, which included *āsanas*, *prāṇayāma* and meditation, I knew I was positively affecting my own healing. This is what Sterios (2019) is referring to when he suggests that we let our pain be our guide.

Sample *āsana* practice

Let's look at some of these variations. It is important to note that whether working in a class, or privately with

Chapter seven

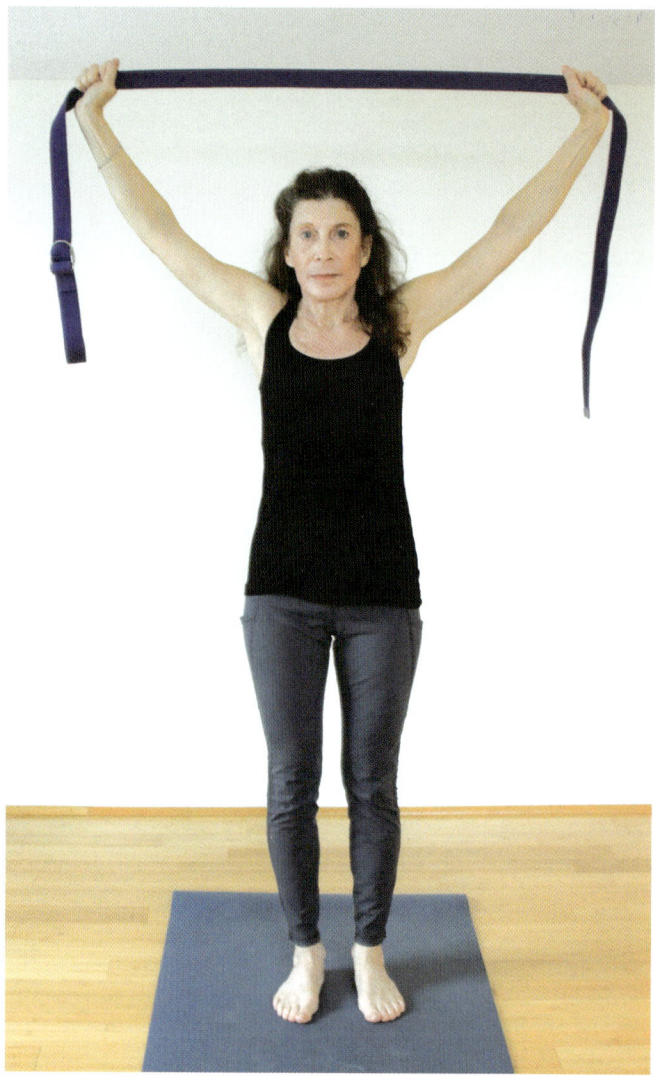

FIGURE 7.1 Author stretching yoga belt overhead while maintain little to no bend in the arms

patients, I always start by setting an intention – going within (preferably closing one's eyes but if uncomfortable, averting them to the ground). This can be done standing or in *sukhāsana*, easy pose (if sitting). The intention could be for one's health, the health of another, or whatever comes up for that person. During the course of the practice, I suggest recalling that intention no matter where they are in their practice. This seems to aid in maintaining *dṛṣṭi* (focus) and serves as a reminder to re-center oneself in mind, body, and spirit. So, once that intention is established, warm-ups begin. It might start with the shoulders using the yoga belt. Figure 7.1 illustrates what this might look like if there is no shoulder injury present. If there is, then this can be done in front of the shoulder while still adducting the rhomboids. Figure 7.2 illustrates what this looks like from the side and taken further if capable of moving the arms behind the back. It is suggested to do this about x10 and then roll the shoulders in one direction and then the other.

In Figure 7.3, I keep one arm bent (shoulder level) and stretch the anterior deltoid of the opposite arm back while keeping my torso stationary. Again, this can be repeated alternating each shoulder x10 or more, depending on ability.

Next I might suggest downward facing dog (DFD) (*adho mukha śvānāsana*) using the chair (Figure 7.4). This can be done as illustrated, using the highest point of the chair or facing the seat towards the person, allowing for a stretch at a lower level. I emphasize that when at home, this can be done at a counter, or if doing computer work (without standing desk) to do this at the desk. I also talk about doing this against a car when breaking from a long road trip.

A sampling of *āsanas* for seniors

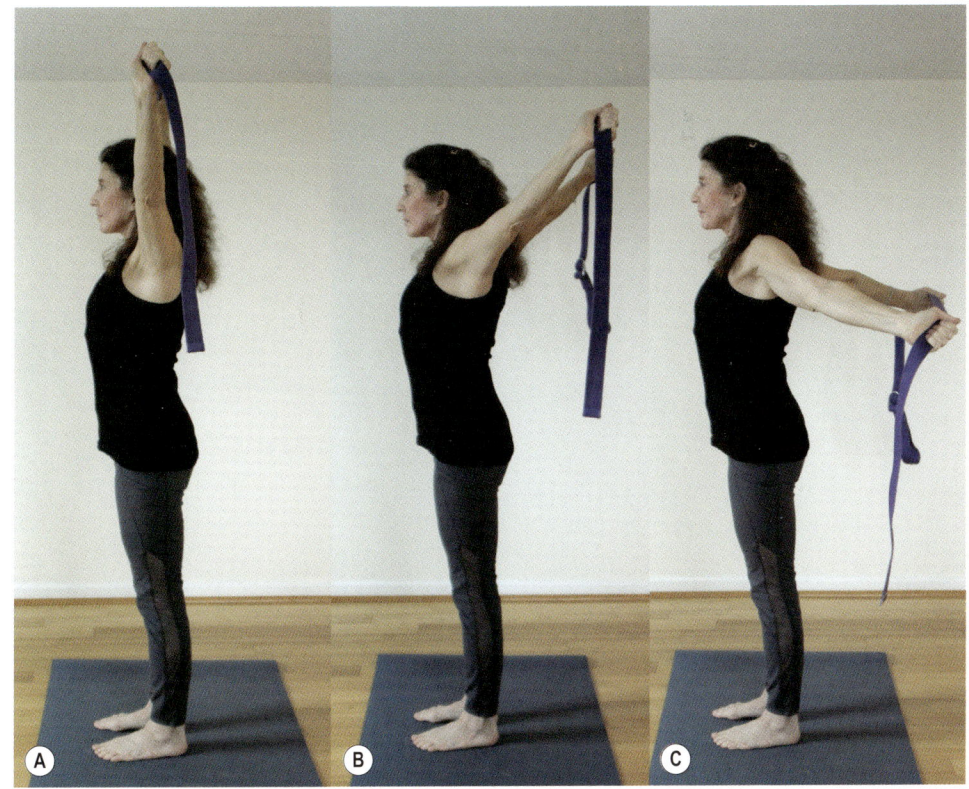

FIGURE 7.2 Author uses yoga belt to stretch the scapular area

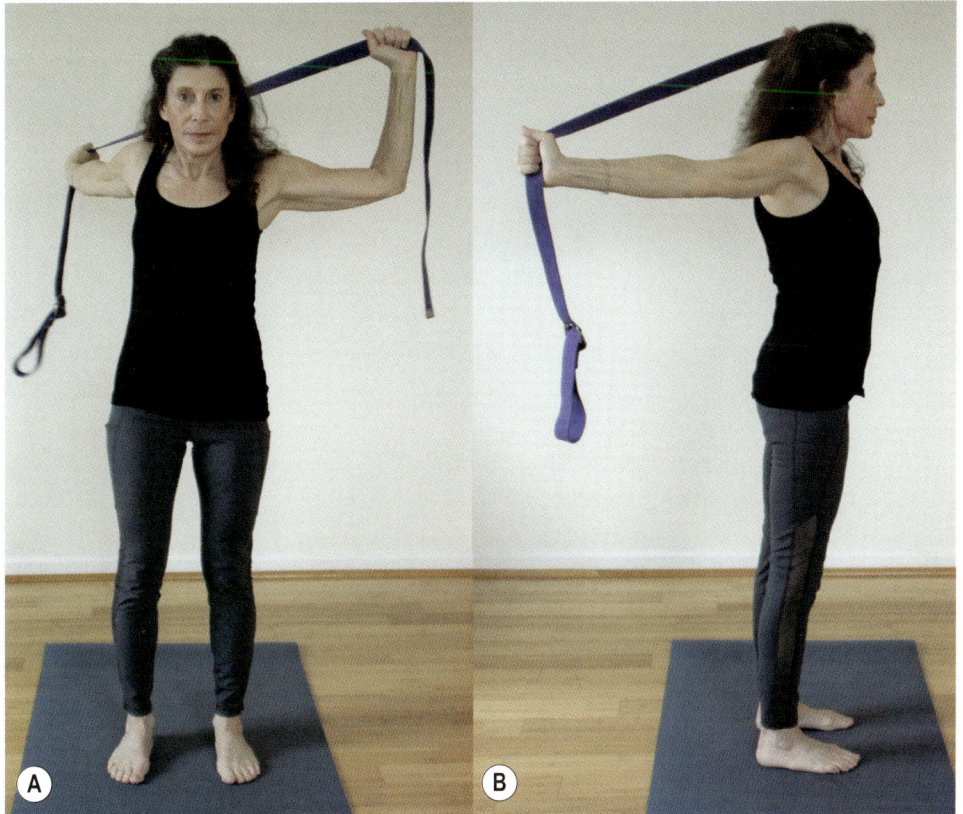

FIGURE 7.3 (**A**) Author stretches right arm behind while leaving left arm stationary and bent at elbow. (**B**) Side view

Chapter seven

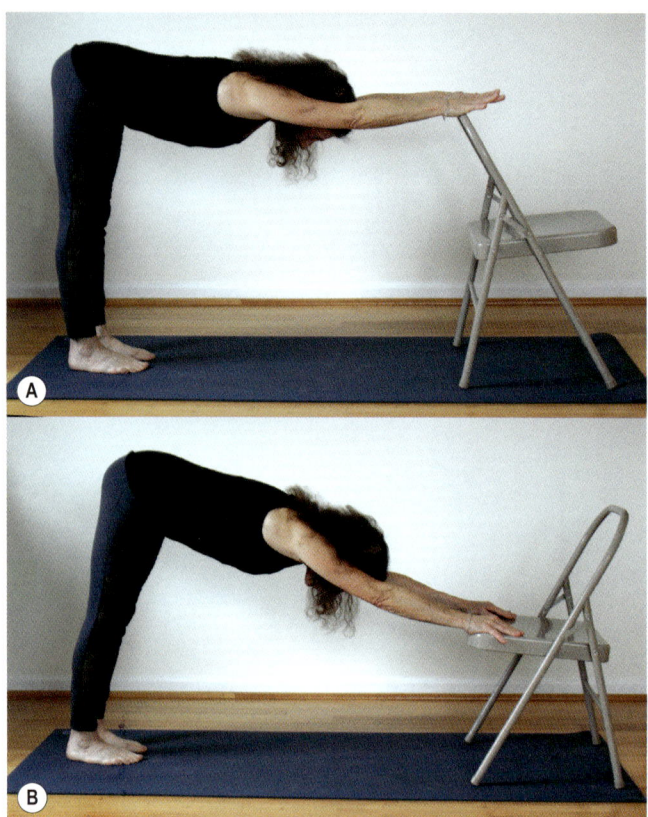

FIGURE 7.4 *Adho mukha śvānāsana* (using the chair at varying levels)

Figure 7.5 illustrates using the chair to do DFD, plank pose, upward facing dog (UFD, *ūrdhva mukha śvānāsana*) and then returning to DFD. You can see how important it is to have proper form (keeping shoulders directly over the wrist in plank and tucking the elbows into the sides when coming into UFD. This actually might be considered a *vinyasa* flow but that is not the aim here. The idea is to go slowly and steadily through these poses. Sometimes, if someone has wrist issues then the fists are closed for this series, or UFD and DFD might be done sitting (not illustrated here).

Figure 7.6 indicates Warrior 1 (*vīrabhadrāsana I*) again using the chair. Note that if uncomfortable keeping both hands up, it is recommended that for balance, that you maintain one arm in contact with the top of the chair. Next (Figure 7.7), I suggest that the arms open like wings with palms turned up (to protect the rotator cuff) (A, B) and then turn the arms downward pivoting into Warrior 2 (*vīrabhadrāsana II*) and if comfortable, reverse Warrior 2 (C, D). Note that the chair is always Fig. 7.10C available if needed for balance and comfort. Here it is available as a prop if needed.

Figure 7.8 indicates these same poses but sitting on the chair as Voelker would teach this pose. Note that in Fig. 7.8A the left hand holds onto the back of the chair for increased ROM and stability. This is a fine way to practice and depending on the ability of the person practicing this pose, the chair might be a much better option. Again, it depends.

Figure 7.9 illustrates using the chair as a prop for *trikoṇāsana*. Note all the variations: one might be perfectly satisfied to stop at Fig. 7.9B, making sure to roll the anterior deltoid back in order to open up the chest wall. Often, I suggest that my students get into this pose by thinking about being a tea pot (Fig. 7.9A) where the arm extends outward while keeping the opposite hand on the hip and then moving more fully into the position. This aids in keeping people in one plane so hips don't jut out when leaning forward and extending (Fig. 7.9D). Again, this same series could be done in a chair (Voelker style). Naturally this pose is held for several moments and then done on the other side. You can repeat this pose as often as you like. I generally do these series x3 on each side. This offers consistency, memorization, and internal digestion of the feeling in a pose. Sterios (2019) likened stretching into a pose as 'softening'. I loved that comparison as it communicates the movement at a cellular level.

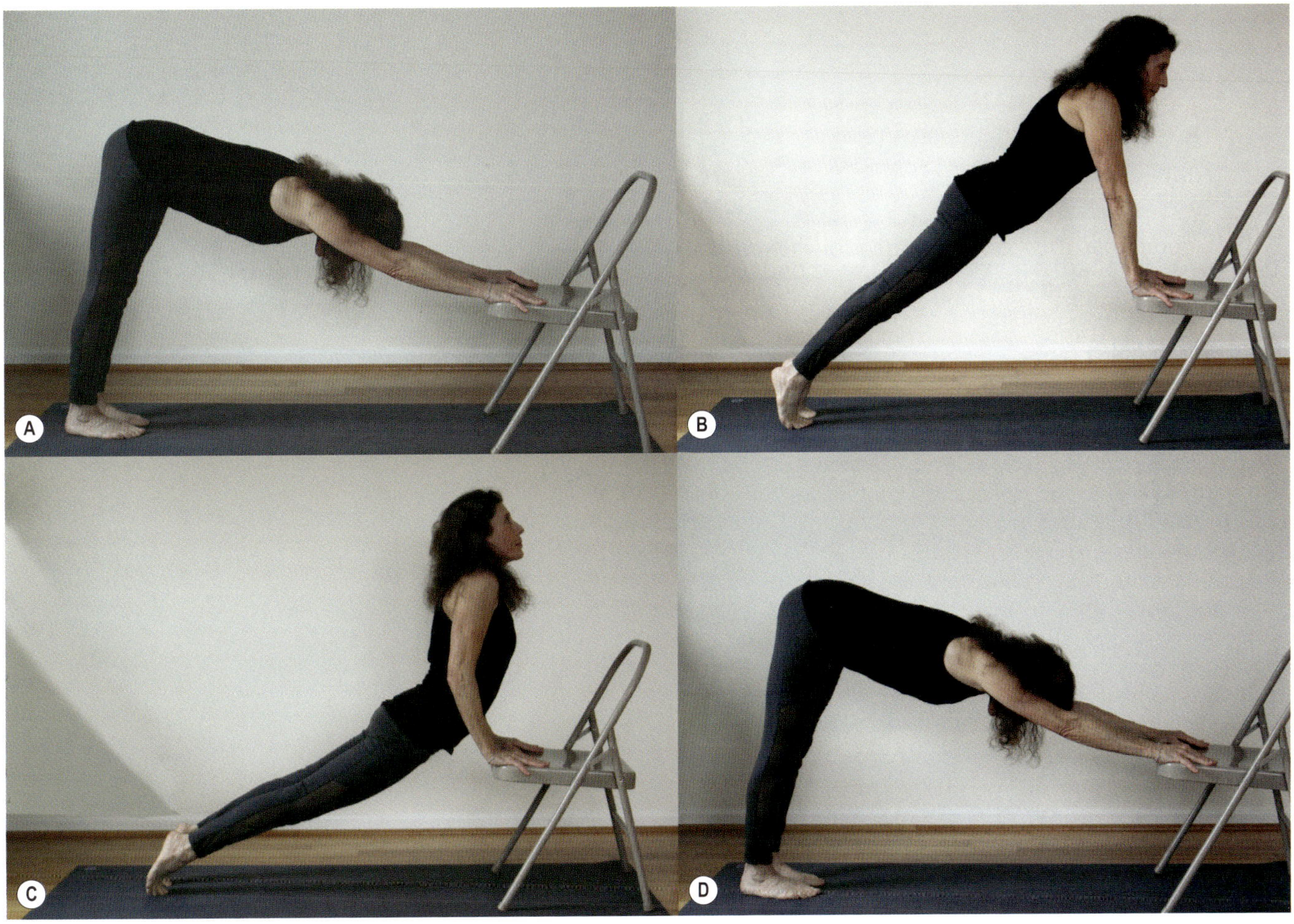

A sampling of āsanas for seniors

FIGURE 7.5 Author in DFD, plank, UFD and back to DFD

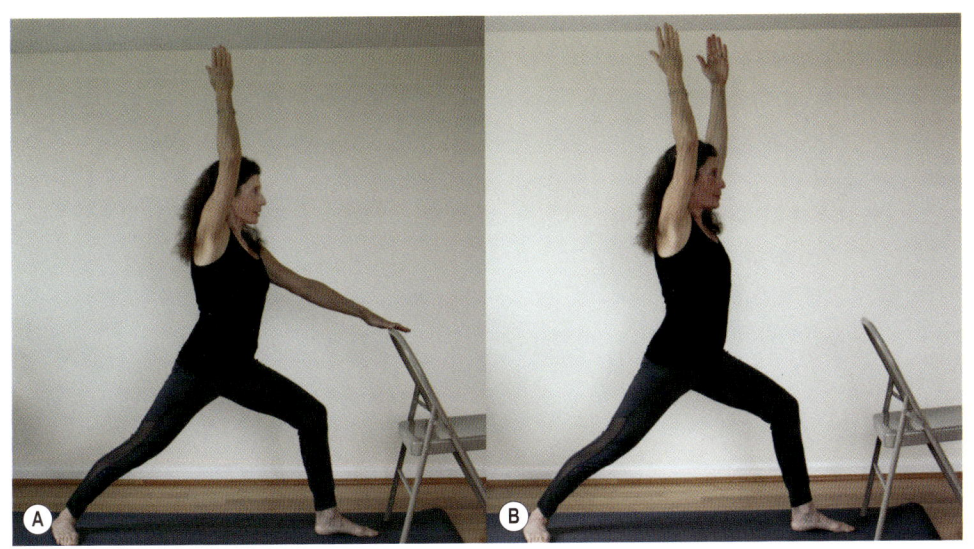

FIGURE 7.6 Author in *vīrabhadrāsana I* using the chair

Chapter seven

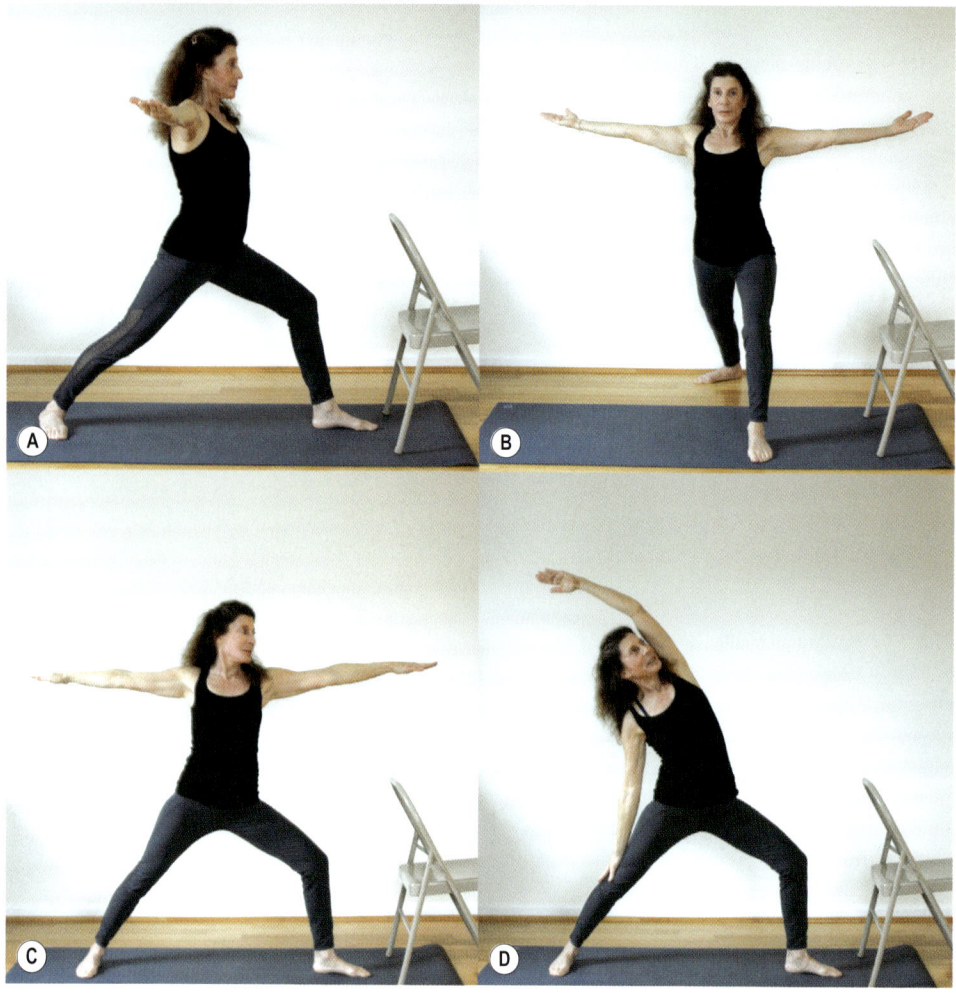

FIGURE 7.7 Author moving into *vīrabhadrāsana I* and *II*, using the chair as a prop, if needed

Using a chair for *supta pādāṅguṣṭhāsana* (Figure 7.10) is one of my senior yoga classes' favorites. We liken ourselves to the Ziegfield Follies or the Rockettes at Radio City Music Hall in New York City. Whether we do this sitting (Figure 7.10) or standing (Figure 7.11) (rather than reclining on the mat), the benefits are enormous. Note that when sitting on the chair and using the yoga belt (Fig. 7.10B), the elbows are brought back towards the shoulders, the leg automatically ascends and so a modified heron pose (*krounchāsana*) is employed. After opening the left leg to the side (Fig. 7.10C), one lets go of the chair seat (held with right hand) and if secure, one glances over the right shoulder extending the arm out from shoulder level. Next, the leg is brought back to the midline (Fig. 7.10D) and then crossed over the right leg (Fig. 7.10E). Once secure, the left arm releases behind you and you look over the left shoulder (Fig. 7.10E). This entire sequence can be repeated several times on each side. Thus, the Rockette analogy.

A sampling of *āsanas* for seniors

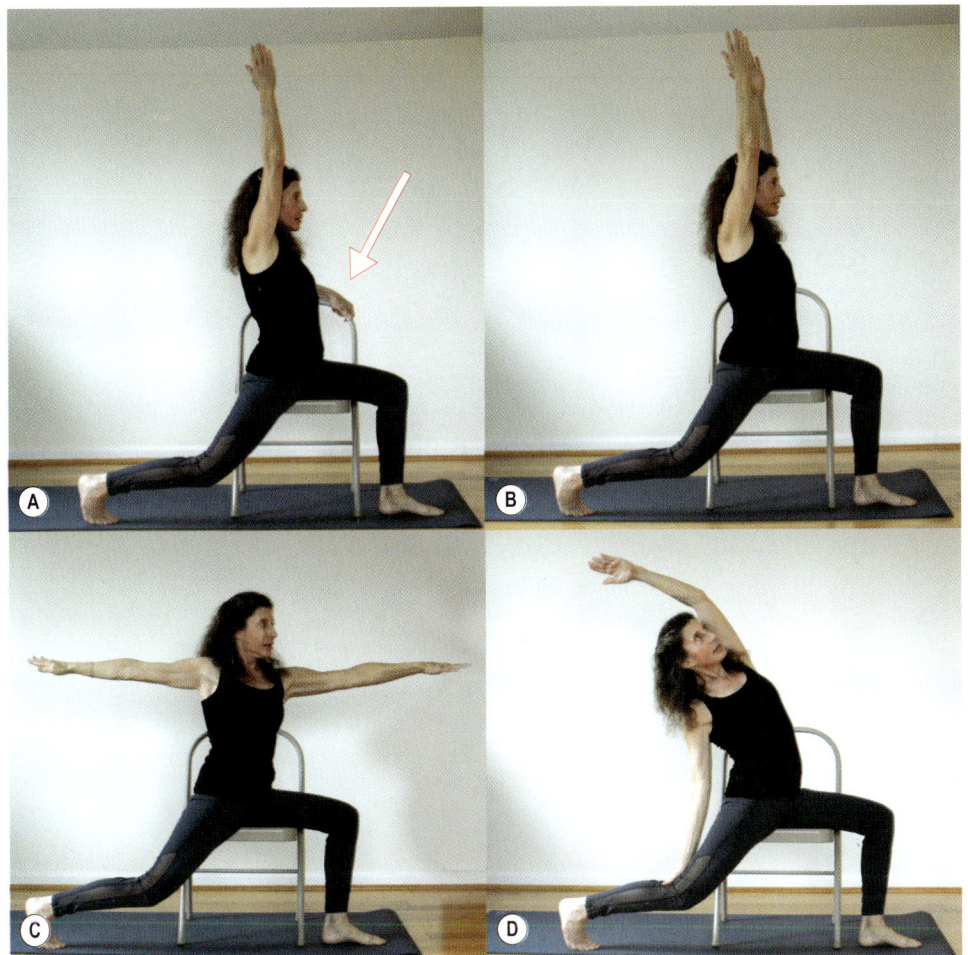

FIGURE 7.8 Author sitting on the chair in *vīrabhadrāsana* I and II and reverse *vīrabhadrāsana* II (Warrior 2)

Hip strengtheners are so important, especially as we age. Many of the people that I work with have had hip replacements, knee replacements, and shoulder replacements. Some are practically bionic. In Figure 7.12, hip work is demonstrated using the chair. Figure 7.12A shows what this looks like, but when practicing with the chair it is recommended that the chair be in front of you (Fig. 7.12B). Naturally if this is not an option, this can be done sitting on the chair (Fig. 7.12C). If one cannot get the ankle to the knee, then the ankle is crossed over the opposite ankle. And naturally if you want to get into the iliotibial (IT) band even further, you can work your hands down the sides of the chair and/or squat further.

Even advanced poses like Baby Dancer (*naṭarājāsana*, Fig. 7.13) can be achieved using the chair. Naturally, this can also be done sitting on a chair in varying modifications depending on the degree of ability. *Vṛkṣasāna* (tree pose) can also be done sitting on the chair (Fig. 7.14) (Voelker's method) or using the chair as a prop (Fig. 7.15). Note the variations in arm and feet positioning in Figure 7.14. It is important to understand how to modify a pose for those who might be less able. Figure 7.16 illustrates side angle pose using the chair (Fig. 7.16A) as well as binding with or without a belt (Fig. 7.16B, C). Figure 7.16D illustrates *uppa vista konāsana* done on a chair (wide legged pose). Figure 7.16E shows 'rock the baby.' This is sometimes employed after the *supta pādāṅguṣṭhāsana* series (see Fig. 7.10).

Chapter seven

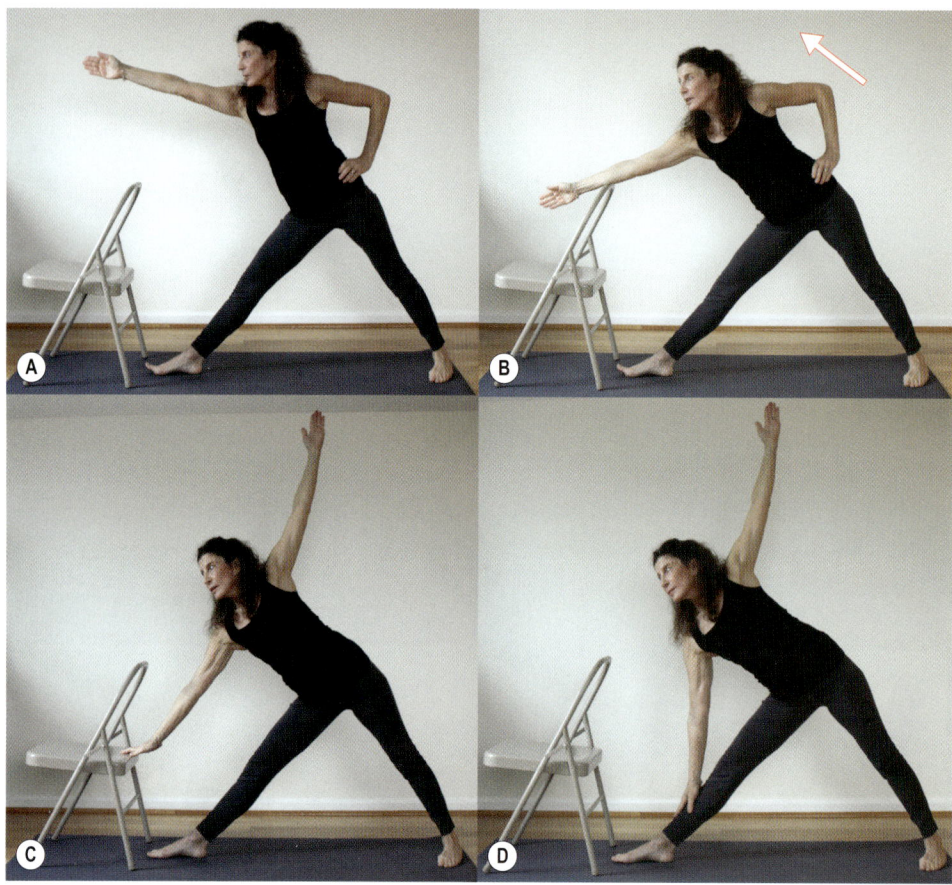

FIGURE 7.9 Author demonstrating *trikoṇāsana* using the chair as a prop

Figure 7.17 illustrates airplane pose sitting on the chair (Fig. 7.17A–C). After numerous standing poses, it helps to get back on the chair. This series of airplane pose and side stretches (Fig. 7.17 D, E) are done as we move onto the chair for the last 15 minutes of class. Depending on the class we can move into more calming poses or ramp it up by using weights.

I started employing this during my Silver Sneaker Yoga teaching but was relieved to discover that my chair yoga teacher, Lakshmi Voelker, also used weights in her trainings. Figure 7.18 illustrates using weights (partially standing, Fig. 7.18A, B) and/or sitting. Figure 7.18C indicates one arm forward the other back towards the shoulder. This may be practiced with both arms for several repetitions. Note in Figure 7.18D, it is recommended to only use one weight while keeping arms as close to the ears as possible before releasing the weight behind (Fig. 7.18E) for tricep extension. There are multiple upper body postures that one can offer, but Figures 7.18 and 7.19 illustrate some that my senior classes particularly like (and ask for). Again, I tend to repeat these movements no more than x8, in order not to exhaust the muscle. Some practice these movements without any weight at all. Figure 7.19 is borrowed from Silver Sneaker yoga but here a light weight is used as the arm circles in one direction (upward) and then the opposite (downward). Based on how strenuous this might be (the circular arm movement), I might suggest practicing these only x5 per side. The same is true for Figure 7.20 as these may be taxing without weights. I always err on the side of caution.

A sampling of āsanas for seniors

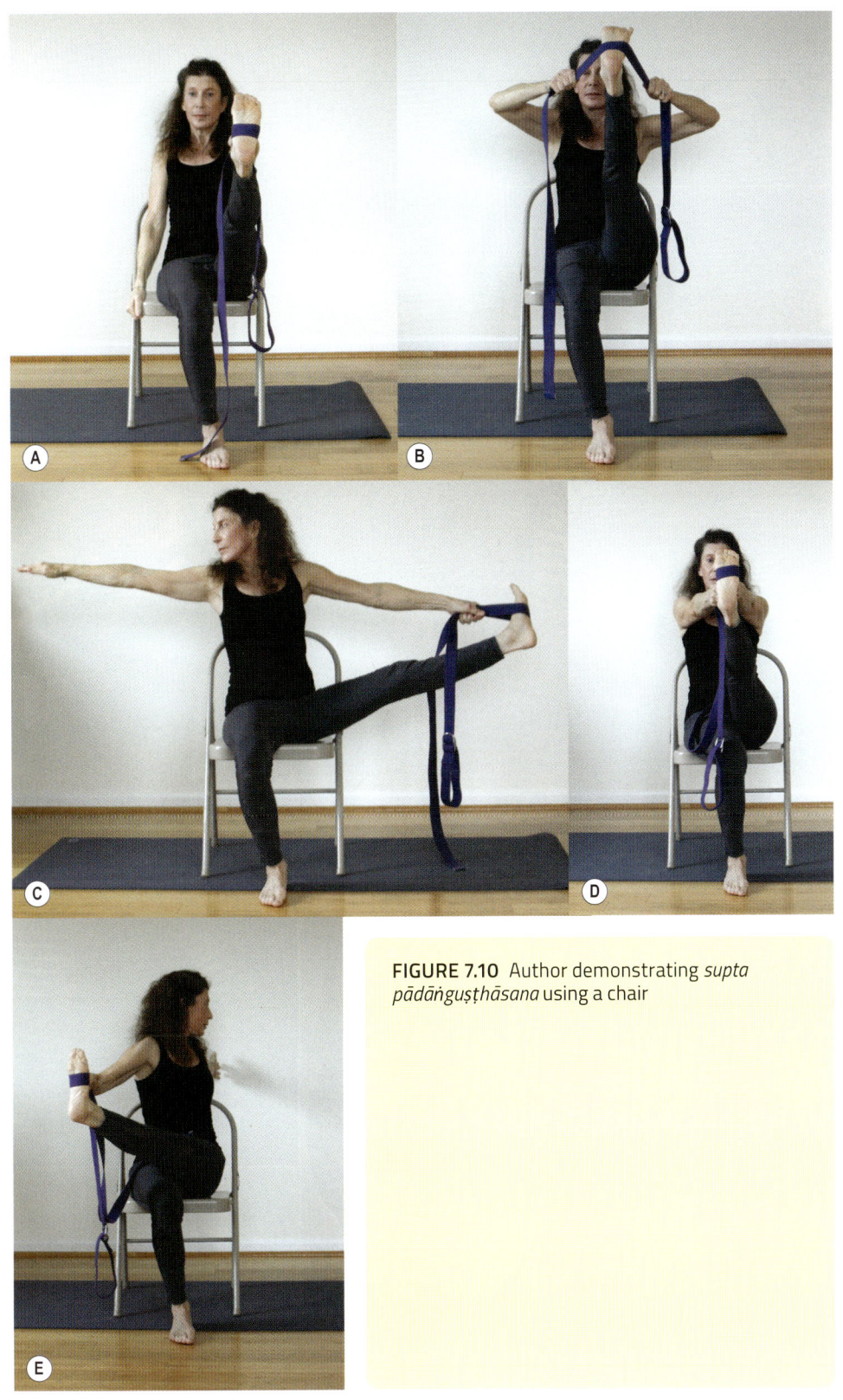

FIGURE 7.10 Author demonstrating *supta pādāṅguṣṭhāsana* using a chair

Chapter seven

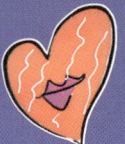
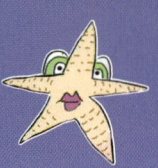

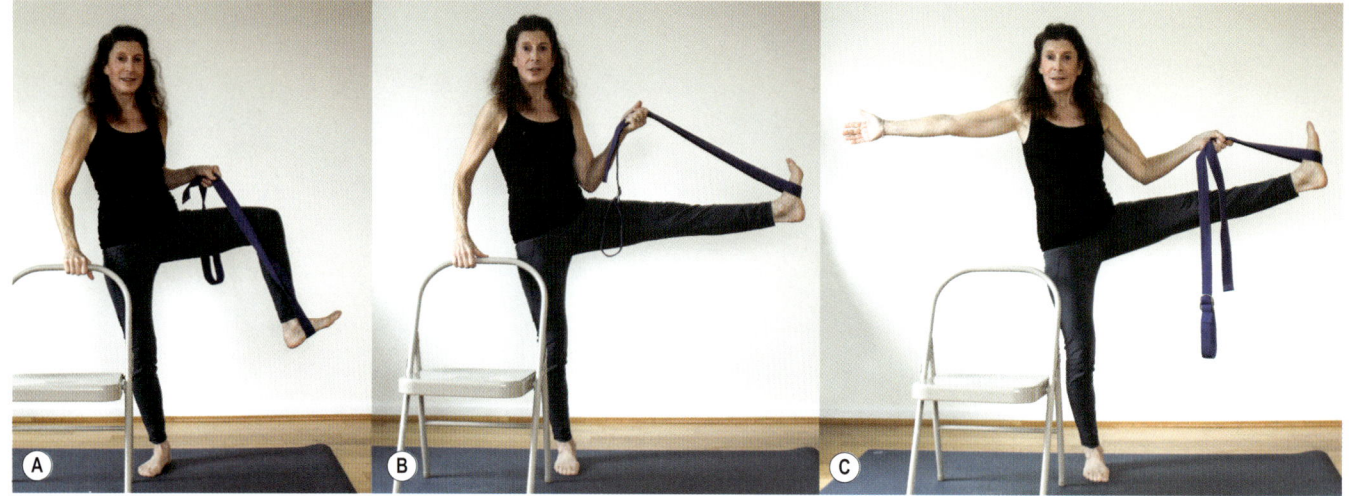

FIGURE 7.11 Author demonstrating *supta pādāṅguṣṭhāsana* standing at a chair

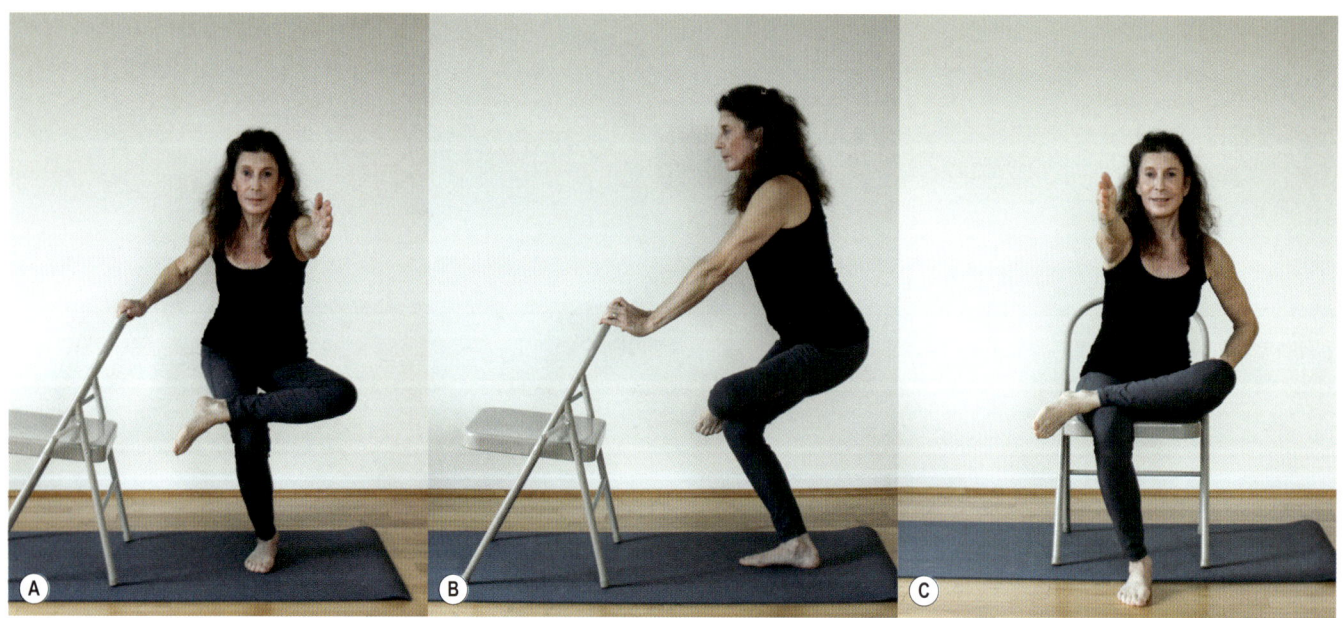

FIGURE 7.12 Author demonstrating iliotibial band modifications with the chair

A sampling of *āsanas* for seniors

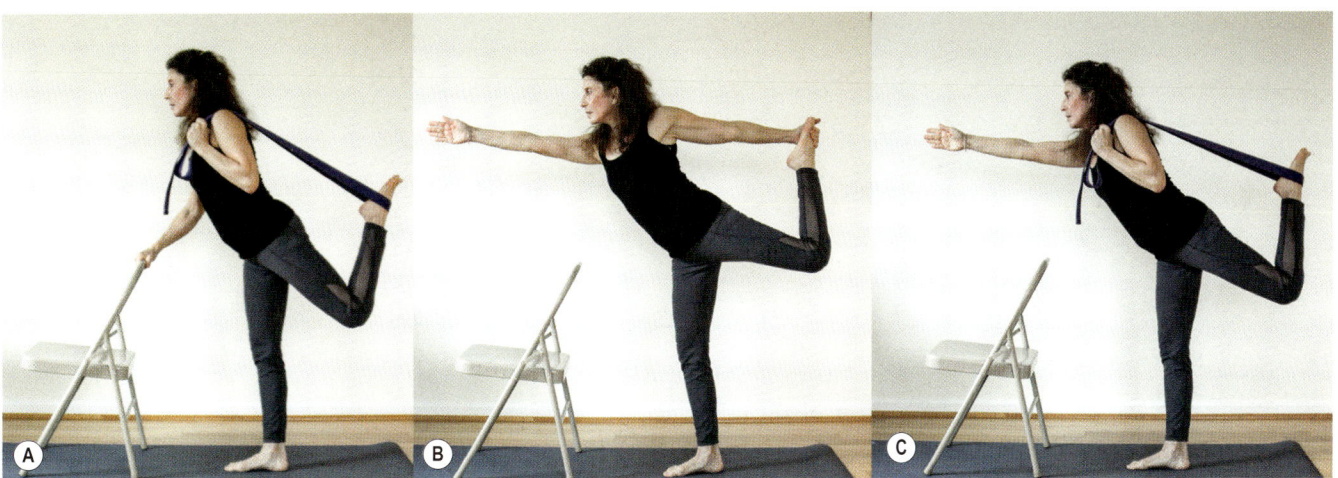

FIGURE 7.13 Author demonstrating baby dancer (*nāṭarājāsana*)

Finally, I might add a bit of core work to help strengthen the lower back muscles. A strong lower back is key to functioning, especially for many of my seniors. There are two ways to do this: (1) this core exercise is accomplished by placing a ball behind the mid-back, and pressing the back into the chair (note: to perform this exercise the chair must have a cushioned back, otherwise the ball will fall through); (2) as in Figure 7.21, I illustrate doing this same exercise by placing the ball between the knees and sitting upright. Holding onto the chair with the hands, lift either one leg or both (harder) in order to work the abdominal muscles (Fig. 7.21A, B). Last but not least, if the chair has a back as illustrated in Figure 7.21C and D, I suggest massaging the mid-back, sacral and scapular area with the ball. Next, whichever of those three points felt best, I suggest choosing that position and placing the ball into that area of the back to begin relaxation (on the chair) in *śavāsana* (corpse pose). Note that there might be many more poses that precede *śavāsana*, but the ones illustrated herein are just a sampling of what a yoga sequence might look like with seniors, no matter their age. Once again, modifications are always offered based on individual functioning and ability.

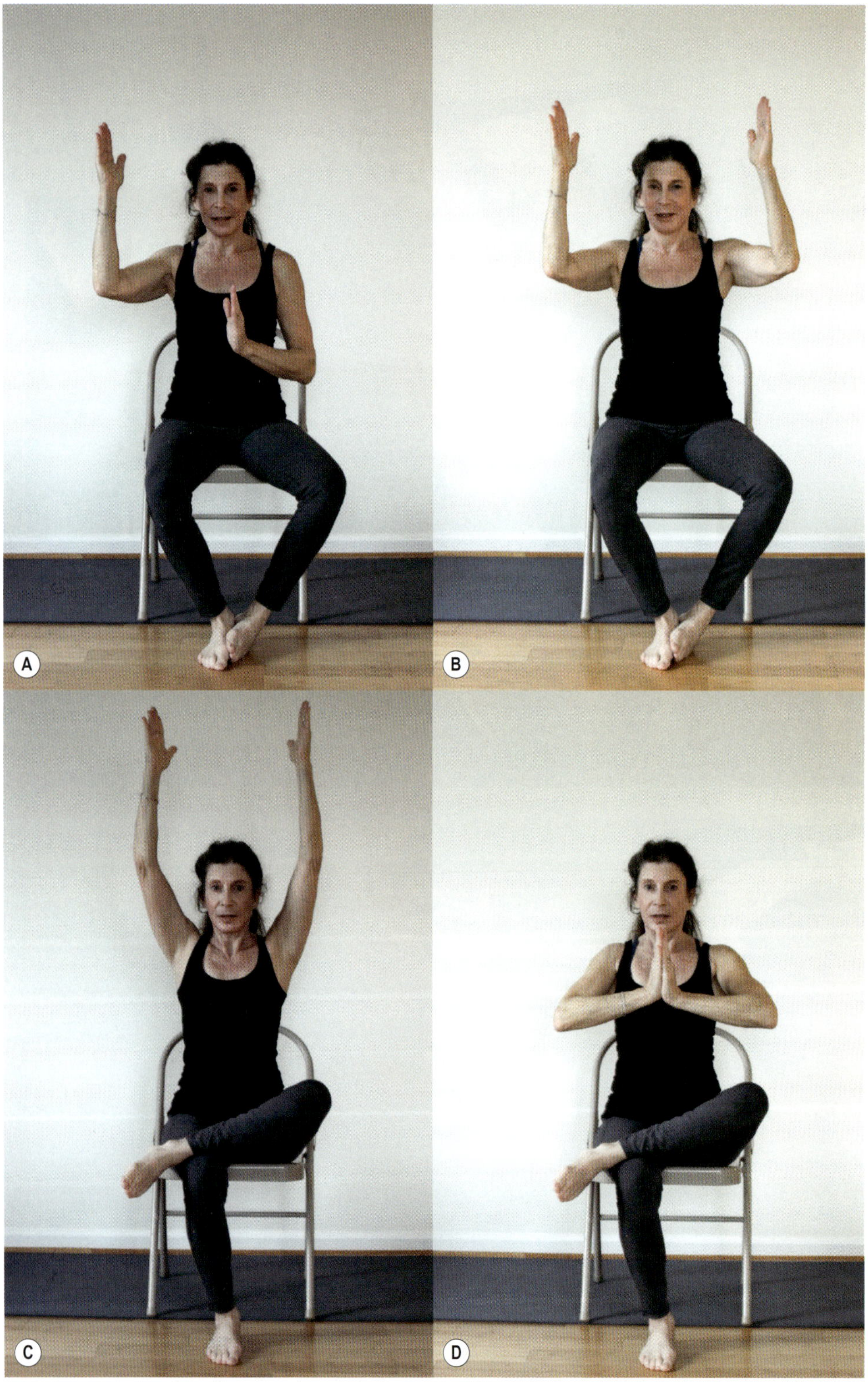

Chapter seven

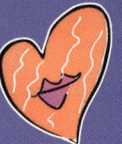
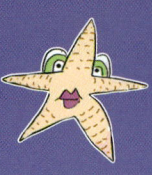

FIGURE 7.14 Author in *vṛkṣasāna* (tree pose) offering modifications for varying abilities

A sampling of āsanas for seniors

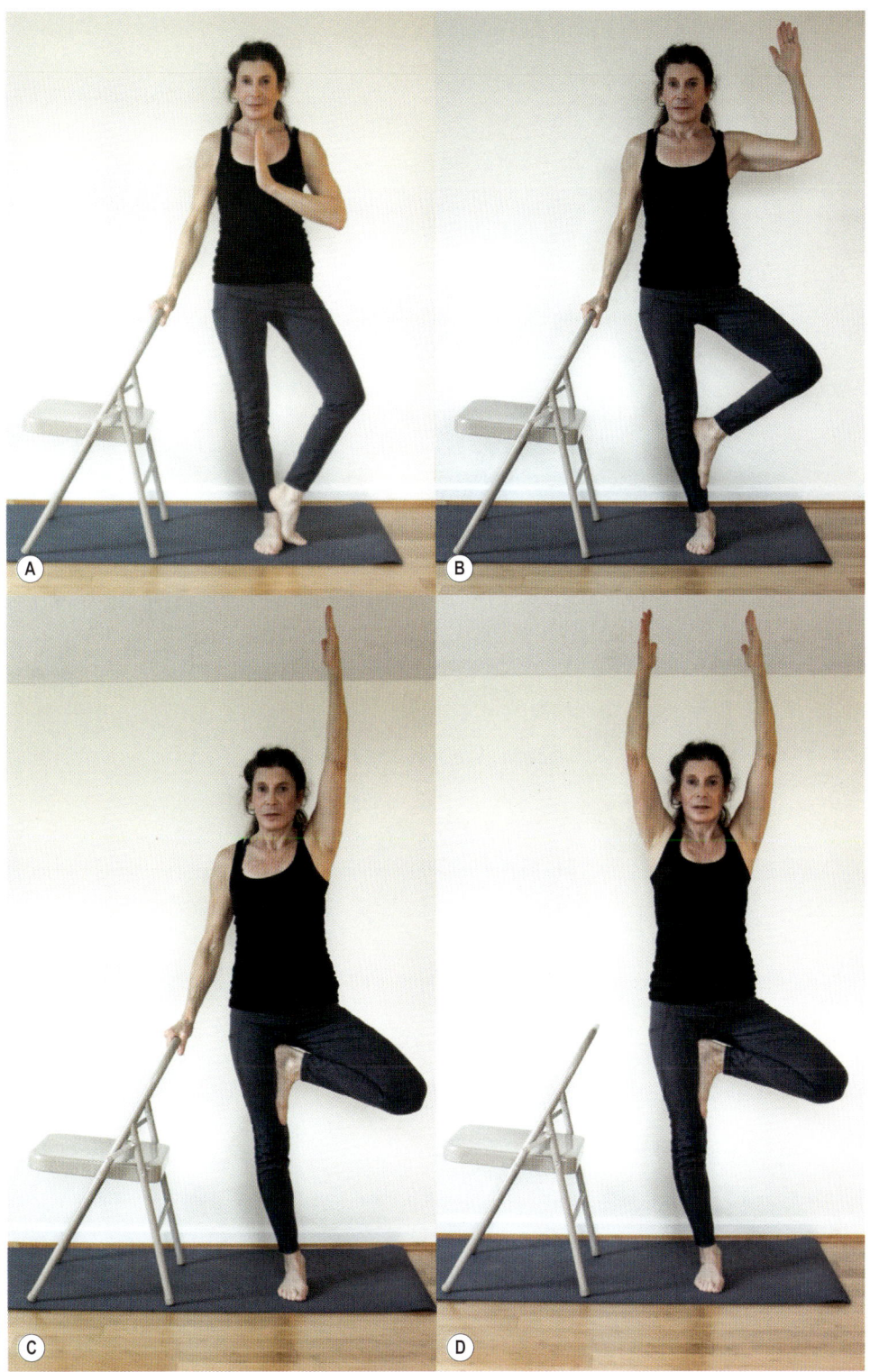

FIGURE 7.15 Author in *vṛkṣasāna* (tree pose) modified poses

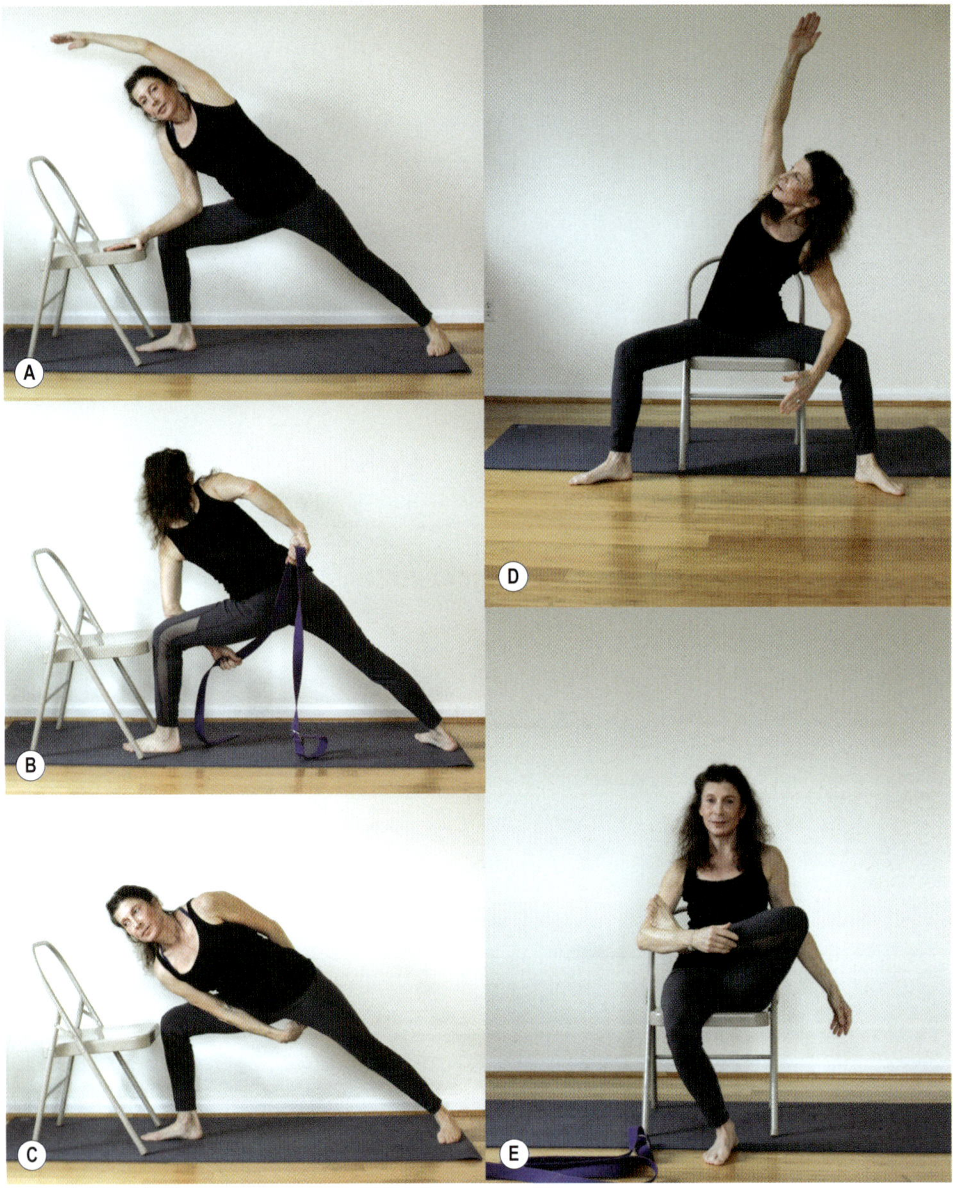

Chapter seven

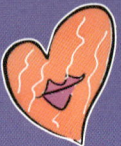
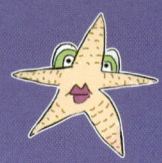

FIGURE 7.16 Author demonstrating side angle pose (*utthita parsvakonāsana*)

A sampling of āsanas for seniors

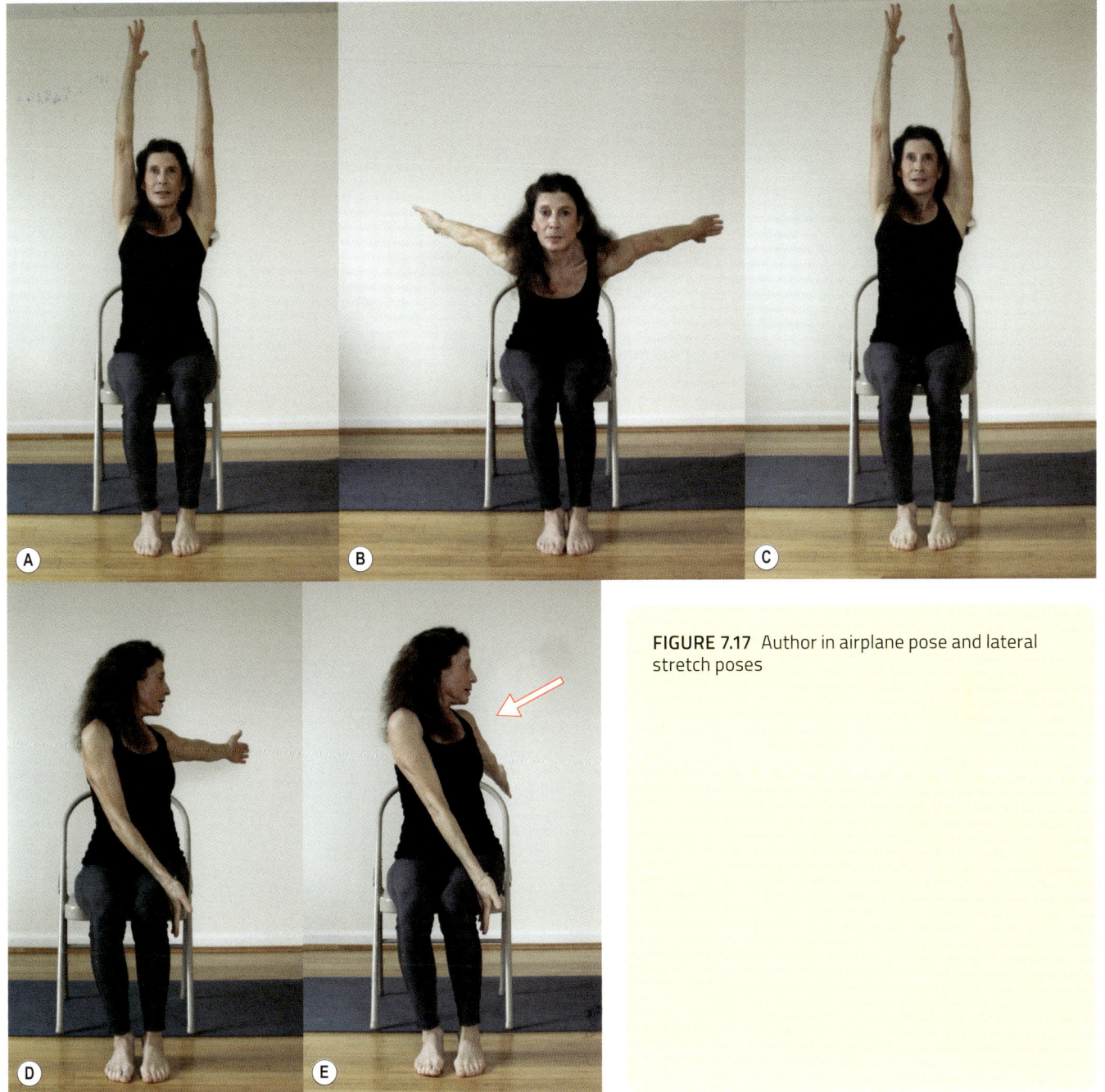

FIGURE 7.17 Author in airplane pose and lateral stretch poses

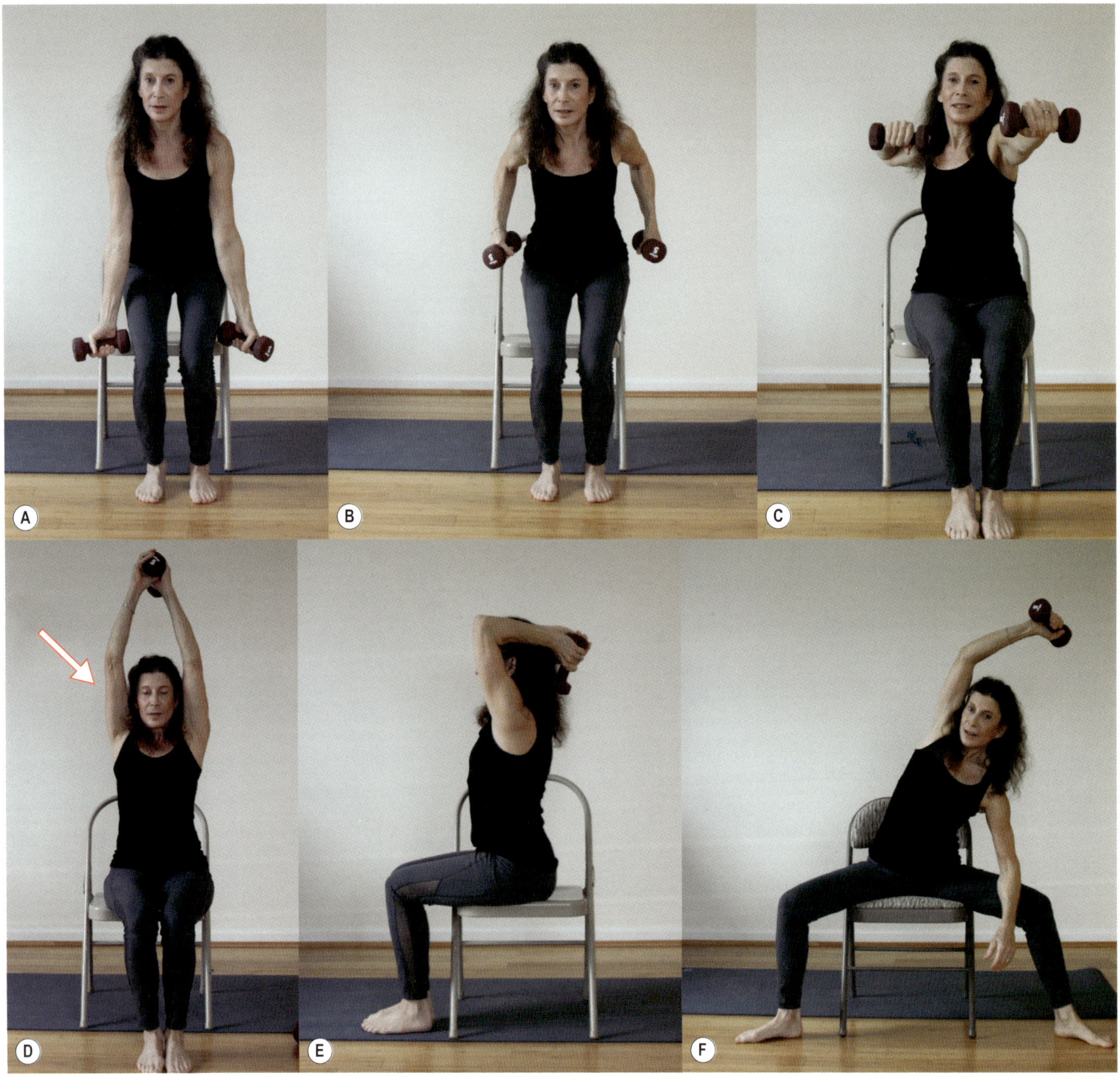

Chapter seven

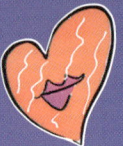
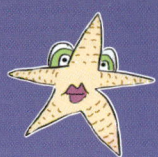

FIGURE 7.18 Author using weights, standing and on a chair

A sampling of *āsanas* for seniors

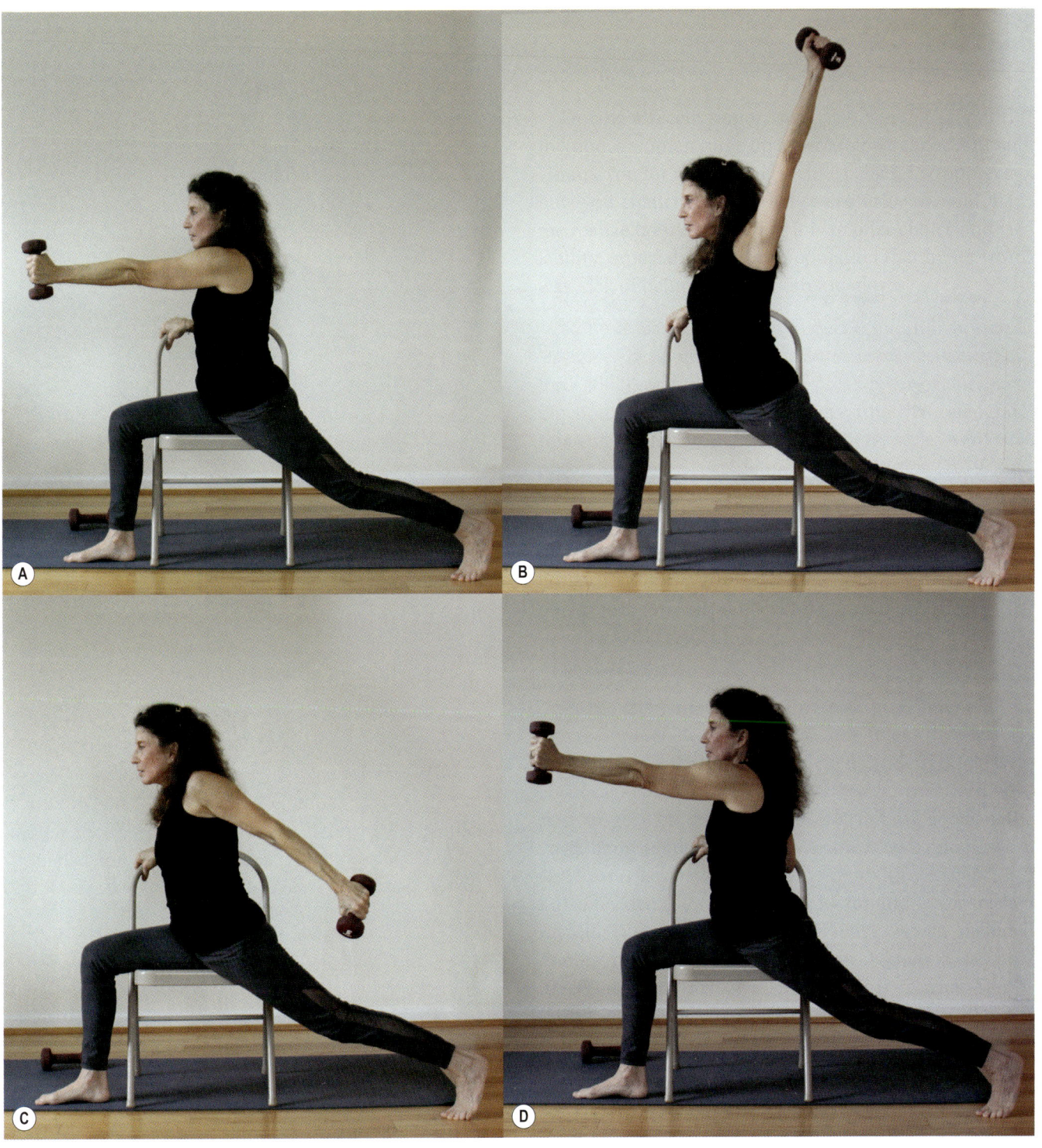

FIGURE 7.19 Author using weights in modified *vīrabhadrāsana II* (Warrior 2)

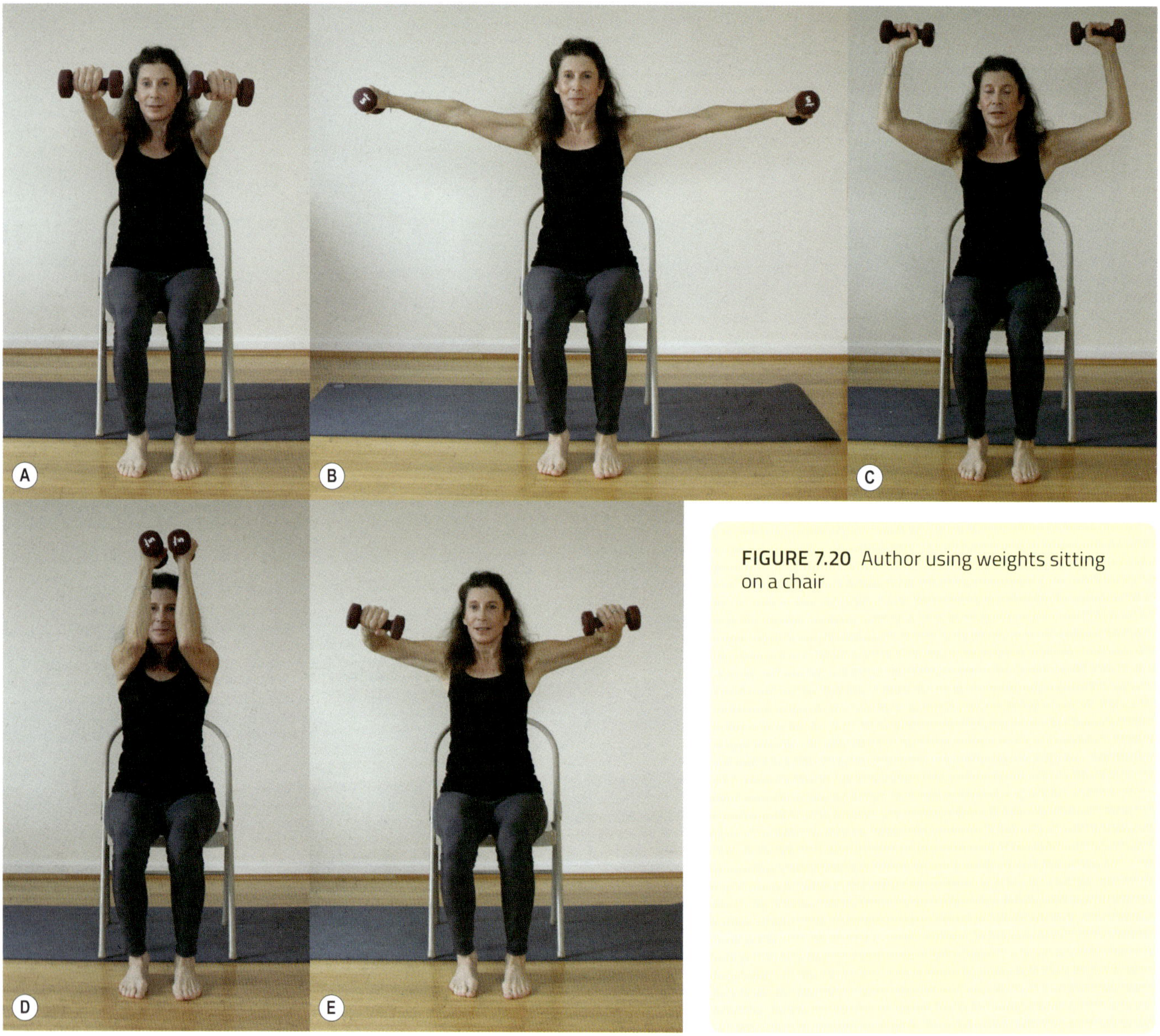

Chapter seven

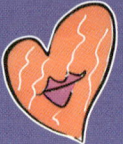
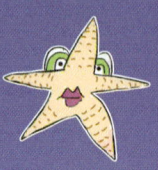

FIGURE 7.20 Author using weights sitting on a chair

Bonus poses

Sometimes, my seniors like using the large balls for stretching at the beginning of the class. If there is sufficient wall space, I teach them how to roll onto the ball and stretch their backs. For safety, I suggest keeping one arm on the wall (Fig. 7.22A, B) before trying to extend without wall support (Fig. 7.22C). This offers an idea of how to safely ease people down onto the ball. I have also used the ball as a prop in other ways during the class. As always, make sure that you are able to do anything that you are planning to teach.

While headstand is not something that I teach in a senior yoga class, this version of using chairs, blankets and a wall is a very safe method that places no undue pressure on the head (Figure 7.23). Since the head securely drops between the blankets on the chair, there is no weight on the neck or head. Some people prefer this version of headstand, and others need a lot of help getting into this

A sampling of *āsanas* for seniors

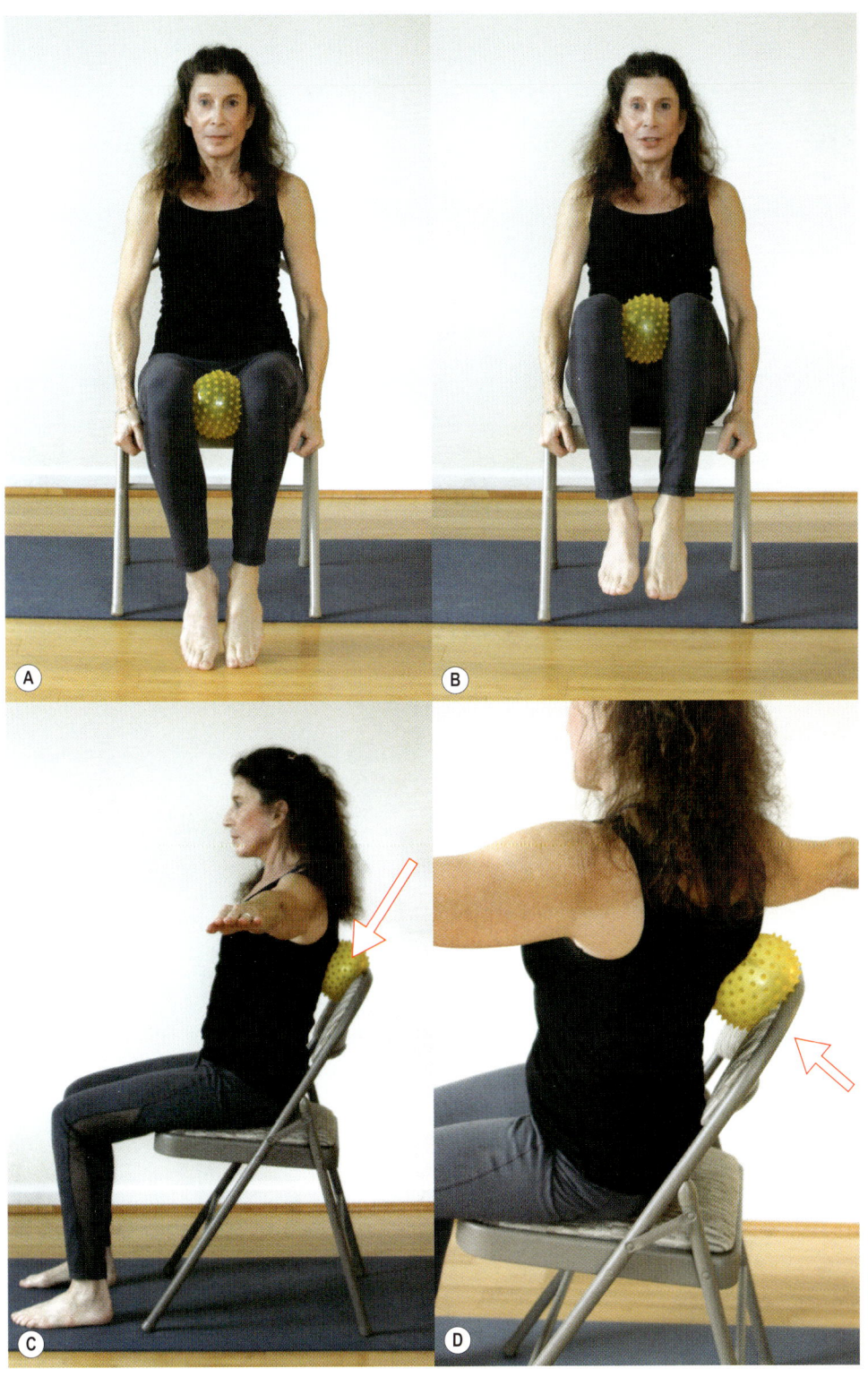

FIGURE 7.21 Author using small ball for core exercise, massage, and *śavāsana*

Chapter seven

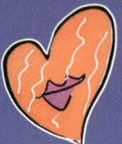
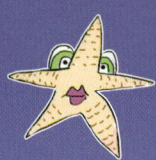

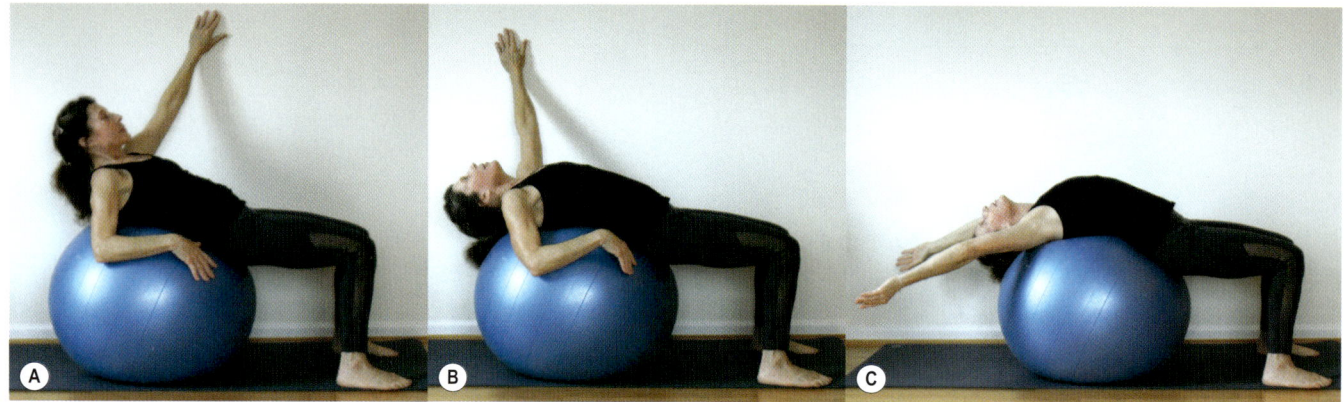

FIGURE 7.22 Author on the medicine ball

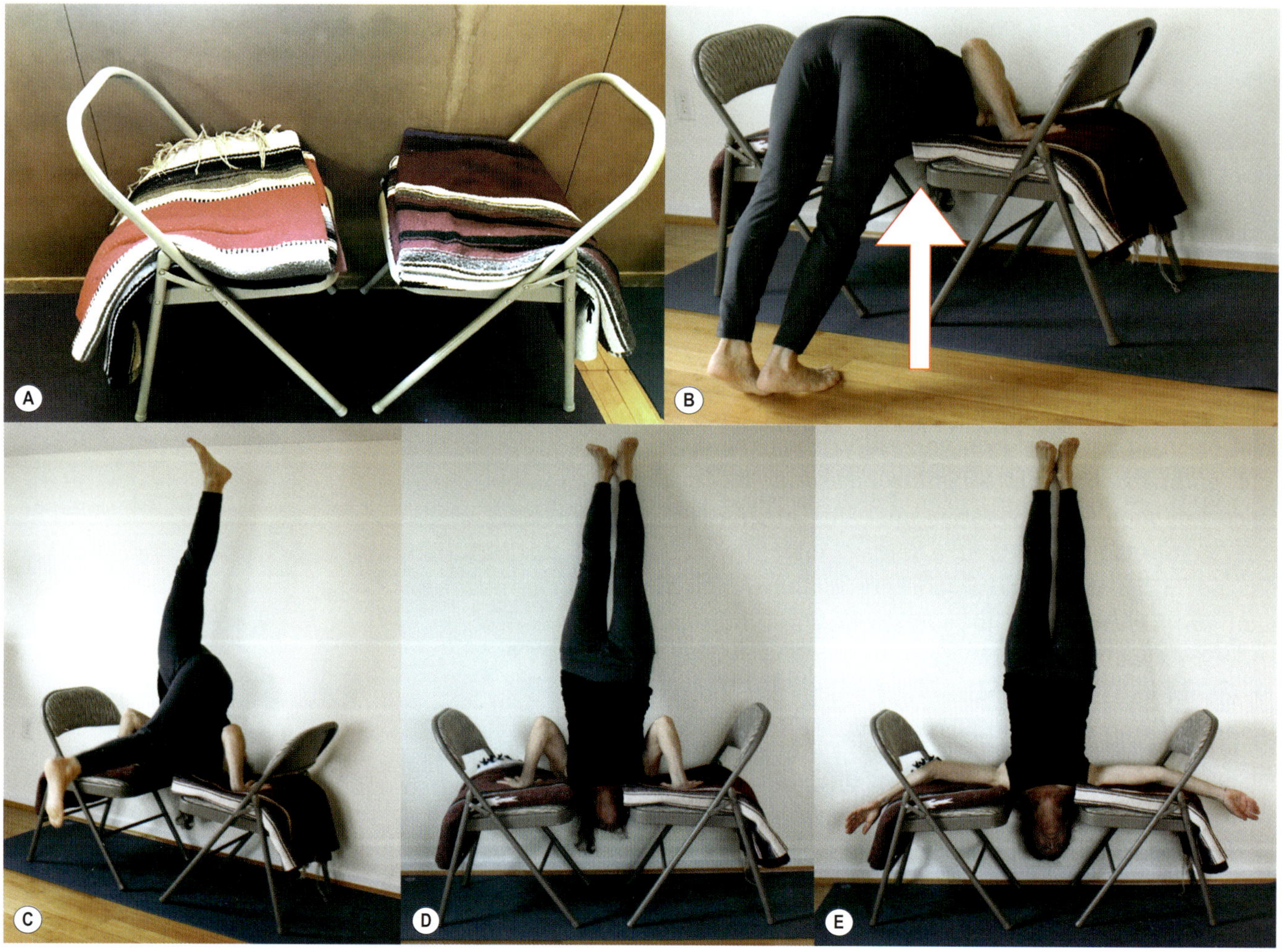

FIGURE 7.23 Author in headstand using chairs, blankets and the wall as props (method taught by Sri François Raoult)

A sampling of *āsanas* for seniors

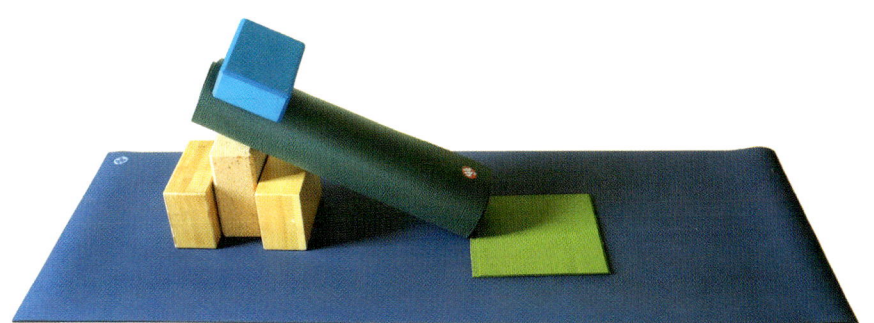

FIGURE 7.24 Set up for *śavāsana* for person with COPD (when no blankets were available)

position. Once learned, it can be very freeing and akin to hanging upside down in a yoga swing, my daily go-to adjustment. I learned this chair/headstand method from my teacher, Sri François Raoult. 'Keeper of the *asāna*,' I still hold out to him for all *asāna* corrections.

While some might balk at using weights with seniors and/or any of these poses offered in this chapter, my method helps build bone mass, stamina, confidence, balance and above all, *sanga*.

As a society, we do too much sitting. According to Colangelo (2003), 'Sitting in chairs limits range of motions, especially in the hips and knees, thus exposing them to malnourishment… wear and tear… pain… and even artificial replacement'. Some have even likened sitting as the 'new cancer': hence the standing desk was created. Colangelo went on to write that when Swami Venkatesananda was asked what the unhealthiest thing was that we exposed our bodies to on a daily basis, his retort was 'furniture' (Colangelo 2003: 202).

In a recent gentle yoga class that I taught, a woman had chronic obstructive pulmonary disease (COPD) and could not lie prone, so I used the set-up in Figure 7.24. Because the teaching facility lacked blankets, this was how I constructed her mat using blocks and an additional mat. I offer this because sometimes, you just have to be creative and use whatever you have at hand. This final image is a reminder to be creative and use whatever you have to safely offer your people what they need. I am confident in my ability to think on my feet, and most of all tune my internal dial towards the needs of others as a therapist and teacher. That is my aim as I move myself and others toward a trajectory of wellness.

In closing this book, I am reminded of Henry James (1917) who said, 'We work in the dark, we do what we can. Our doubt is our passion, and our passion is our task. The rest is the madness of art'. So, as we move out of darkness and help create light for others, we experience a secondary gain, we light our own ways. May your path be illuminated by your innermost light, and guide your internal compass towards that aim. For in that space, both healer and patient mutually benefit from the course. That is true union, this is art, this is yoga.

References

Amy M (2019) Personal communication.

Colangelo J (2003) Embodied Wisdom: What Our Anatomy Can Teach Us About the Art of Living. New York, NY: iUniverse, Inc.

Iyengar BKS (2005) Light on Life: The Yoga Journey to Wholeness, Inner Peace and Ultimate Freedom. Emmaus, PA: Rodale Press.

James H (1917) The Middle Years. New York, NY: Charles Scribner & Sons.

Lasater HJ (1995) Relax and Renew: Restful Yoga for Stressful Times. Berkeley CA: Publishing Group West.

Sanford M (2008) Waking: A Memoir of Trauma and Transcendence. Emmaus, PA: Rodale Press.

Sterios P (2019) Grace and Gravity: How to Awaken your Subtle Body and the Healing Power of Yoga. Boulder, CO: Sounds True.

Voelker L (2020) Lakshmi Voelker Chair Yoga. Available at: https://getfitwhereyousit.com/

APPENDIX A Professional practice considerations

A little ancient history

In Western society, art therapy has been acknowledged as a healing profession since around 1940 (Borowsky Junge 2010). But the history of yoga therapy precedes it via *The Bhagavad Gita* (Sargent 2016). *The Bhagavad Gita* was written somewhere between 400 and 200 BCE and was first translated in 1795 CE from the Sanskrit by Sir Charles Wilkins (there have been numerous translations since). *The Bhagavad Gita* (often referred to as *The Gita*) is truly the first fundamental tale about managing anxiety. *The Gita* is one of the most influential treatises in Eastern philosophy. The setting takes place in a battlefield and has been interpreted as an 'allegory for the ethical and moral struggles of the human life' (Violatti 2013). Thus, this would be angst at its finest, but resolved via this ancient therapeutic tale contained in 700 verses. This ancient Indian text is about the search for peace, quietude, and permanence in a world of rapid change, and how to integrate spiritual values into an ordinary life. And isn't that not much different from today's existence and search for meaning?

According to Mason and Birch (2018), 'Yoga is a comprehensive mind–body practice that is particularly effective for self regulation, mood management, fostering resilience, and promotion of wellbeing… [with the] … potential as a key component of integrative and complementary mental health… now being recognized internationally'.

Scope of practice regarding yoga therapy and art therapy

The use of any of the yoga therapy and art therapy exercises represented in this guide should be based on your patient's individual needs. These exercises should not be viewed as a 'be all and end all' prescription on how to treat a patient who presents with a specific range of problems. Specific diagnoses and cases are presented as examples for the reader to draw on when working with similar patient diagnoses.

Clinicians should be mindful that working with patients requires self-compassion, and an attitude of responding to their needs through present moment awareness, rather than based on prescriptive techniques. With this in mind, these exercises are presented as guidelines to use along with your own therapeutic intuition, based on your patient's needs.

For beginning practitioners, these exercises should aid you in building a database of knowledge to draw upon when developing patient treatment. It should be noted that each therapist approaches therapy with their own foundation of psychological/physiological interventions, whether it be psychiatric/medical intervention, psychotherapy, cognitive behavioral therapy (CBT), dialectic behavioral therapy (DBT), psychoanalytic or other methodologies. Your individual background can only augment your own intuitive style in working with your patients.

Finally, it should be noted that using the methods described herein does not allow you to call yourself either a yoga therapist or an art therapist. Both fields require extensive training and are protected by their educational requirements.

To learn more about the field of yoga therapy (worldwide), go to: https://www.iayt.org/page/AccredStds

To learn more about the art therapy field (within the US), go to: https://arttherapy.org/becoming-art-therapist/

Privacy issues

Confidentiality relating to therapy records and personal information is subject to both ethical and legal protection. It is important to ensure that respect for confidentiality of personal information acquired in the course of treatment is given the highest priority. (For my 'Authorization to release confidential information' form, see Appendix D). All patient cases have been disguised and I have obtained written releases to ensure that patient identity will be protected and that any material will remain confidential.

APPENDIX A

Art therapy: history, standards and regulations

According to the American Art Therapy Association (AATA, www.arttherapy.org), art therapy is, 'an integrative mental health and human services profession that enriches the lives of individuals, families, and communities through active art-making, creative process, applied psychological theory, and human experience within a psychotherapeutic relationship'.

Art therapy is facilitated by a professional art therapist and effectively supports personal and relational treatment goals as well as community concerns. Art therapy is used to improve cognitive and sensorimotor functions, foster self-esteem and self-awareness, cultivate emotional resilience, promote insight, enhance social skills, reduce and resolve conflicts and distress, and advance societal and ecological change. This approach uses the art creation as a form of psychotherapy for people experiencing trauma or illness, seeking personal development, or struggling to deal with the day-to-day act of living. Through the act of creating art and thinking about the process and medium, people are able to develop skills that increase cognitive ability, increase awareness of self and others, and help them cope with the distressing symptoms or limitations imposed by disability or disease.

Art has been used since the beginning of human history as a medium for communicating thoughts and ideas. The oldest cave painting was found in the El Castillo cave in Cantabria, Spain and dates back 40,000 years to the Aurignacian period. Though researchers are uncertain as to the exact purpose of cave drawings, it has been theorized that they were likely used as part of religious ceremonies or to reach out to others in the area (New York Times 2014).

Moving forward through history, art became an instrument for self-expression and symbolism. However, it wasn't until the 1940s that the therapeutic use of art was defined and developed into a distinct discipline. The discipline arose independently in the USA and Europe.

In England, the first person to refer to the therapeutic applications of art as art therapy was Adrian Hill. While being treated in a sanatorium for tuberculosis, this artist suggested participating in art projects to his fellow patients (London Art Therapy Centre 2018). This was just the beginning for Hill and he discusses much of his work as an art therapist in his book *Art Versus Illness* (Hill 1945).

Edward Adamson expanded on Hill's work and worked with him to introduce this new therapy to long-term UK patients in mental hospitals, starting with the Netherne Hospital in Surrey, UK. Adamson continued establishing programs in facilities until he retired from the industry in 1981. Adamson also created an open studio where patients could freely create art without comment or judgment from others. He was a proponent of 'non-interventionist' art therapy where patients simply created art for self-expression rather than for psychological interpretation by a clinician. This work was documented in his book *Art as Healing* (Adamson 1981).

Adamson collected over 100,000 pieces of art made by patients and displayed them. His intent was to foster a greater understanding of the creativity and contributions of the mentally ill by sharing the fruits of their labor with the public at large. Out of the mass of artwork he collected over the decades, only 6,000 pieces remain, and many are on display at the Wellcome Library Collection in London, UK.

The two pioneers of art therapy in the United States (although helmed from Europe) were Dr Margaret Naumburg and Edith Kramer. In the mid-1940s, psychologist Margaret Naumburg began referring to her work as art psychotherapy. Unlike Hill, Naumburg believed that art led to unconscious association. The artwork was considered 'symbolic speech' that the therapist encouraged the patient to expand on, interpret and then analyze.

My mentor, Edith Kramer, was of Austrian descent and studied under Anna Freud. She also studied art, painting, drawing and sculpture in Vienna, and was an exceptional artist. After becoming a US citizen in 1944,

Professional practice considerations

she founded the art therapy graduate program at New York University and served as the Adjunct Professor of the program from 1973 to 2005. During that time she was also the Assistant Professor of the art therapy graduate program at George Washington University in Washington DC.

By the middle of the 20th century many hospitals and mental health facilities began including art therapy programs after observing how this form of therapy could promote emotional, developmental and cognitive growth in children. The discipline continued to grow from there, becoming an important tool for assessment, communication and treatment of children and adults alike.

In 1992, when I was Education Chair of the American Art Therapy Association, I rewrote the educational standards with Drs Holly Feen-Calligan and Mary St. Clair. Since then, the minimum entrance requirement to the field is a Master's Degree in Art Therapy. Currently, the Art Therapy Credentials Board (ATCB.org) is a standalone organization that both registers and board certifies (ATR = Art Therapist Registered, BC = Board Certified) art therapists in the USA.

Yoga therapy: history, standards and regulations

The International Association of Yoga Therapists (IAYT), of which I am a member and certified yoga therapist (C-IAYT), wrote a position paper which was published on 1 July 2012 entitled *Educational Standards for the Training of Yoga Therapists: Definition of Yoga Therapy*. In this position paper, the IAYT acknowledged that yoga, a 5,000-year-old practice, is a scientific system of self-investigation, self-transformation and self-realization. It acknowledged that the teachings were rooted in the Vedas and grounded in classical texts and oral traditions. The position paper went on to say:

The yoga tradition views humans as a multidimensional system that includes all aspects of body, breath, mind, intellect, and emotions and their mutual interaction. Yoga is founded on the basic principle that intelligent practice can positively influence the direction of change within these human dimensions, which are distinct from an individual's unchanging nature or spirit.

(IAYT 2012)

Yoga therapy was differentiated as the appropriate application of these teachings in a 'therapeutic context'. The goals of yoga therapy include to:

- Eliminate, reduce or manage symptoms that cause suffering.
- Improve functioning.
- Prevent reoccurrence of the underlying causes of the illness.
- Move toward improved health and well-being.

More importantly, the paper went on to delineate yoga therapy from yoga teaching. Requirements of yoga therapy require 'specialized training', which as a trained yoga therapist is quite rigorous, and differs strongly from the training to become a registered yoga teacher.

The IAYT Board approved the *Educational Standards for the Training of Yoga Therapists* in 2012. Updates were made in 2016 and again in 2017 after receiving input from many member schools (IAYT 2017). The net result was consensus on competency-based educational standards that focus on entry-level requirements for the training of yoga therapists and include a definition of yoga therapy, and admission and training requirements. The goal was to define the foundational knowledge and skills required for the safe and effective practice of yoga therapy.

Minimum requirements to become a yoga therapist include:

- 200 hours of teacher training, such as a Yoga Alliance 200-hour registered school program (RYS 200), or its equivalent.

APPENDIX A

- In addition to minimum yoga teacher training, students must have completed the following, which can be accomplished concurrently: 1 year of teaching experience, with specifics to be determined by the school; and 1 year of personal practice, with specifics to be determined by the school.

An entry-level yoga therapy training program must be at least 800 hours total and taught over a minimum of 2 years. Schools may choose to allow more time for completion of the 800 hours. The 800 hours does not include the admission requirements.

Competency requirements to become a yoga therapist include:

- A minimum of 120 hours of yoga foundations.
- A minimum of 155 hours of biomedical and psychological foundations.
- A minimum of 140 hours of yoga therapy tools and therapeutic skills.
- A minimum of 205 hours of practicum providing yoga therapy.
- A minimum of 30 hours of professional practice.

The Yoga Alliance legal advisors determined that many states were seeking to tax and regulate yoga and yoga studios (including certification programs, schools and studios) in order to protect the public who receive treatment from yoga therapists. Yoga Alliance therefore brought in Attorney Kristi Kung to head their legal team. Her clearly written legal statement on behalf of Yoga Alliance asserts that yoga's therapeutic benefits have become increasingly accepted by the public as well as health professionals, while no clear definition or scope of practice exists (Yoga International 2020).

Consistent with the procedures in the Code of Conduct, the Yoga Alliance Registry will revoke a registrant's right to use the RYS and RYT Registry Marks for violating this policy.

A yoga teacher or yoga therapist's lack of training or understanding in physiology, anatomy, pathology or mental health could possibly cause more harm than good to clients/patients. Many noted yoga therapists have stepped forward to express the opinion that the division is a positive step toward ensuring that (hatha) yoga teaching and yoga therapy have clear and concise boundaries, and that those offering these services are well trained and credentialed.

For more information and opinions on the decision, there is much information at yogaalliance.org and IAYT.org. In the meantime, if you are interested, you may want to look at the publications, websites, and resumés of individuals to determine whether they comply with these newly established guidelines.

To call oneself a yoga therapist (C-IAYT), yoga teacher (RYT-200, E-RYT, RYT 500, E-RYT 500) or Yoga Alliance Continuing Education Provider (YACEP) requires extensive training just like any other discipline and/or professional field.

In summary, I hope this provides the reader with a rudimentary idea of the scope of practice, educational requirements, history, regulations, certifications and/or licensing behind the therapeutic fields covered in this book.

References

Adamson E (1981). Art as Healing. Newburyport, MA: Red Wheel/Weiser.

Borowsky Junge M (2010) The Modern History of Art Therapy in the United States. Springfield, IL: Charles C Thomas.

Hill A (1945) Art Versus Illness: The Story of Art Therapy. Crows Nest, Australia: Allen & Unwin.

IAYT (2017) Educational Standards for the Training of Yoga Therapists. Available at: https://cdn.ymaws.com/www.iayt.org/resource/resmgr/accreditationmaterials/2017_11_Updates-Ed_Stds/2017_IAYT_Educational_Standa.pdf

London Art Therapy Centre (2018) Adrian Hill, Tuberculosis and

Professional practice considerations

Art Therapy. Available at: https://arttherapycentre.com/blog/adrian-hill-uk-founder-art-therapy-morgan-bush-intern/

Mason H and Birch K (2018) Yoga for Mental Health. Edinburgh, UK: Handspring Publishing Ltd.

New York Times (2014) Cave Paintings in Indonesia May Be Among the Oldest Known. Available at: https://www.nytimes.com/2014/10/09/science/ancient-indonesian-find-may-rival-oldest-known-cave-art.html

Sargent W (2016) The Bhagavad Gita. New Delhi, India: Aleph.

World History Encyclopedia (2020) Bhagavad Gita Definition. Available at: https://www.ancient.eu/Bhagavad_Gita/

Yoga International (2020) Understanding Yoga Alliance's Policy on Yoga Therapy. Available at: https://yogainternational.com/article/view/understanding-yoga-alliances-ruling-on-yoga-therapy

APPENDIX B Health history form

Creative Arts Therapy Practice

Your answers on this form will help your yoga practitioner to better understand your medical concerns and conditions before starting yoga. This form is to ascertain any medical information that might be pertinent to your treatment and will be placed into your file. If you are uncomfortable with any question, you need not answer it. If you cannot recall specific details, please provide your best guess. Thank you!

Name				
Address				
Age				
Date of birth				
Phone				
Email				
How would you rate your health?	Excellent	Good	Fair	Poor
Main reason for participation in yoga or therapy				
Have you ever practiced yoga and if so, for how long?				
Other concerns				

APPENDIX B

Review of symptoms, please check all that apply:

Constitutional: Recent sweats/fever	Eyes/ENT: Changes in vision
Unexplained weight loss	Difficulty hearing
Unexplained fatigue/weakness	Ringing in ears
Cardiovascular: Chest pains/discomfort	Nasal/sinus congestion
Palpitations	Difficulty swallowing
Shortness of breath	Musculoskeletal: Muscle/joint pain
Breast issues: Lump/nipple discharge	Recent back pain
Respiratory: Cough/wheeze/coughing blood	Skin: New or changed mole/rash
Heartburn/reflux	Headaches
Blood in stool (bowel movement)	Memory loss
Nausea/vomiting/diarrhea	Fainting
Abdominal pain	Anxiety/stress
Painful or bloody urine	Sleep problem
Leaking urine	Lymphatic: Unexplained lumps
Night-time urine frequency change	Easy bruising/bleeding
Discharge: Penis/vaginal bleeding or other concerns	Cold/heat intolerance
	Increased thirst or appetite

In the past month, have you had little interest or pleasure in doing things or felt down, depressed or hopeless?

    Yes   No   Sometimes

Medications, dosages, times of day

Allergies or adverse reactions to medicines

Health history form

Personal medical history

Heart disease (specify type)

Asthma/lung disease

Diabetes

Other (specify)

High cholesterol

Thyroid problems

Cancer (specify type)

Surgical history

Please list dates and prior operations

Date/Type

Date/Type

Date/Type

Date/Type

Date/Type

Family history

Please indicate the current status of your immediate family members and their relationship to you (parent, sibling, grandparent, aunt or uncle) with any of the following conditions

Alcoholism

Cancer (specify type)

Heart disease

Depression/suicide

Genetic disorders

APPENDIX B

Family history continued

Diabetes

High cholesterol

High blood pressure

Stroke

Bleeding or clotting disorder

Asthma

Other concerns

Social history

Cigarette smoking

Never   Quit (date?)   Current smoker   Packs per day/years

Other tobacco   Interested in quitting?

Pipe   Cigar   Snuff   Chew   Yes   No

Do you drink alcohol?   Is your alcohol use a concern to you or others?

No   Yes   Number of drinks/week   No   Yes

Recreational drug use?   Have you ever injected drugs?

No   Yes   No   Yes

Are you sexually active?   No   Yes

                                                              Personal identification

If yes, sexual partner's identification

Male   Female   Bisexual   Gay   Male   Female   Bisexual   Gay

Queer   Non-binary   Trans   Queer   Non-binary   Trans

Health history form

Social history

Type of birth control if used

Are you satisfied with your weight?

No   Yes

Caffeine intake

None   Coffee   Tea   Soda cups/day?

Do you eat or drink four servings of dairy or soya supplements per day, or take calcium supplements?

No   Yes

How do you rate your diet?

Excellent   Good   Fair   Poor

Do you exercise daily?

No   Yes

What kind of exercise?

How long (minutes)?

How often do you exercise and why?

If you bike, do you wear a helmet?

No   Yes

Do you use seat-belts consistently?

No   Yes

Is violence at home a concern for you?

No   Yes

Have you ever been abused?

No   Yes

Do you have a gun in your home?

No   Yes

Have you completed a 'living will' or Durable Power of Attorney for Health care?

No   Yes

APPENDIX B

Socioeconomic history

Occupation

Employer

Highest educational degree

Marital status   Single   Partner   Married   Divorced

                   Separated   Widowed   Living together

Spouse/partner's name

Do you have children?   Yes   No   How many?

Who lives at home with you?

Women's health history

Number of pregnancies   Number of deliveries   Number of abortions

Number of miscarriages   Age at onset of menstruation   Age at menopause (if applicable)

I am aware that Dr EG Horovitz is here to serve me by sharing knowledge of yoga and health. I understand that the practice of yoga involves physical movement and exercise which may from time to time be strenuous, and that such practice carries some risk of injury. I also understand that I must judge my own capabilities with respect to practicing yoga with Dr Horovitz. By participating in classes, I agree to take full responsibility for not exceeding my limits in the practice of yoga and for any injury I may incur in the practice of yoga. I acknowledge that it is my responsibility to inform Dr Horovitz *immediately* if an injury occurs during class. I understand that, from time to time, she may physically adjust my form during a yoga posture. If I do not want such physical adjustments, I will so inform her. I also acknowledge that if I do not wish to receive physical adjustments, it is my responsibility to inform Dr Horovitz when an adjustment has gone as far as I desire at that time. I hereby waive and release any claim that I might have at any time for injury of any sort against Dr Horovitz.

I have carefully read, fully understand, and agree to all the above.

Signature   **Date**

APPENDIX C Stages of development

Eras/ages	Erikson et al (1959)	Piaget (1971, 1973)	Kohlberg (1981)	Lowenfeld and Brittain (1975)	Fowler (1995)	Gantt and Tabone (1998)	Horovitz
Infancy (0–1.5 yrs)	Basic trust vs basic mistrust (hope)	Sensorimotor stage		Scribble stage: beginning of self-expression (0–2 yrs)	Stage 0: primal or undifferentiated (0–2 yrs)	Rating 0: cannot be rated	
Early childhood (2–6 yrs)	Autonomy vs shame and doubt Initiative vs guilt (purpose)	Preoperational or Intuitive	Preconventional level 1. Heteronomous morality	Preschematic stage: First representations (4–7 yrs)	Stage 1: intuitive–projective (3–7 yrs)	Rating 1: scribbles/masses Rating 2: geometric shapes (4–6 yrs)	
Childhood (7–12 yrs)	Industry vs inferiority	Concrete operational	2. Instrumental exchange, conventional level 3. Mutual interpersonal relationships	Schematic stage formed concepts (7–9 yrs) Gang age: dawning realism (9–12 yrs)	Stage 2: mythic-literal (mostly in school children)	Rating 3: latency, age/logical and proportionate	
Adolescence (13–21 yrs)	Identity vs role confusion (fidelity)	Formal operational	4. Social system and conscience	Pseudonaturalistic stage: age of reasoning (12–14 yrs) Adolescent art: period of decision (14–17 yrs)	Stage 3: synthetic-conventional (12–adulthood)	Rating 4: adolescence/realism	Adult stage: formation in the world (8–adulthood)
Young adulthood (21–35 yrs)	Intimacy vs isolation (love)		Postconventional principled level 5. Social contract, individual rights		Stage 4: individuative–reflective (mid 20s – late 30s)	Rating 5: adult/some artistic sophistication	Artistic stage: formed art any age (generally in adolescence through adulthood)
Adulthood (35–60 yrs)	Generativity vs stagnation (care)				Stage 5: conjunctive (mid-life crisis)		
Maturity (60+ yrs)	Integrity vs despair (wisdom)		Universal ethical principles		Stage 6: universalizing (enlightenment)		

APPENDIX C

References

Erikson E, Paul IH, Heider F, Gardner RW and Klein GS (1959) Identity and the Life Cycle. New York, NY: International Universities Press.

Fowler J (1995) Stages of Faith: The Psychology of Human Development and the Quest for Meaning. New York, NY: Harper.

Gantt L and Tabone C (1998) The Formal Elements of Art Therapy: The Rating Manual. Morgantown, WV: Gargoyle Press.

Kohlberg L (1981) Essays on Moral Development, Vol. I: The Philosophy of Moral Development. San Francisco, CA: Harper & Row.

Lowenfeld V and Brittain WL (1975) Creative and Mental Growth, 6th Edn. New York, NY: MacMillan.

Piaget J (1971) Biology and Knowledge. Edinburgh, UK: Edinburgh University Press.

Piaget J and Inhelder B (1973) Memory and Intelligence. London: Routledge and Kegan Paul.

APPENDIX D Practice information

Dear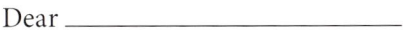

Welcome to my practice. I appreciate your giving me the opportunity to be of help to you.

Sometimes, I take notes during our meetings. You may find it useful to journal outside of our meetings.

By the end of our first or second session, I will tell you how I see your case at this point and how I think we should proceed. I view therapy as a *partnership* between us. You define the problem areas to be worked on, I use some special knowledge to help you make the changes you want to make.

Art therapy/yoga therapy and psychotherapy is not like visiting a medical doctor. It requires your very active involvement. It requires your best efforts to change thoughts, feelings, and behaviors. For example, I want you to tell me about important experiences, what they mean to you, and what strong feelings are involved. This is one of the ways you are an active partner in therapy. An important part of your therapy will be practicing new skills that you will learn in our sessions.

I may ask you to practice outside our meetings, and we will work together to set up homework assignments for you. I might ask you to do exercises, keep records, and read to deepen your learning. You may have to work on relationships in your life and make long-term efforts to get the best results. These are important parts of personal change. Change will sometimes be easy and quick, but more often it can be slow and frustrating. There is no instant, painless cure and no 'magic pill.' However, you can learn new ways of looking at your problems that will be very helpful for changing your feelings and reactions.

About confidentiality

I will treat with great care all the information you share with me. It is your legal right that our sessions and my records about you be kept private. That is why I ask you to sign 'Informed Consent' and 'Authorization to Release Confidential Information' forms before I can talk about you or send my records about you to anyone else. In general, I will tell no one what you tell me. I will not even reveal that you are receiving treatment from me. In all but a few rare situations, your confidentiality (that is, our privacy) is protected by federal and state laws and by the rules of my profession. Here are the most common cases in which confidentiality is not protected:

1. If you make a serious threat to harm yourself or another person, the law requires me to try to protect you or that other person.

2. If I believe a child has been or will be abused or neglected, I am legally required to report this to the authorities.

3. Sometimes, I consult other therapists or other professionals about my patients. This helps me in giving high-quality treatment (we call this peer supervision). These persons are also required to keep your information private. Your name will never be given to them, some information will be changed or omitted, and they will be told only as much as they need to know to understand your situation.

4. It may be beneficial for me to confer with your primary care physician with regard to your psychological treatment or to discuss any medical problems for which you are receiving treatment. In addition, if you are a Medicare patient, I am required to notify your physician by telephone or in writing, concerning services that are being provided by me unless you request that notification not be made.

About our appointments and upcoming vacations

The very first time I meet with you, we will need to give each other much basic information. For this reason, I usually schedule 1 hour for this first meeting. Following this, we will meet for a 55-minute session once a week. We can schedule meetings for both your

APPENDIX D

and my convenience. I will tell you at least a month in advance of my vacations or any other times we cannot meet. Please check my events calendar to be abreast of times I am lecturing on the road. http://www.yogartherapy.com/

An appointment is a commitment to our work. We agree to meet here and to be on time. If I have to cancel 24 hours before our appointment then your next appointment is free. I also assure you that you will receive the full time agreed to. If you are late, we will be unable to meet for the full time, because it is likely that I will have another appointment soon after yours. A cancelled appointment delays our work. I will consider our meetings *very important* and ask you to do the same. Please try not to miss sessions if you can help it. If you must cancel and if possible, please give me 72 hours' notice. Your session time is reserved for you. You will be charged the full fee for sessions cancelled with less than 24 hours' notice, for other than the most serious and/or medical reasons. Except for unpredictable emergencies (or because of a situation that would be seen by both of us as an unpredictable emergency), I will charge you the regular fee for any missed sessions.

Again, if I have to cancel an appointment, then your next session is free.

Fees, payments and billing

Payment for services is an important part of any professional relationship. My current regular fees are as follows. You will be given advance notice if my fees should change.

- Regular therapy services: _____ for the therapeutic hour (55 minutes), depending on assessments.
- Please pay for each session at its end. After our first meeting, my fee is _____ per hour.

I have found that this arrangement helps us stay focused on our goals, and so it works best. It also allows me to keep my fees as low as possible, because it cuts down on my bookkeeping costs. I suggest you make out your check before each session begins, so that our time will be used efficiently.

If you prefer to use a credit card, I accept credit using the Square App and PayPal.

Of course, there is no charge for calls about appointments or similar business.

Extended sessions

Occasionally it may be better to go on with a session, rather than stop or postpone work on a particular issue. When this extension is more than 15 minutes, I will tell you, because sessions that are extended beyond 10 minutes will be charged on a prorated basis.

Other services

I realize that my fees involve a substantial amount of money, although they are well in line with similar professionals' charges. For you to get the best value for your money, we must work hard and well.

Depending on your financial circumstances and total medical costs for any year, psychotherapy may be a deductible expense; consult your tax advisor. Cost of transportation to and from appointments and fees paid may be deductible from the client's personal income taxes as medical expenses.

If you think you may have trouble paying your bills on time, please discuss this with me. I will also raise the matter with you so we can arrive at a solution.

I look forward to working with you.

Practice information

Informed consent to treat – important

Client Name _____

Date _____

This notice of privacy practices describes how we may use and disclose your protected health information (PHI) to carry out treatment, payment or healthcare operations and for other purposes that are permitted or required by law. It also describes your rights to access and control your protected health information. 'Protected health information' is information about you, including demographic information, that may identify you and that relates to your past, present or future physical or mental health or condition and related healthcare services.

Please read and sign at the end stating you have fully read and understood the information below.

Confidentiality

Dr Horovitz follows all ethical standards prescribed by state and federal law. She is required by practice guidelines and standards of care to keep records of your counseling. These records are confidential with the exceptions noted below. Discussions between a therapist and client are confidential. No information will be released without the client's written consent unless mandated by law. Possible exceptions to confidentiality include, but are not limited to the following situations: child abuse; abuse of the elderly or disabled; abuse of patients in mental-health facilities; sexual exploitation; AIDS/HIV infection and possible transmission; criminal prosecutions; child custody cases in which the mental health of a party is in issue; situations where the therapist has a duty to disclose or where, in the therapist's judgment, it is necessary to warn or disclose; fee disputes between therapist and client; a negligence suit brought by the client against the therapist or the filing of a complaint with the licensing or certifying board.

If you have any questions regarding confidentiality you should bring them to the attention of the therapist when you and the therapist discuss this matter further. By signing this Informed Consent Form, you are giving consent to the undersigned therapist to share confidential information with all persons mandated by law and also releasing and holding harmless the undersigned therapist from any departure from your right of confidentiality that may result.

Duty to warn/duty to protect

If my therapist believes that I am (or my child is, if child is the client) in any physical or emotional danger, I hereby specifically give consent to my therapist to contact any person who is in a position to prevent harm to me or another, including, but not limited to, the person in danger. I also give consent to my therapist to contact the following person(s), in addition to any medical or law enforcement personnel deemed appropriate:

_____

Incapacity or death

I understand that in the event of death or incapacitation of the undersigned therapist it will be necessary to assign my case to another therapist and for that therapist to have possession of my treatment records. By my signature on this

APPENDIX D

form, I hereby consent for another mental-health professional to take possession of my records and provide me copies at my request, and/or to deliver those records to another therapist of my choosing.

Consent to treatment

By signing this form, I acknowledge that I have read, understood and agree to the terms and conditions contained in this form. I have been given appropriate opportunity to address any questions or request clarification for anything that is unclear to me. I am voluntarily agreeing to receiving mental-health assessment, treatment and services for me (or my child, if said child is the client) and I understand that I may stop such treatment at any time.

Signature / date _____

Practice information

Authorization to release confidential information

Name of patient _____

Date of birth _____

I understand that the purpose of this release is to assist with my treatment by improving communication between professional service providers or agencies. To further this goal, I authorize specific clinician Dr Ellen Horovitz to release the below-specified information regarding me/the patient to the individual(s) listed below, and to receive information from them. I have been informed of the risks to privacy and limitations on confidentiality of the use of electronic means of information transfer, and I accept these.

Information to be discussed marked X in the boxes below

Any items not to be released are scored through

☐ ☒ Treatment plan   ☐ ☒ Progress notes   ☐ ☒ Genogram and psychosocial history

☐ ☒ Compliance with treatment   ☐ ☒ Treatment summary   ☐ ☒ Psychological evaluation

☐ ☒ Medications   ☐ ☒ Other _____

This information is to be disclosed to this person(s), who have the indicated relationship to me/the patient:

Name of person _____

Relationship _____

I understand that I may revoke this release at any time, except to the extent that it has already been acted upon. This release will expire: ☐ one year from this date, ☐ upon my discharge from treatment by Dr Horovitz, or ☐ under these circumstances: _____

Signature of client / printed name / date _____

Signature of parent/guardian/representative / printed name / relationship / date _____

☐ Copy for patient/parent/guardian

☐ Copy for provider/therapist

APPENDIX D

Art therapy research release

Client name _____

Date _____

I understand that by signing this document, I give my permission to Dr Ellen Horovitz to do the following (*please check all that apply*):

❐ Photograph my artwork and / or myself

❐ Display with identifying patient information removed

❐ Use my artwork in teaching, research, publication or educational presentations

❐ Use session dialogue in teaching, research, publication or educational presentations

I understand that this agreement is valid for the following time period (if defined by client) _____

I understand that all measures will be made to ensure that my identity will be protected and that confidential material will remain confidential. I understand that if at any time that I choose to withdraw my permission, I can do so by contacting Dr Horovitz and my request will actioned immediately. I understand that if this work has been already shared for research, teaching, publication or educational presentations, my withdrawal of permission cannot be retroactive.

Signature of client / printed name / date _____

Signature of parent/guardian/representative / printed name / relationship / date _____

APPENDIX E Cognitive art therapy assessment

This procedure has been developed to complement rather than duplicate the multidisciplinary teams' clinical findings. It concentrates on methods whereby art therapy can prove the participant's personality in a unique manner.

It offers open-ended creative activities with pencil, paint, and clay. The dual appeal both towards regression and towards progress to formed expression inherent in all art activities is utilized. In addition, the three media's propensity to elicit specific kinds of behavior is an essential source of information.

- Typically, **line drawing** elicits intellectually controlled expression, as well as storytelling that may be factual or dominated by fantasy.
- **Paint** raises the emotional key and invites the expression of affect and moods. This might lead to a loosening of controls and/or to flooring of the ego with raw affect.
- **Clay** invites regression to playful behavior that easily takes on oral, anal, phallic or genital character. Clay also readily elicits sustained efforts at constructive integration, even in severely disorganized people.

Set-up

The procedure should be planned to last at least a full hour, 1½ hours are preferable. The session is, on the whole, conducted as a model art therapy session. Art materials should be set up in advance. This should include:

1. Soft pencil, eraser and white 8" × 11" bond paper.
2. Complete set of poster paint not including orange and violet and also omitting green and brown — set out in an ice cube tray or similar container that allows mixing paints. Two yellows and both ultramarine and turquoise shades of blue for mixing green. Two compartments filled with white to allow mixing lighter colors. An additional empty tray for mixing additional colors. 18" × 24" paper.
3. Ceramic clay, simple clay tools (they can be improvised — sharpened pencils, tongue depressors, etc), container for mixing clay slip, container for water, hand lotion. Paraphernalia for protecting participants and environment must not be forgotten (aprons, newspaper, sponges, etc.)

Procedure

The administrant states, '*You have a choice to draw, paint or make whatever you want from clay. You can do all three. With which (medium) would you like to start?*'

As the subject chooses his/her art materials, the art therapist will ask whether, where, and how he/she has previously used the materials. The art therapist does not interfere while the subject draws. Later on, the art therapist may offer comment, suggestions, advice, or active help when appropriate.

For the art therapist to consider when writing up results

Focus of observation

1. Drawing: (a) developmental stage, (b) motor coordination, (c) perceptual problems, (d) reality perception, (e) thought disorder, (f) family dynamics.
2. Color effect, mood response to the excitement of color (anxious, eager).
3. Can handle the excitement of color, overwhelmed, color preference, response.
4. The miracle of mixing green, emotional response, can the client use the newly mixed colors? Do they understand the principle in mixing colors?
5. Clay: capacity for integration, propensity for specific kinds of regression (undifferentiated, playful, oral, anal, aggressive, phallic, etc.), capacity to reintegrate after initial regression.

Quality of the artwork

1. No product: withdrawal / playful experimentation, play / destructive behavior.

APPENDIX E

2. Product in the service of defense: banal common stereotype / personal stereotype / bizarre stereotype / doing and undoing.

3. Product in the service of primitive discharge: chaotic / aggressive / obliterating.

4. Attempt at formed expression: successful (a product with evocative power, inner consistency) / nearly successful / failed (when and how did it fail?).

5. Comparison of the artwork in the three media offered: similarity / dissimilarity / incongruence.

6. Is there any material that stimulates extraordinary process or regression?

Formal qualities of artwork

- Empty / full, dull / original, fragmented / integrated, static / in motion, rigid / fluid, frantic, bizarre, etc.
- Color over form; form over color.
- Skill, talent.

Subject matter

What themes emerged? Note whether there was any contradiction between overtly stated subject matter and the message conveyed by the work itself.

The client's attitude

- General: cooperative, withdrawn, rebellious, suspicious, ambivalent, clinging, integrating, charming, distractible, anxious, intensity, etc. (changes?).
- Towards their work: highly invested, indifferent, proud, denigrating, self-destructive.
- Towards the art materials: preferences, dislikes.
- Towards suggestions and/or help: oblivious, negative, oh yes! (understanding) / dependent but able to integrate help, dependent (bottomless pit of needfulness).

Important points to consider

- Did any learning take place?
- Any indication of capacity to master inner resources in art?
- Do observations concur with or contradict team's findings?
- Did art activity contribute to expression of material not otherwise accessible?
- Could art activities contribute to ego strength?

Guidelines for evaluation procedures

Focus of observation in each of the three media

The chronological age must always be taken into consideration when evaluating developmental stage. Both art process and art product should be observed. Observations of artwork in one medium will sometimes complement or contradict findings in another medium. Note unevenness of performance, sequence of work done.

I. Drawing

A. Developmental stage of drawings:

1. Scribble.

2. Capacity to produce controlled configurations — circle, triangle, square, etc.

3. Early representation of the human figure — predominance of head and limbs, omission of trunk.

4. Later representation — trunk appears, limbs form, whole people

5. Spatial representation — no directness, baseline, fold-over, overlapping, attempts at visual perspective.

Signs of constitutional problems can be seen more clearly in drawing than in work with the other materials. However, they should be noted wherever they appear.

- Eye-hand coordination?

Cognitive art therapy assessment

- Problems with fine motor control? Ability to control pencil.
- Form perception — ability to produce the basic forms (circle, square, cross, triangle, letters, numbers).
- Left—right dominance established?
- Reversals or confused directions?
- Space discrimination — foreground/background difficulty?
- Ease or awkwardness in handling the art material.

B. Facets of personality:

- Use of total space, placement of people and objects; directness (framing?, objects afloat?, objects unrelated?).
- Size of elements and their relations to each other (this must be considered in relationship to chronological age of participant).
- Body image intact; omissions; fragmentations; distortions; bizarre elements.
- Faces, facial features complete, omissions, distortions; bizarre element; expressions.
- Drawing stroke-pressure, broken lines, tentative quality, modulation, continuity, etc. This must be considered in relation to the subject's chronological age.
- Omissions, shadings, erasures, transparencies, overemphasis? When corrections are made note whether there is improvement; repetition of the same mistake: deterioration?
- Emotional content — joyful, free, pressured, aggressive, boxed-in, etc.
- Personal expression or stereotype?

II. Painting

A. Developmental stage of painting:

- Kinesthetic pleasure — squiggle; selection of specific color not important.
- Single areas of massive color; color blobs.
- Separation into different areas of color.
- Color and line combine in representational work and in designs.
- Color modulation through mixing and sensitivity to color relationships. Intellectual comprehension of the principle of mixing color.

B. Facets of personality:

- Reaction to paint; strongly attracted to color; able to handle it; reluctant to use it; overwhelmed by it?
- Does color dominate form, swallow, or drown it?
- Is color subordinate to form and subject matter?

C. Specific color preferences and their possible symbolic meaning:

- Hot or cool colors predominate? Dark colors, pastel colors, muddy colors?
- Is there a balance between hot and cool colors?
- Where are emotionally loaded colors placed (in sky, ground, middle area)?
- Overlay, painting one color over another (hiding)?
- Free intermingling of colors or separation of colors?
- Indiscriminate mixing — desire to smear, loss of control, mud?
- Exploration of combinations of color?
- Sequence of color use.
- Response to the miracle of green, brown, and other mixed colors.
- Ability to use colors that are mixed.
- Does mood change with color change?
- Brush stroke, pressure, broken lines, scattered, movement, predominance of vertical and horizontal or curved line.
- Personal expression or stereotype?
- Paint as a way of access to fantasy life?

APPENDIX E

III. Clay

A. Developmental stage of clay modeling:

1. Clay used playfully; what kind of play?
2. Clay — patted down flat — flat representational work; gingerbread people.
3. Clay — squeezed, punched; small differentiated shapes stuck together.
4. Use of whole hand — ball, upright forms reminiscent of block building.
5. Sculptural form attained: figures assembled from their various parts; simply stuck together; well joined to make a whole. The sculpture is conceived as a whole from the beginning.
6. Face: features incised in clay; stuck onto the clay; conceived as structure. Note particularly nose (hole, stuck-on protrusion, protruding element of face).

B. Facets of personality:

- Enjoying the 'feel' of clay? Afraid, repelled by it? Open to experimentation?
- Capacity for integration? Specific kinds of regression (undifferentiated, playful, oral, anal).
- Ability to regress and finally re-integrate? Immediately re-integrate?
- Ability to learn and later recall (after some brief instruction) how to work with clay.
- Structural elements – faulty connection between parts? Holes, tunnels, hiding place, lack of stability, balance, noting upright, relationship of parts to each other?
- Emotional content of clay work – playful, imagination, fantasy, bizarre qualities, rigidity, stereotype, aggressive, jabbing?
- If clay is painted, realistic, symbolic color, bizarre colors?

General assessment as seen through art activity

1. Outstanding developmental capacities, deficits, deviations, visual-motor functioning. Developmental stage as seen in artwork. If deficits, is it possible that they are constitutional and/or emotional, cultural?
2. Self-image: sexual identity, self-esteem, ego ideals.
3. Perception of self in relation to others. Individuation, strong emotional attachments, symbiosis?
4. Sense of reality. Distortions of self and body parts, depersonalization?
5. Thought processes, ability to conceptualize, memory, judgment, concrete or abstract thinking?
6. Defenses — and dangers defended against.
7. Capacity for other gratifications — not art but playful manipulation of materials.
8. Potential to learn, to master, to function on a higher level, environmental, or cultural factors that might be influential.
9. Temperamental assessment as seen in art session, mood quality — exuberant, hesitant, overwhelmed by anxiety, etc.
10. Activity level — hyperactive, deliberate, reflective, attention span approach or withdrawal? Adaptability or construction.
11. Capacity for ego gratification through art. Capacity for ego maturation through art.

APPENDIX F Directional movements of the spine and their application

Directional movements of the spine and their application			
	Intention	Example	Application
Forward bending	To stretch the lower back		To release lower back tension (in combination with back bending and twisting)
	To stretch the structures of the upper back, shoulder girdle and neck		To address upper back and neck tension
	To stretch the hamstrings		To stretch the hamstrings and release lower back tension
Back bending	To expand and stretch the chest		To reverse slouching and relieve tension in the chest area To deepen breathing To facilitate "heart opening"
	To stretch the solar plexus, abdomen, front of hips and thighs		To address tension in the hip flexors and thighs
	To strengthen the musculature of the back		To strengthen the back to release lower back tension To stabilize the lower back before going into deep LB, TW, or unsupported BB
Twisting	To rotate the spine		To build strength and flexibility in deep and superficial spinal and abdominal muscles To bring balance to asymmetrical muscular development

APPENDIX F

	Directional movements of the spine and their application *continued*		
	Intention	**Example**	**Application**
Twisting	To adjust the relationship between the shoulder girdle and the spine		To address upper back and neck tension To address asymmetries of the shoulder, upper back and neck
	To adjust the relationship between the pelvic girdle and the spine		To release lower back tension To address asymmetries of the hips, pelvis and legs
Lateral bending	To laterally stretch the torso from the shoulder to the hip joint		To restore balance to the asymmetries of the spine, shoulders and pelvis To stretch and strengthen the musculature of shoulder joints and upper back To expand the ribcage and facilitate deeper breathing
	"Pelvic opening"		To stretch and strengthen the musculature of hip joints, front of the pelvis and inner thighs

Directional movements of the spine and their application

	Intention	Example	Application
Axial extension postures	To bring the spine into maximum vertical alignment, integrating the spinal curves without strain or compression		To improve postural alignment and overall structural integration To strengthen the diaphragm and abdominal muscles
	To extend the arms and legs, facilitating the extension of the spine		To create space in the shoulder and hip joints and improve circulation

This appendix is based on Sequence Wiz handouts.

APPENDIX G Movement observation sample

Movement observation sample

	Pose	Observe
1	Static supine observation	Ask client to compare the right and left sides of the body (mentally) Note if it matches your observation
2	Pelvic tilt	Depth and location of breath Head, shoulders, lower back, pelvis, knees, feet position Ability to do the pelvic tilt on exhale
3	Apanasana	Ability to contract the abdomen on exhale Neck/shoulder position Trajectory of leg movement (compare)
4	Various leg movements	Ability of neck/shoulders to stay relaxed Imbalanced development in adductors/abductors, hip flexors/glutes, deep rotators
5	Various arm movements	Range of motion of neck and shoulders How arm movement affects the positioning of the lower body
6	Chakravakasana	Pelvic lumbar rhythm Position of the head, elevation of the shoulders, position of the elbows Mobility of the thoracic curve

APPENDIX G

Movement observation sample *continued*

	Pose	Observe
7	Bhujangasana	Ability to use upper back muscles, symmetry of development Position of the head, ability to turn it; position of the shoulders Hip position (in relation to the floor); leg/foot position (symmetry)
8	Vajrasana	Origin of movement; ability to use upper back muscles Range of motion in the shoulders Position of the knees/feet (compare R/L), weight distribution (R/L)
9	Virabhadrasana 1	Try different arm adaptations to observe the positioning of the lower back, upper back, neck, hips and knees and range of motion in the shoulders
10	Uttanasana	Check alignment on the way down and up; positioning of the head, angle of the knees, overall range of motion and comfort level
11	Utthita trikonasana	Check the range of motion and symmetry of the torso, hip position, lumbar curve, range of motion in the shoulders and neck

Movement observation sample

	Pose	Observe
Movement observation sample *continued*		
12	Prasarita padottanasana	Check alignment on the way down and up; positioning of the head, angle of the knees and hips, overall range of motion and comfort level
13	Static standing observation	Ask client to compare the right and left sides of the body (mentally) Note if it matches your observation

In every pose observe:
Connection between breath and movement/breathing pace/ease of inhalation relative to exhalation/body awareness/understanding of the pose/range of motion/habitual movement patterns/ability to follow instructions/ability to stay focused

This appendix is based on Sequence Wiz handouts.

PERMISSIONS

Introduction, Figure 1 Bad apples, illustration by author. (From the collection of Christopher Kisiel, chef and owner of Bad Apples.)

Introduction, Figure 5 Meditation. (From Paolo E. Marino, with permission.)

Figure 2.5 Goniometer evaluation chart from the Washington State Department of Social and Health Services (www.dshs.wa.gov).

Figure 2.6 The kośhas by Paolo E. Marino.

Figure 3.1 Sight for sore eyes, by the author. (From the collection of David Klein MD, with permission.)

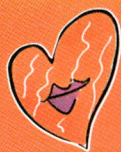

INDEX

Note: Page number followed by f indicates figures

A

Abhiniveśa, meditating on, 50
Adho mukha śvānāsana, 55, 61, 87f, 186f
Adolescence and culture, 113
Age progression and artistic development in children stages, idea on, 66
Agoraphobic patient, case study on, 64
Allostatic load, 57
Aloneliness, concept of, 113
American Art Therapy Association, 20, 206
American Diabetes Association, 115
American Psychiatric Association (APA), 35, 131
Anāmaya kosa, 45
Anubis clay sculpture, 107, 107f
Anubis sketch, 107, 107f
Anxiety, mandalas and coloring in reducing, 72–73, 73f
Apāna vāyu mudrā
    importance, 25
    instruction for, 26
Ardha matsyendrāsana, 115, 118f, 128f
Aromatherapy, role, 60
Art development comparison chart, stages, 37–40
Artistic development with art samples, stages, 38–40f
Art materials. *See also* Yoga therapy session
    for office, basic compendium, 66–67
    in therapy session, 65–67
Art therapist
    art materials for office, 66–67
    digital software programs development, 67–68
    guidelines for, 25
    need of resourcefulness, 63
    skills of, 65
    texting and telehealth, HIPAA-compliant software importance, 74–75
    therapeutic attitude and body language, 26–29
    on therapeutic hours, 24
Art therapy
    advantage, 19
    assessment and efficacy, 37–40
    chanting of *Aum*, 25
    daily incorporation, 19
    environment provided, 21–22
    ethical boundaries and therapeutic bond, 19–21
    guidelines for therapist, 25
    history, standards and regulations, 206–207
    patient dis-ease understanding, 22
    ritual of invitation, 24
    rules establishment and etiquette for groups, 24
    setting up studio, 22
    therapeutic attitude and body language, 26–29
    therapeutic clean-up and studio maintenance, 23
    therapeutic hours, issue, 22–23
    in treatment, 21
    using *mudras* and *bhavana*, 25–26
    vacation planning for therapist, 23
    and yoga therapy, patient's involvement, 20, 155–156
Asāna, 81, 85, 97
    Ardha matsyendrāsana, 115
    Bhujangāsana, 115
    Dhanurāsana, 115
    Halāsana, 115
    Nādi sodhana pranayama, 115
    Pachimotanāsana, 115
    Setu bandha sarvāngāsana, 117
    Tādāsana, 115
    Vajrāsana, 115
    Vrksasāna, 115
A's genogram, 102f
Ashtanga yoga, 115–116
Attention deficit disorder (ADD), 92–93
    case study
        background and history, 93
        family session, 95–99
        yoga therapy and KFD assessment, 94–95
Attention deficit-hyperactivity disorder (ADHD), 92–93
    case study
        artistic level of development, 106
        background and history, 101–102
        court date, 103–105

developmental and psychological assessments, 105–106
intake with father and stepmother, 103
partner yoga therapy session, 107–108, 108f
recommendations, 109
session summations, 106–107
technology, 102–103
Aum, chanting of, 25, 53
Autonomous nervous system (ANS), 20, 27, 116
Avidya, meaning of, 50

B

Baby dancer, 193f
Bellows breath, steps for, 56, 57f
Belly breath, 86f
Bender Gestalt Visual Motor Integration Test II, 105
Berenstain Bear family, 100f
Better Mind app, usage, 32, 72, 102
Bhāvanā, 95, 97
 importance, 26
 meaning, 52
Bhujangāsana, 115
Biopsychosocial care model, 57
Bipolar disorder
 case study
  addiction and yoga, 131–133
  background and history, 77–78, 133–134
  drug and alcohol rehabilitation, 138–139
  further progress, 79–83
  sessions, 78–79, 135–138
Bitilasāna, 79
Brain
 levels of, 92
 wave chart, 129f
Breath and creative exercise, 57
Breathing techniques, practice, 25
Breath of joy, 136f
Breathwork/*pranamaya*, benefits, 45, 72

C

Capterra, telehealth site, 74
Center for Epidemiologic Studies Depression Scale, Revised (CESD-R), 35, 36f
Chakravakasana, 99f, 127f
Children and family systems, 77
Chronosytem patterning of environmental events and transitions, 58, 58f
Clay kneading effect, on patients. *See also* Yoga therapy session
 agoraphobic patient, 64
 pressured speech patient, 63
Clay mirrors, 98f
Clearing space, importance, 50–52
Cognitive behavioral therapy (CBT), 132, 140, 205
Coherent breath, 86f
Compass pose, 128f
Co-OperBands in yoga, usage, 21
Co-OperBlankets in yoga, usage, 21
Copaiba oils, usage, 60
Creative Arts Therapy Practice, 211–216
Cross-sex hormone therapy, 148
Culture and adolescence, 113

D

Depression, Stress and Anxiety Scale (DASS-21), 27, 81, 83, 106f, 117, 119
Depression
 or anxiety, yoga strategies, 45
 treatments, yoga in, 20–21
 case study
  couple's therapy, 157–164
Dhanurāsana, 115
Dhi Rhi Ha, 79, 80f
Dialectic behavioral therapy (DBT), 205
Digital applications, in art therapy, 67–68
Digital image, in artwork creation, 67
Downward facing dog (DFD), 87f, 184
Dry art materials, usage, 65
Dynamic stretching, 44

E

Eating Attitudes Test-26 (EAT-26), 125
Eka pāda rājakapotāsana, 58, 59f
Electronic medical record (EMR), 31
Empathy, 91–92
E's genogram, 94f
Essential Anatomy 5, 32
Essential oils in therapy, usage, 60–61
Exercises with F and R, 161f

INDEX continued

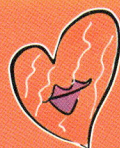
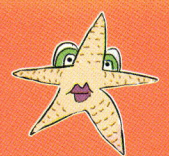

F
Face-to-face (F2F) relationships, 145
Facial feminization surgery (FFS), 147
Family session with child, case study on, 68–70
Family yoga therapy, 99f
Flexibility training, methods used, 44
FOMO (fear of missing out), 113
Formal Element Art Therapy Scale (FEATS), 93
    Assessment, 37
Frankincense, usage, 60
F's dream fugue state sketch, 165f
F's genogram, 158f
F's shoulder injury, 159f

G
Gamma-aminobutyric acid (GABA), 54
Gang Age of Development, 106
Gender dysmorphia, 140
Gender identity, 140
Genogram Analytics software, 31
Genogram applications
    case study for, 32–36
    importance, 31
    information, assessments, anatomy and physiology, 31–36
God gene, 132
Goniometer
    evaluation chart, 42–43f
    important tips for using, 41
    for measuring musculoskeletal injury, 41
    techniques for using, 41
Graphics and photography programs, in artwork creation, 67

H
Halāsana, 115
Health Assessment and Pain Assessment forms, 27
Heart rate variability (HRV), 91
Heron pose, 128f
Hidradenitis suppurativa (HS), 113
High lunge, 127f
HIPPA-compliant software programs, importance, 73–74
Horovitz-adapted formal elements chart, for non-standardized assessments, 37f
Hula hooping, 54
Hyperbaric oxygen therapy (HBOT), 132

I
Ideogram of Om (Aum), 25
Index card exercise, 70f
Integrated Movement Therapy, 93
International Association of Yoga Therapists (IAYT), 20, 73, 207

J
Japanese spiraling method of kneading clay, 63f
Jehovah's Witness, 83, 84
Joint flexibility
    definition, 41
    improvement, role, 44
Journaling
    art making, 68–70
    exercise, effects of, 70

K
Kapalābhāti breath, role, 54
Kapalābhāti padmasana, steps of, 54–55
Kinetic family drawing (KFD), 93, 135
    assessment, 34-35, 34f, 94–95
Krama exhale, 86f, 118f
Krama inhale, 86f, 118f
Kriyā, 53
K's genogram, 83, 84f
K's invisible string bracelet, 90, 90f

L
L in *savāsana*, 178f
L in *supta pādāngusthāsana, 178f*
Lotus, 87f
L's angel, 178f
L's genogram, 142f, 172f
L's Self-box, 145f

M
Major Depressive Disorders, 35
Mandalas and coloring in reducing anxiety, 72–73, 73f
Mental hygiene arrest (MHA), 77
MetroFax app, application, 74
Mirror neurons, 91–92
Mood management. *See also* Yoga therapy session

INDEX continued

regulation, 19
visual imagery, 62–65
yogic breathing and meditation techniques, 54–57
Morris-Payne technique, aim, 41
Mother and E's yoga sequence, 100f
Mountain pose *(tadāsana)*, 28f
M's genogram, 134f
Mudrā, 52
Musculoskeletal injury (MSI) prevention, goniometer in, 41

N
Nadi sodhana pranayama, 86f, 115
Naukasana, 115

O
Oppositional defiant disorder (ODD), 119
Oversharenting, 113

P
Parasympathetic nervous system (PNS), 35
Paripoorna matsyendrāsana, 62f
Parsvokanasana, 128f
Participants intention for yoga practice, 24
Partner breathing, 108f
Partner twist, 108f
Partner *vrikasana*, 108f
Paschimottanasana, 120f
Polyvagal theory, 21, 156
Poses, modifications and sequencing of, 57–60
Post-traumatic stress disorder (PTSD), 68, 141
Pranamaya breathing practice, 45
Pranamaya kosa, affect, 45
Pratiloma ujjayi, 136f
Pressured speech patient, case study on, 63
Proprioceptive neuromuscular facilitation (PNF), 44
Protractor goniometer, application, 41
Psychological assessments
importance, 32, 35
on patient, case study, 27–29
Psychological testing, smartphone for, 32

R
Range of motion (ROM), measurement, 41
Recapping and assigning homework, importance of, 70–72
Reward deficiency syndrome (RDS), 132
Right brain theory, 156
R's genogram, 114f
R's mask, 82, 82f

S
Safe container creation, for patients, 19–20
Sankālpa, meaning, 53
Savāsana, 115, 118f
Separation anxiety
case study
background and history, 83–84
sessions, 84–90
symptoms of, 83
update, 90
Setu bandha sarvāngāsana, 115, 118f
Side angle pose *(utthita parsvakonāsana)*, 196f
Skill-building, enhancement, 65
SmartLine, application, 74
Smartphone for psychological testing, 32
SOAP note, 31
Software importance, in yoga therapy, 74–75. *See also* Yoga therapy and art therapy techniques
Software in medical art therapy, 67
Somatic integration and yoga therapy, 91
Somatics, defined, 91
Spence's Children Anxiety Scale (SCAS), 103, 105, 106f
Sphinx pose, 120f
Stair-step breath
steps for, 56
usability, 24
Standards of care (SOC), 141
Static and dynamic stretching, for flexibility, 44
Stroke
case study, 171–178
Studio, clean-up and maintenance, 23–24
Systematizing genogram, 31

T
Tapas, meaning, 51
Telehealth site, application of, 72–73

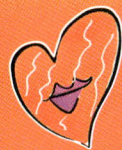
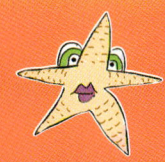

INDEX continued

Temple pose, 108f
Texting and telehealth, HIPAA-compliant software importance, 74–75
Therapist and patient, relationship, 20–21
Transcranial magnetic stimulation (TMS), 132
Transgender to transsexual case study
    background and history, 141–143
    facial feminization surgery, 147–149
    sessions, 143–145
    surgery and telehealth yoga, 145–147, 146f
Traumatic brain injury (TBI), 37, 133
Treatment, yoga therapy and art therapy introduction, 21
Tree pose, 176f
T's mask, 82, 82f
Type 1 diabetes mellitus (T1DM) case study, 113
    background and history, 113–115
    house fire, 119–121
    present situation, 130
    sessions, 117–119, 121–130
    yoga and diabetes, 115–117

U
Uppavista konasana, 100f

V
Vesicoureteral reflux disorder, eating disorder and PTSD case study, 165–170
Vesicular transporter gene (VMAT2), 132
Vijnanamaya kosa, affect, 45
Virabhadrasāna, 79, 127f
Vrksasāna (tree pose), 195f
Virabhdrāsana, 187f
Vrkshasana, 99f, 115

W
Warm-up techniques, 52–54
Warrior 1 to triangle pose, 120f
Wet art materials, disadvantage, 65
World Professional Association of Transgender Health (WPATH), 148

Y
Yoga, 85, 86f
    and addiction, 131–133
    for agoraphobic patient, 64
    ardha matsyendrāsana, 118f, 128f
    Ashtanga, 115–116
    breath of joy, 136f
    chakravakasana, 127f
    compass pose, 128f
    and diabetes, 115–117
    family session artwork post, 96f
    heron pose, 128f
    high lunge, 127f
    krama exhale, 118f
    krama inhale, 118f
    parsvokanasana, 128f
    paschimottanasana, 120f
    practice
        benefits and healing process, 19
        effect on mind and body, 44–45, 49
    pratiloma ujjayi, 136f
    savasana, 118f, 120f, 128f
    setu bandha sarvāngāsana, 118f
    sphinx pose, 120f
    tadasana, 118f, 127f
    telehealth, 145–147, 146f
    therapy, 94–95
    therapy session, partner, 107–108, 108f
    virabhadrasana, 127f
    warrior 1 to triangle pose, 120f
Yoga therapy
    and art therapy techniques
        advantage, 19
        chanting of Aum, 25
        daily incorporation, 19
        environment provided, 21–22
        ethical boundaries and therapeutic bond, 19–21
        guidelines for therapist, 25
        patient dis-ease understanding, 22
        ritual of invitation, 24
        rules establishment and etiquette for groups, 24

INDEX continued

setting up studio, 22
therapeutic attitude and body language, 26–29
therapeutic clean-up and studio maintenance, 23
therapeutic hours, issue, 22–23
in treatment, 21
using *mudras* and *bhavana*, 25–26
vacation planning for therapist, 23
at distance, telehealth format, 74

history, standards and regulations, 207
session
    art materials, in therapy session, 65–67
    mandalas and coloring in reducing anxiety, 72–73, 73f
    modification for, 57–60
    mood management, visual imagery, 62–65
    sequencing, 61–62
    texting and telehealth, HIPAA-compliant software importance, 74–75

Yoga therapy and art therapy
    privacy issues, 205
    scope of practice regarding, 205
Yoga therapy with older adults, 153–155
Yogic practice, goals of, 54
Yogic tools, establishment, 61
Young children, session time in therapy, 22–23